CONTROL OF OVULATION

CONTROL OF OVULATION

Proceedings of the Conference held at
Endicott House, Dedham, Massachusetts, 1960

Edited by

CLAUDE A. VILLEE

HARVARD MEDICAL SCHOOL
BOSTON, MASSACHUSETTS

SYMPOSIUM PUBLICATIONS DIVISION

PERGAMON PRESS

OXFORD · NEW YORK · LONDON · PARIS

1961

PERGAMON PRESS LTD.
Headington Hill Hall, Oxford
4 and 5 Fitzroy Square, London, W.1

PERGAMON PRESS INC.
122 East 55th Street, New York 22, N.Y.
Statler Center 640, 900 Wilshire Boulevard, Los Angeles 17, California

PERGAMON PRESS S.A.R.L.
24 Rue des Écoles, Paris Ve

PERGAMON PRESS G.m.b.H.
Kaiserstrasse 75, Frankfurt am Main

Library of Congress Card No. 60-14946

Printed in Great Britain by John Wright and Sons Ltd., at The Stonebridge Press, Bristol

PREFACE

ALTHOUGH recent years have seen major advances in all aspects of endocrinology, some of the most exciting ones have been in our understanding of the mechanisms controlling ovulation. In addition to a clarification of the roles of steroid hormones and the pituitary gonadotropins in this process, evidence has accrued that certain regions in the hypothalamus, and perhaps in other regions of the central nervous system, have a primary function in controlling ovulation, probably by way of the pituitary. On February 26–28, 1960, a group of investigators met at Endicott House, Dedham, Massachusetts, under the sponsorship of Harvard University and the Association for the Aid of Crippled Children, New York City, to review and evaluate the experimental evidence upon which the current concepts of the mechanisms controlling ovulation are based. The results of some current attempts to inhibit or prevent ovulation by the administration of analogs of the steroid hormones were also discussed in detail.

Some thirty endocrinologists, biochemists, physiologists, neurologists, anatomists, obstetricians and gynecologists from the United States, England, and the Continent were invited to participate in this conference. The twelve papers given at the conference have been published with the minimum of scientific editing necessary to bring them into a consistent form. The discussion following each paper was recorded by a stenotypist and edited by each discussant. The task of the editor was greatly facilitated by the generous co-operation of the authors and discussants in returning their corrected manuscripts promptly.

The conference was planned by a committee composed of Drs. Roy O. Greep, Duncan E. Reid, and Claude A. Villee of Harvard University with Mr. Leonard W. Mayo and Mrs. William F. FitzGerald of the Association for the Aid of Crippled Children as consultants. Funds to underwrite the costs of the conference were provided by a grant from the Association which is interested in conferences of this type as part of its program in medical and social research related to the prevention of disabling diseases and conditions of children and youth.

CLAUDE A. VILLEE

Boston, Massachusetts

CONTENTS

PAGE

List of Contributors ix

The Role of the Pituitary Gonadotropins in Induction of Ovulation in the Hypophysectomized Rat 1
Frances Carter, Marion C. Woods and Miriam E. Simpson
Discussion by Knobil

Follicular Development, Ovular Maturation and Ovulation in Ovarian Tissue Transplanted to the Eye 24
R. W. Noyes, T. H. Clewe and A. M. Yamate
Discussion by Hammond

The Role of Steroids in the Control of Mammalian Ovulation 37
Gregory Pincus and Anne P. Merrill
Discussion by Barraclough, Breneman, Chang, Folley, Greep, Hisaw, Knobil, McArthur, Meyer, Nalbandov, Nelson, Noyes, Pincus, Segal, Simpson and Sturgis

The Pituitary Stalk and Ovulation 56
Geoffrey W. Harris
Discussion by Critchlow

Interactions between the Central Nervous System and Hormones Influencing Ovulation 79
Charles H. Sawyer and M. Kawakami
Discussion by Hansel

The Preoptic Region of the Brain and its Relation to Ovulation 101
John W. Everett
Discussion by Barraclough, Folley, Hansel, Harris and Segal

Mechanisms Controlling Ovulation of Avian and Mammalian Follicles 122
Andrew V. Nalbandov
Discussion by Hisaw, Meyer and Nalbandov

Ovulation in the Domestic Fowl 133
Richard M. Fraps

PAGE

Hormonal Augmentation of Fertility in Sheep and Cattle 163
John Hammond, Jr.

Discussion by Breneman, Chang, Folley, Ganong, Greep, Hammond, Harris, Hisaw, Knobil, Meyer, Nalbandov and Pincus

The Induction of Ovulation in the Human by Human Pituitary Gonadotropin 192
Carl A. Gemzell

Discussion by McArthur, Reid, Segal and Villee

Factors Influencing Ovulation and Atresia of Ovarian Follicles 213
Somers H. Sturgis

Discussion by Gemzell, Greep, Hertz, McArthur and Pincus

Inhibition of Ovulation in the Human 222
John Rock

Discussion by Hisaw and Nelson

Subject Index 245

LIST OF CONTRIBUTORS

Edward B. Astwood, Department of Medicine, New England Center Hospital, Boston, Massachusetts

Charles A. Barraclough, Department of Anatomy, University of California Medical Center, Los Angeles, California

W. R. Breneman, Department of Zoology, Indiana University, Bloomington, Indiana

Min Chueh Chang, Worcester Institute for Experimental Biology, Shrewsbury, Massachusetts

Vaughn Critchlow, Department of Anatomy, Baylor University, Houston, Texas

John W. Everett, Department of Anatomy, Duke University, Durham, North Carolina

Mrs. William FitzGerald, Consultant, Association for the Aid of Crippled Children, New York

S. John Folley, The National Institute for Research in Dairying, Shinfield, Reading, England

Richard M. Fraps, Agricultural Research Service, Beltsville, Maryland

William F. Ganong, Department of Physiology, University of California Medical Center, San Francisco, California

Carl Gemzell, Department of Obstetrics and Gynecology, Karolinska Institute, Stockholm, Sweden

Roy O. Greep, Harvard School of Dental Medicine, Boston, Massachusetts

Dwain D. Hagerman, Department of Biological Chemistry, Harvard Medical School, Boston, Massachusetts

John Hammond, Jr., School of Agriculture, Cambridge University, Cambridge, England

William Hansel, New York State College of Agriculture, Ithaca, New York

Geoffrey W. Harris, Department of Neuroendocrinology, The Maudsley Hospital, London, England

Roy Hertz, Endocrinology Department, National Institutes of Health, Bethesda, Maryland

Frederick Hisaw, Biology Laboratories, Harvard University, Cambridge, Massachusetts

Ernest Knobil, Department of Physiology, Harvard Medical School, Boston, Massachusetts

Charles W. Lloyd, Department of Obstetrics and Gynecology, Upstate Medical Center, Syracuse, New York

Janet McArthur, Department of Obstetrics and Gynecology, Harvard Medical School and Massachusetts General Hospital, Boston, Massachusetts

Roland K. Meyer, Department of Zoology, University of Wisconsin, Madison, Wisconsin

Andrew V. Nalbandov, Department of Animal Science, University of Illinois, Urbana, Illinois

Warren O. Nelson, The Population Council, Inc., The Rockefeller Institute, New York

Robert W. Noyes, Department of Obstetrics and Gynecology, Stanford University School of Medicine, Palo Alto, California

Gregory Pincus, Worcester Institute for Experimental Biology, Shrewsbury, Massachusetts

Duncan E. Reid, Department of Obstetrics and Gynecology, Harvard Medical School, and Boston Lying-in Hospital, Boston, Massachusetts

John Rock, Rock Reproductive Study Center, Brookline, Massachusetts

Charles H. Sawyer, Department of Anatomy, University of California Medical Center, Los Angeles, California

Sheldon Segal, The Population Council, Inc., The Rockefeller Institute, New York

Miriam E. Simpson, Institute of Experimental Biology, University of California, Berkeley, California

Somers H. Sturgis, Department of Obstetrics and Gynecology, Harvard Medical School, and Peter Bent Brigham Hospital, Boston, Massachusetts

Claude A. Villee, Department of Biological Chemistry, Harvard Medical School, Boston, Massachusetts

THE ROLE OF THE PITUITARY GONADOTROPINS IN INDUCTION OF OVULATION IN THE HYPOPHYSECTOMIZED RAT*

FRANCES CARTER, MARION C. WOODS and MIRIAM E. SIMPSON
Institute of Experimental Biology and Departments of Anatomy
University of California
Berkeley and San Francisco

THE experimental induction of ovarian follicular development constitutes no problem. Growth of follicles has been induced in many species by homologous and heterologous gonadotropins. Luteinization of follicles can also be accomplished with relative ease, but ova are too often enclosed.

Monkey

This was our experience (van Wagenen and Simpson, 22, 26, 27) in efforts made to induce ovulation in the primate (*Macaca mulatta*). Immediate success was attained in causing follicular growth but the conditions for induction of ovulation were more difficult to determine. Once conditions of timing and dosage were mastered, ovulation was induced after administration of follicle-stimulating hormone (FSH) and interstitial cell-stimulating hormone (ICSH) derived from sheep pituitaries, as well as by monkey pituitary extracts. Ovulation resulted more consistently after administration of preparations from monkey pituitaries, either with or without supplementation by human chorionic gonadotropin (HCG). Both immature and adult females ovulated after injection of appropriate dosage for 7 to 9 days. Adults were injected during the first half of the cycle (from day 5 to 15). Ovulations were multiple in all adults but not in all prepuberal animals. Whether this constitutes a significant difference in the response of the immature monkeys is not yet certain. These observations in the monkey have been adequately documented in the literature.

Similar procedures have been followed by Gemzell *et al.* (8, 8a) and by Rosemberg *et al.* (18) with success in the human female, and recently by Knobil *et al.* (12) in the hypophysectomized monkey. However, these studies

* Aided by grants A-800 and RG-4339 from the United States Public Health Service, and by a grant from the Committee on Research, Council of Pharmacy and Chemistry, American Medical Association, and from the Population Council, Inc., New York City.

in primates share the defects common to all efforts which have been made in the last 30 years to obtain an understanding of the pituitary factors necessary for ovulation (9, 10, 19, 20, 29). The presence of a pituitary in the recipients complicates the response of normal animals to any gonadotropin administered. All efforts have been handicapped by the lack of pure gonadotropins. In the studies of van Wagenen and Simpson, to which reference has just been made, neither hypophysectomized monkeys nor single pure gonadotropins were available. The products from sheep pituitaries which were injected were prepared by repeated ammonium sulfate fractionation of 40% ethanol extracts of whole glands. The preparations from monkey pituitaries were lyophilized 40% ethanol extracts of anterior lobes. No further purification could be undertaken at the time due to the scarcity of material. It was therefore evident that we were not ready for sufficiently exacting experiments in the primate.

Hypophysectomized Rat

Meanwhile studies were in progress in which hypophysectomized rats were being used as the experimental animal (2). These animals were available in adequate numbers, and their use avoided the confusion introduced into interpretation of the results by contributions from the recipient's pituitary. These studies, like those in the primate, were subject to the criticism that no completely pure pituitary gonadotropins were available, so that the proportion of the two pituitary gonadotropins, FSH and ICSH, tentatively regarded as essential for ovulation, could not be precisely determined. An attempt will be made, however, to define the status of our knowledge regarding the pituitary factors necessary for ovulation in the rat as determined with the purest sheep pituitary FSH and ICSH now available.

In the rat, as in other species investigated, there was no difficulty in developing follicles, or in luteinizing them, but conditions necessary to cause release of ova were more exacting. When these conditions were determined for the hypophysectomized rat, it was found that superovulation was typical, a characteristic observed repeatedly in experimental induction of ovulation with exogenous gonadotropins in normal animals of many species. The shedding of a number of ova greater than that characteristic for the species is in itself an abnormal phenomenon, and the question must be raised eventually as to the significance of the number of ova shed, though no attempt will be made here to evaluate this matter.

In order to analyze which pituitary hormones are needed, and in what proportion they must be present, it was necessary first to determine a set of conditions under which ovulation might reliably be obtained in the hypophysectomized rat. These standard conditions were determined by the use of a follicle-stimulating preparation from sheep pituitaries which was obtained by repeated refractionation of an 0.8 saturated ammonium sulfate (AS) fraction from which a number of fractions had already been removed at lower AS concentrations (Table 1). Such preparations are commonly called "FSH", because instigation of follicular growth is their predominant biological characteristic. No corpora lutea are produced until many multiples

TABLE 1. AMMONIUM SULFATE METHOD FOR FRACTIONATION OF GONADOTROPINS FROM 40% ETHANOL EXTRACT OF DRIED WHOLE SHEEP PITUITARIES

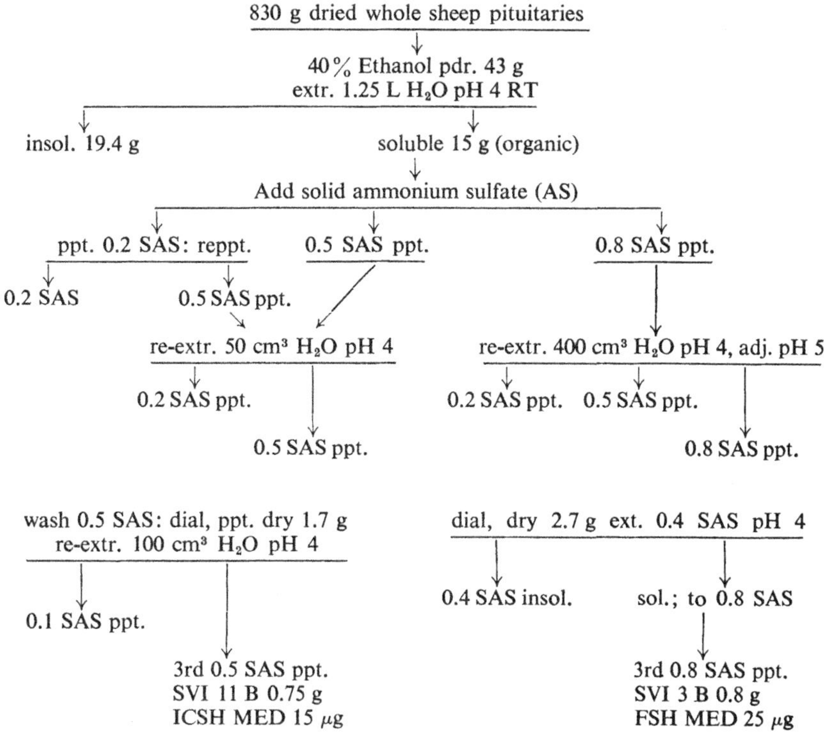

of the minimal effective dose are given. Since microscopic evidence of repair of the interstitial tissue was found on injection of this preparation at 10-fold the dose giving follicular development it was characterized as containing 10% ICSH.

In experimental induction of ovulation in the hypophysectomized rat, both dosage and timing of administration of the hormones are of utmost importance. Rats hypophysectomized at 26 to 29 days of age were used in experimentation 7 days after the operation, which allowed time to determine completeness of hypophysectomy on a body weight basis, to insure elimination of circulating endogenous hormones, and to establish a reasonably uniform degree of atrophy of the reproductive tract. Table 2 shows the standard conditions adopted for induction of ovulation. Adequate follicular development had to be induced, and for this, subcutaneous injection of FSH once daily for 4 days was found to be satisfactory; during this period a total of 4 RU FSH (4 times the minimally effective dose) was injected. Many healthy medium to medium large, or fully developed (large) follicles were then present. The interstitial tissue was deficient, as only 4 RU FSH had been given, and it would be necessary to inject 10 RU or more of this FSH preparation before interstitial cells would be repaired. Ovulation did not

TABLE 2. STANDARD CONDITIONS FOR INDUCTION OF OVULATION IN HYPOPHYSECTOMIZED RATS

Total dose, subcutaneous		No. of rats	Number ovulating	Ova in oviducts	Ovaries	
Preparatory days 1–4	Supplement late day 4				Wt.	Histology
RU	RU				mg	
4	—	10	0	—	39	mml F IT deficient
4	8	34	28 82%	27 (3–65)	61	1F IT partial repair young CL

follow this preparatory treatment without supplementary hormonal administration. However, it could readily be induced by giving an injection of twice the total preparatory dose (8 RU, likewise subcutaneously) late on the day of the 4th injection (6 hr after the last preparatory dose). Observations of the ovaries and oviducts to determine the incidence of ovulation were made 24 hr after this supplementary injection. Under these circumstances young corpora lutea were present in the ovaries in 82% of the 34 rats so treated. Multiple ova were shed, and an average of 27 were present in the oviduct.

Figure 1 shows the multiplicity of corpora lutea, interspersed with some follicles which did not rupture. The large number of ova shed is indicated by the clumps of granulosa cells in the loop of oviduct shown. Figure 2 shows a group of ova in a distended loop of oviduct. Figure 3 shows that ova sometimes still lingered in the bursa at time of autopsy.

The corpora lutea present 24 hr after the last injection were still not completely formed, the predominating cell, the granulosa lutein cell, not having developed much cytoplasm (FIG. 4). Rupture points were seen occasionally but these close quickly in the rat (FIG. 5).

The treatment almost always developed multiple follicles. The proportion of follicles releasing ova, together with the proportion of rats in the group which ovulated were used as a measure of the efficacy of treatment. With the particular FSH preparation shown in Table 2 the number of ova released varied from 3 to 65, the average being high (27) so this was considered an effective treatment. (At least a few of the multiple follicles stimulated always enclosed ova with luteinization of their walls. Therefore a higher proportion of follicles releasing their ova was evaluated as a better response, although, as pointed out previously, the normality of superovulation may itself be questioned.) Figure 6 shows some apparently normal follicles which did not ovulate within 24 hours. It had been determined previously, however, that the differences in number of ova shed between 18 and 24 hours was no greater than the variation between animals, and that a longer period before autopsy (28, 32, 40 hours) merely resulted in greater maturity of the corpora lutea, and enclosure of the remaining ova in luteinized bodies.

When the corpora lutea were allowed to complete their development under the influence of lactogenic hormone, they could be shown to be functional. The corpora lutea after administration of 2 IU daily of lactogenic hormone* for 10 days were large and compact (FIG. 7) and the uteri of such animals were able to produce placentomata around threads inserted through the endometrium (Table 3).

TABLE 3. FUNCTIONAL CAPACITY OF CORPORA LUTEA INDUCED IN HYPOPHYSECTOMIZED IMMATURE RATS BY FSH OR BY FSH+HCG AND MAINTAINED FOR 10 DAYS BY LACTOGENIC HORMONE. PLACENTOMA REACTION

Ovulatory treatment (4 days)*	No. of rats	Placentoma	Ovarian weight
			mg
FSH 4 RU + FSH 8 RU day 4	6	100%	85
FSH 4 RU HCG 1 RU + FSH 8 RU day 4	3	100%	122

* Followed by lactogenic hormone: 2 IU daily 10 days, threads in endometrium 5th day.

As the FSH preparation used initially in determining the standard conditions for induction of ovulation contained ICSH, it was important to determine the significance of each of the two gonadotropins present. Attention was first directed to the adequacy of FSH unsupported to induce ovulation, for which purpose FSH preparations of increasing purity and potency were compared in regard to this capacity. The FSH preparations used were

* The lactogenic hormone (prolactin) used in these studies was a gift from the Endocrinology Study Section, National Institutes of Health.

assayed carefully in hypophysectomized immature rats. The end point, or RU, in the assay was the minimal dose which would cause resumption of follicular growth (Table 4).

TABLE 4. ASSAY FOR PITUITARY FOLLICLE-STIMULATING HORMONE (FSH) IN HYPOPHYSECTOMIZED FEMALE RATS (AFTER SIMPSON, 21)

Strain, Long-Evans. $\bar{H}$ 26–28 days, 7 days PO.
Inject SQ, 1 × day, 3 days Autopsy 72 hr.
RU: Minimal total dose, in a graded series of doses, giving microscopic evidence in two-thirds of the animals of growth of follicles from control size (< 375 μ) to beginning antrum formation (450–500 μ).

The purified FSH preparations were made from sheep pituitaries by 40% ethanol extraction of whole glands followed by fractional ammonium sulfate precipitation, anion-exchange chromatography on DEAE-cellulose and further ammonium sulfate fractionation.

The best preparations had minimal effective doses (RU) for FSH ranging from 4.0 down to 1.7 μg, when given subcutaneously over a 3-day-period, and did not show contamination with ICSH by interstitial cell repair until 25 to 70 times this dose was injected by the intraperitoneal route (IP), likewise for 3 days. As can be seen (Table 5), the process of purification

TABLE 5. PURIFICATION OF SHEEP FSH (AFTER SIMPSON, 21)

Procedure	Yield mg/kg wet gl	MED FSH μg	Multiple IT repair
		SQ	IP
Frozen pituitary Acetone-dried	250×10^3	*ca.* 2500	0.4 ×
40% EtOH, pH 7, 25°C	8000	250	1 ×
AS Fractionation	300–400	15	5 ×
DEAE-cellulose	30–40	2.9	35 ×
AS 0.6–0.7 sat	12–15	1.7	70 ×

reduced the MED for FSH from 2.5 mg in the original glands to 1.7 μg in the final product. Whereas the original glands gave interstitial repair at 0.4 the MED for FSH the final product could be given at 70-fold the MED before evidence of presence of ICSH was obtained.

The favorable comparison with potency of other purified sheep FSH preparations is shown in Table 6 (3–5, 11, 15, 17, 25, 30, 31). To be noted particularly is the relative potency for FSH, and the contamination with ICSH present in the NIH-FSH-Sl standard. By the assay method used here this preparation had an MED of ≥ 50 μg and showed contamination with ICSH at 5-fold this dose. It may be noted that Velardo in the recent report on induction of ovulation in hypophysectomized rats (28) used this standard, a preparation which is less potent and more contaminated with ICSH than the gonadotropin used in establishing the standard conditions described here. The FSH used in determining standard conditions was made in 1939 and is comparable in method and preparation and potency to that listed as the first item in Table 6.

TABLE 6. COMPARISON OF FOLLICLE-STIMULATING HORMONE (FSH) PREPARATIONS FROM SHEEP PITUITARY MADE IN DIFFERENT LABORATORIES (AFTER SIMPSON, 21)

Preparation		Unitage		Multiple giving	
Author + year	Method	MED μg F in $\bar{H}$ SQ	Multiple of Armour std.	Repair IT in $\bar{H}$ IP	VP 100% in $\bar{H}$ SQ
Jensen, Simpson, Tolksdorf, Evans 1939	40% EtOH; AS	25	6	10	
Conrat, Simpson, Evans 1940	40% EtOH; AS	2.5–3	55	40	
Li, Simpson 1949	aq. ext.; AS	≳100	*ca.* 1.4	≳20	
Raacke, Lostroh, Li 1958	Electrophoresis	25	6		50
Ellis 1958	NIH-SI AS DEAE-C Electrophoresis	≳50 4 (g)	2.7 20 (40)	5	 35
Steelman, Segaloff 1957	EtOH; DEAE-C	*ca.* 4	35		
Woods, Simpson 1959	40% EtOH; AS DEAE-C; AS	15 1.7	10 73	5 70	18 85

TABLE 7. EFFECT OF FURTHER PURIFICATION OF FSH ON ITS ABILITY TO INDUCE OVULATION IN HYPOPHYSECTOMIZED RATS, UNDER STANDARD CONDITIONS OF DOSAGE AND TIMING

Total dose, subcutaneous		MED and % ICSH contamination of FSH preparation used					
days 1–4	day 4	25 μg	5%	4 μg	4%	1.7 μg	1.5%
RU	RU	Ovaries mg	Ova	Ovaries mg	Ova	Ovaries mg	Ova
FSH 4	—	33	— 0/8	35	— 0/8	30	— 0/9
FSH 4	FSH 8	55	29 4/9	54	6 12/34	45	10 10/19

The sheep FSH from DEAE-cellulose columns, given at the same total unitage, and under the same time relationships used in determining standard conditions, resulted in ovulation less reliably than did the original preparation containing 10% ICSH. Pilot experiments (Table 7) show the ovulatory response from three FSH preparations of increasing purity, as indicated by lower MED (25 μg down to 1.7 μg) and decreasing percentage of ICSH contamination (5%, 4% and 1.5%, respectively). The results from use of these purified fractions did not equal that obtained from the original less purified preparation; in fact, only about one-third to one-half of the rats ovulated.

Several possible explanations for the discrepancy between these and earlier results can be offered. In the first place, the rate of absorption and excretion of the more purified preparations may differ from that of cruder ones. Several means for obtaining prolonged action were tried, such as multiple injections and injection of FSH in solutions containing gelatin or serum albumin, but no clear evidence was obtained that this was an important factor. The possibility that pituitary tropic hormones other than gonadotropins may be involved in induction of ovulation also must be considered. This seems improbable, however, as the only important biologically active contaminant of FSH preparations is ICSH. Even the starting material for all preparations, the 40% ethanol extract of whole sheep pituitaries which had an MED for follicle development of 0.250 mg, contained less than 0.1% growth, thyrotropic and adrenocorticotropic hormones. It did contain a small amount of lactogenic hormone (0.075 IU/mg) but lactogenic hormone has been tested as an ovulatory supplement in rats (as well as monkeys) and no effect in inducing ovulation has been demonstrated. Purified preparations of FSH with potency of 25 μg down to 1.7 μg contained less than 0.1% of all the other tropic hormones: growth, thyrotropic, adrenocorticotropic and lactogenic hormones.

The most obvious explanation of the reduced efficacy of more highly purified FSH preparations was that the ICSH content had been depleted too far. Attention was therefore turned to whether the ovulatory stimulus from purified FSH was improved by addition of ICSH. Reconstitution of the fraction of ICSH found in the original preparation, by addition of 10% by unitage of ICSH, was the first approach.

As the ICSH added was a highly purified product a word should be said regarding its chemical fractionation and assay. These preparations were all standardized in hypophysectomized immature rats by determining the minimal dose (RU) which would repair the deficient interstitial cells (Table 8).

The ICSH was prepared by methods similar to those used in purifying FSH from a starting material of 40% ethanol extract from whole sheep pituitary. The steps in the procedure, the potency of the preparation, and the multiple of the MED which showed evidence of FSH contamination are

Ovaries of rats hypophysectomized at 26–29 days of age and treated one week later, for 4 days, with gonadotropins to induce ovulation. H and E stain. (Magnifications × $\frac{1}{2}$)

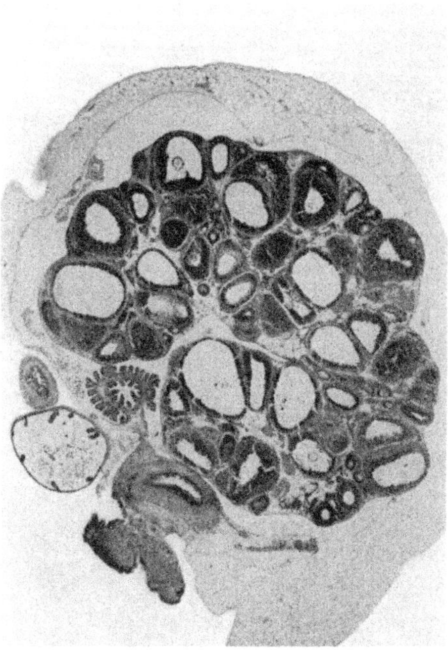

FIG. 1. Whole ovary, in bursa, showing multiple corpora lutea of ovulation, residual large follicles, some with luteinized walls enclosing their ova. A few ova, still surrounded by granulosa cells, may be seen free in the bursa or within a distended loop of oviduct. ×27.

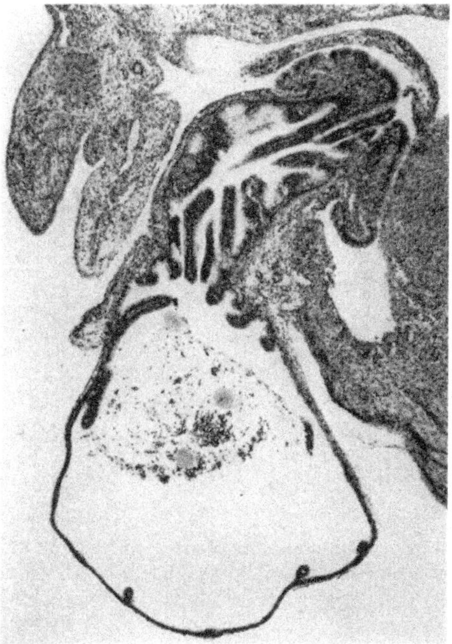

FIG. 2. Fimbriated end of oviduct and distended loop of oviduct, with ova. ×91.

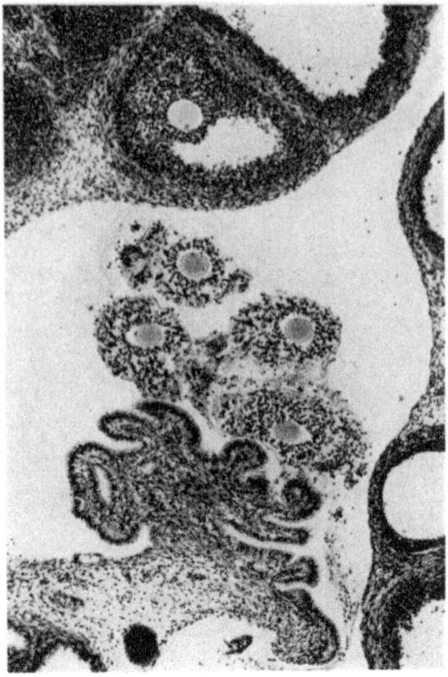

FIG. 3. Ova surrounded by granulosa cells, still free in the bursa and approaching the fimbriated end of the oviduct, 24 hr after injection of the ovulatory supplement. × 125.

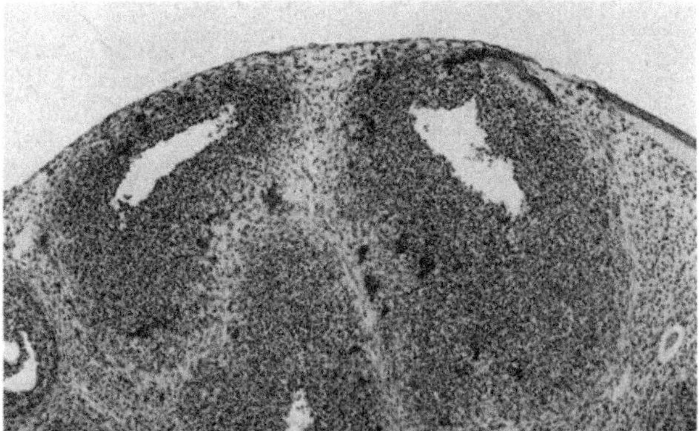

FIG. 4. Numerous young corpora lutea of ovulation, surrounded by capillaries which have not yet penetrated very deeply into the granulosal walls. × 125.

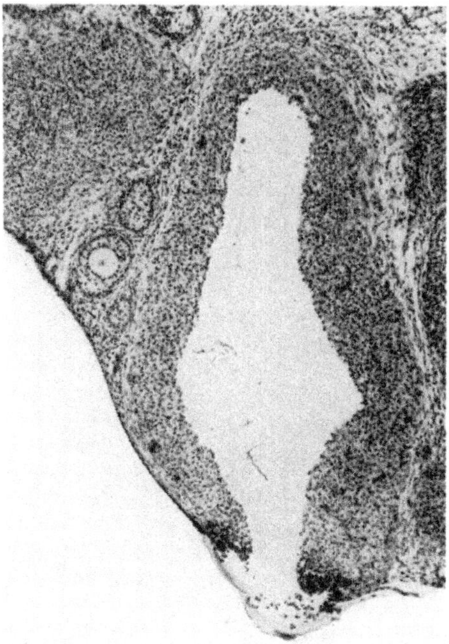

FIG. 5. Young corpus luteum showing rupture point. × 125.

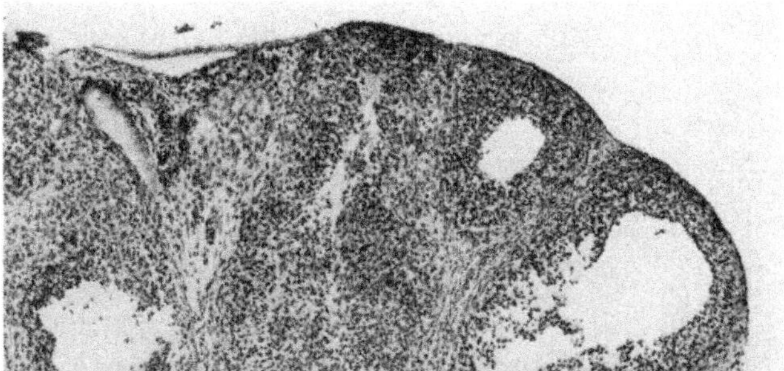

FIG. 6. Young corpus luteum, with residual large follicles. × 125.

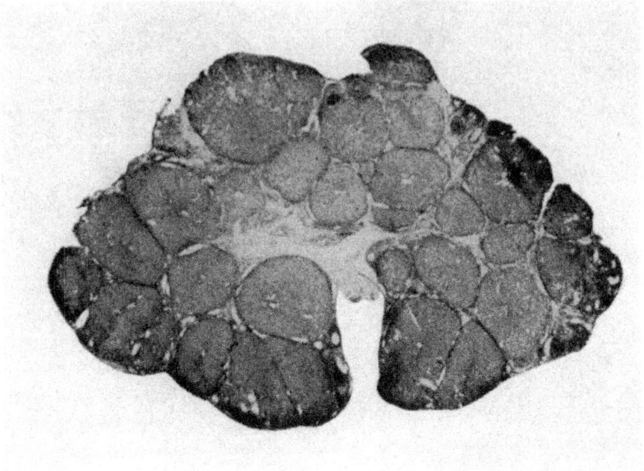

FIG. 7. Corpora lutea maintained for 10 days by 2 IU lactogenic hormone daily, following induction of ovulation by 4 RU FSH in 4 days with a supplementary injection of 8 RU FSH late on the 4th day. Frozen section. H and E. ×27.

given in Table 9. Judged by the assay procedure described the best preparations had an MED of 1 μg and did not lead to resumption of follicular development at 6000-fold this dose. No other pituitary tropic hormones were present in significant amounts in these ICSH preparations.

TABLE 8. ASSAY FOR PITUITARY INTERSTITIAL CELL-STIMULATING HORMONE (ICSH) IN HYPOPHYSECTOMIZED FEMALE RATS (AFTER SIMPSON, 21)

Strain, Long-Evans. $\bar{H}$ 26–28 days, 7 days PO.
Inject IP 1 × day, 3 days Autopsy 72 hr.
RU: Minimal total dose, in a graded series of doses, giving microscopic evidence in two-thirds of the animals of repair of "deficient" interstitial cells: increased nuclear size, loss of pyknosis; reappearance of rim of eosinophilic cytoplasm.

TABLE 9. PURIFICATION OF SHEEP ICSH (AFTER SIMPSON, 21)

Procedure	Yield mg/kg wet gl.	MED ICSH μg*	Multiple of MED F devel.†
Frozen pituitary			
Acetone-dried	250 × 10³	*ca.* 1000	2.5 ×
40% EtOH, pH 7, 25°C	8000	100	2.5 ×
AS 0.4–0.45 sat.	50–75	5–7.5	75 ×
DEAE-cellulose	10–12	1	> 6000 ×

* IP. † S.Q.

The purity of these preparations can be judged by comparing them with those from sheep pituitaries made elsewhere, shown in Table 10 (13, 14, 23, 24, 30).

The comparison of potency of ICSH with different standard preparations (NIH and Armour) by two different assay methods is given in Table 11. The best preparation was 4 times as potent as the Armour "LH" standard, judged by the repair of interstitial tissue of hypophysectomized female rats, and 5 times as potent by the ventral prostate test in hypophysectomized male rats (21).

Table 12 shows a preliminary effort to determine whether the efficacy of more purified FSH preparations is increased by reinstating the ICSH content to 10%. The two FSH preparations used, with MED's of 5 and 1.67 μg respectively, did not cause ovulation during the preparatory stimulation of follicular growth when given in doses of 4 RU combined with 10% ICSH. When this preparatory treatment was supplemented as before by FSH alone, given at twice the total dose used in the preparatory treatment (or 8 RU FSH), ovulation occurred in most rats and large numbers of ova were shed. A supplement of the combination (FSH+10% ICSH) gave comparable

TABLE 10. COMPARISON OF INTERSTITIAL CELL-STIMULATING HORMONE (ICSH) PREPARATIONS FROM SHEEP PITUITARY, MADE IN DIFFERENT LABORATORIES (AFTER SIMPSON, 21)

Author + Year		Preparation	Unitage (μg)		Multiple of Armour std.		Multiple $\bar{H}$ MED given SQ F dev.
			IT repair $\bar{H}$ ♀ IP	VP 100% SQ	IT rep.	VP	
Li, Simpson, Evans	1940	40% EtOH; AS	7	7			500
Squire, Li	1958–9	aq. ext.; IRC-50	2	$\lesssim$ 2	2.5	$\gtrsim$ 7	> 1000
Ellis	1958	aq. ext.; IRC-50	*ca.* 5	5	1	3	150
Leonora, McShan, Meyer	1958	IR-4B; IRC-50		<60			>20
Woods, Simpson	1959	aq. ext.; AS DEAE-C	3	5	1.7	5	> 1200
		IRC-50; AS (from above)	2		2.5	7	
		40% EtOH AS, DEAE-C	1	3	4	5	> 6000

TABLE 11. COMPARISON OF POTENCY OF ICSH PREPARATIONS MADE IN DIFFERENT LABORATORIES, BY VENTRAL PROSTATE WEIGHT INCREASE OR BY INTERSTITIAL CELL REPAIR, IN HYPOPHYSECTOMIZED RATS (AFTER SIMPSON, 21)

Preparation	Ventral prostate 100% increase* μg	Interstitial cell repair MED rats μg
Armour std. (sheep) LH 227-80	15† (S-D strain) 13 (L-E)	5 (L-E strain)
Ellis (sheep) LH XIII-25-2	5 (S-D)	>5 $\lesssim$ 10 (L-E)
WDI 40C (sheep) WDIII 58A (sheep)	15 (L-E) 2.2 (L-E)	15 (L-E) 1.3 (L-E)

* 21–22 days at $\bar{H}$, onset injection 2 days PO; injections given 1 × day, 4 days, autopsy 96 hr; injection SQ; Greep, PSEBM **46**: 644, 1941.

† Potency reported by Ellis, *J. Biol. Chem.* **233**, 63, 1958, for assay in Sprague-Dawley rats. Steelman and Pohley, *Endocrinology* **53**, 604, 1953 (15 μg, V.P.), for Sprague-Dawley rats.

ovulation, judged both by the proportion of rats ovulating and the average number of ova shed. However, this combined supplement did not appear to be so effective after FSH alone was used in preparation of the follicles; fewer ova were released. From this we proceeded on the assumption that the presence of ICSH is of more importance during preparation of the follicles than it is in the ovulatory supplement.

TABLE 12. PILOT EXPERIMENT. RECOMBINATION OF TWO PURIFIED FSH PREPARATIONS WITH 10% ICSH, IN DIFFERENT PHASES OF THE OVULATORY TREATMENT

Total dose, subcutaneous		MED of FSH preparation used			
days 1–4	day 4	5 μg		1.67 μg	
RU	RU	Ovaries mg		Ovaries mg	
FSH 4 ICSH 0.4	—	53	—	25	—
FSH 4 ICSH 0.4	FSH 8	89	Ova: 58 3 of 3	63	Ova: 15 2 of 3
FSH 4	FSH 8 ICSH 0.8	71	Ova: 6 3 of 3	54	Ova: 5 2 of 2
FSH 4 ICSH 0.4	FSH 8 ICSH 0.8	81	Ova: 31 3 of 3	54	Ova: 17 3 of 3

Table 13 shows a more careful analysis, which confirms the importance of the presence of 10% ICSH during preparation of follicles. Six FSH preparations were tested; for preparation of the follicles each was injected alone in 4 RU total dose, and after addition of 10% ICSH. The respective FSH under examination was given alone as the supplement to all groups. Neither the purified FSH preparations given alone nor those to which 10% ICSH was added caused ovulation without supplementation. FSH alone followed by the respective FSH as supplement on the 4th day gave variable results; some FSH preparations caused all rats to ovulate whereas others resulted in ovulation in as few as 30%. The same FSH preparations, upon the addition of 10% ICSH during the preparatory period caused ovulation in most groups when supplemented by the respective FSH. Both the number of rats ovulating and the numbers of ova shed were in most instances greater than when the follicles had been prepared by FSH without the addition of 10% ICSH. The number of purified FSH preparations used and the size of the groups tested seem adequate to establish that more ICSH is needed during follicular growth than is provided by the purest FSH preparations.

It should not be concluded from the data presented that the proportion of ICSH used (10%) was that most favorable for ovulation. The proportion of FSH and ICSH occurring naturally differs in the pituitaries of various species. The rat pituitary is high in ICSH, certainly far higher than the purified FSH preparations from sheep pituitary. In turning to an analysis

TABLE 13. INDUCTION OF OVULATION BY DIFFERENT PURIFIED FSH PREPARATIONS FROM SHEEP PITUITARY, WITH OR WITHOUT THE ADDITION OF 10% ICSH* IN THE PREPARATORY PHASE OF TREATMENT

Total dose, subcutaneous		MED (RU) and % ICSH contamination of FSH preparation injected											
da 1–4	da 4	25 μg	3%	25 μg	5%	4 μg	4%	2.5 μg	2.5%	2.5 μg	4%	1.7 μg	1.5%
RU	RU	Ovaries mg	Ova	Ovaries mg	Ova	Ovaries mg	Ova	Ovaries mg	Ova	Ovaries mg	Ova	Ovaries mg	Ova
FSH 4	—	40	— 0/6	33	— 0/8	35	— 0/8	20	— 0/9	23	— 0/15	30	— 0/9
	FSH 8	61	24 12/12 100%	55	16 4/9 44%	54	6 12/34 35%	34	9 5/9 55%	50	14 6/21 29%	45	10 10/19 53%
FSH 4 ICSH 0.4	—	50	— 0/6	43	— 0/8	45	— 0/12	20	— 0/8	34	— 0/15	37	— 0/8
	FSH 8	102	52 6/6 100%	62	53 9/9 100%	75	40 16/17 94%	40	14 7/9 78%	67	29 14/15 93%	72	43 9/9 100%

* ICSH (sheep) MED 5 μg in first column, 1 μg in remainder.

of the efficacy of rat pituitary preparations it was also kept in mind that species specificity of the pituitary proteins might constitute an important factor in the ability of the protein hormones to induce ovulation. Saline suspensions of pooled rat anterior pituitaries were tested for ovulatory response in hypophysectomized rats and found to be effective when given even at lower unitage than the sheep preparations (provided, of course, that they were given under the conditions of timing described above which were rigidly maintained in this and all subsequent experiments).

TABLE 14. INDUCTION OF OVULATION BY SALINE SUSPENSIONS OF RAT ANTERIOR PITUITARY, UNDER STANDARD CONDITIONS OF TIMING

Total dose, subcutaneous (RU by assay)		Ovarian weight	Ova in oviducts
days 1–4	day 4		
RU FSH 4 ICSH 16	RU FSH 4 ICSH 16	mg 99	63 (30–98) 3/3
FSH 2 ICSH 8	FSH 4 ICSH 16	113	* 3/3
	FSH 2 ICSH 8	74	* 3/3
FSH 1 ICSH 4	FSH 4 ICSH 16	83	* 3/3
	FSH 2 ICSH 8	73	* 3/3

* Distended oviducts indicating ovulation.

The 40% ethanol extracts of rat pituitary were likewise effective. The unitage administered was, however, of critical importance in determining whether ovulation resulted. When a dose containing 4 × the minimum dose for follicular stimulation was administered, a dose most nearly comparable therefore to the 4 RU dose of sheep FSH though containing 16 times the minimal dose necessary for interstitial cell stimulation, it proved to be too high for ovulation (Table 15). This dose sometimes caused luteinization of the follicle wall with enclosure of ova even before the supplement of twice the total preparatory dose of the same material was given. When a half or a fourth this preparatory dose was given, containing the equivalent of 2 RU FSH + 8 RU ICSH or 1 RU FSH + 4 RU ICSH, normal, large follicles developed which ovulated when supplemented as before.

In order to determine whether these results were peculiar to rat pituitary gonadotropins, an effort was made to reconstitute the proportion in rat pituitary ethanol extracts by use of sheep pituitary gonadotropins. Purified sheep FSH and ICSH preparations were therefore combined in the proportion 1 : 4, and were given at unitages corresponding to those of the rat pituitary preparations (Table 15). Sheep gonadotropins in doses of 4 RU FSH + 16 RU

TABLE 15. INDUCTION OF OVULATION BY A 40% ETHANOL EXTRACT OF RAT PITUITARY, OR BY SHEEP FSH AND ICSH COMBINED IN THE SAME PROPORTION

Total dose, subcutaneous (RU by assay)		Rat pit. 40% EtOH extr. MED: F stim. 75 μg IT repair 20 μg		Sheep pituitary FSH: MED 4 μg ICSH: MED 1 μg	
days 1–4	day 4				
RU	RU	Ovaries mg	Ova	Ovaries mg	Ova
FSH 4 ICSH 16	—	110 Encl.	9 3/3	53 Encl.	— 0/3
	FSH 8 ICSH 32	128 Encl.	9 3/3	76 Encl.	14 3/3
FSH 2 ICSH 8	—	61 1F	3 1/3	36 1F	7 1/12
	FSH 8 ICSH 32	117 CL	35 3/3	60 CL	35 12/12
FSH 1 ICSH 4	—	31 1F	— 0/3	10 mF	— 0/3
	FSH 8 ICSH 32	49 CL	42 3/3	18 mF	— 0/2

ICSH caused luteinization of follicles with enclosure of ova, even before supplementation. Half these unitages, 2 RU FSH + 8 RU ICSH, caused follicular development, but even without supplementation occasionally caused ovulation, as had the rat pituitary extract at this level; optimal conditions for ovulation were attained only when the usual supplement was administered. Mixtures of 1 RU FSH + 4 RU ICSH did not give adequate follicular growth in the first phase of treatment and the supplementary dose was therefore ineffective, so that such mixtures were slightly inferior to the rat pituitary preparations.

Several purified FSH preparations were combined with ICSH in this ratio (1 : 4) and when given at the optimal dose level, 2 RU FSH and 8 RU ICSH, were equally effective in promoting follicular development. When this was followed by the usual supplementary dose of the combination excellent ovulation ensued (Table 16).

TABLE 16. SUPPLEMENTARY TREATMENTS EFFECTIVE IN INDUCING OVULATION, AFTER FOLLICULAR DEVELOPMENT BY PURIFIED SHEEP FSH AND ICSH* PREPARATIONS COMBINED IN THE PROPORTION PRESENT IN A RAT PITUITARY EXTRACT

Total dose, subcutaneous		MED and % ICSH contamination of FSH injected							
days 1–4	day 4	25 μg	10%	4 μg	4%	2.5 μg	2.5%	1.7 μg	1.5%
RU	RU	Ovaries mg	Ova	Ovaries mg	Ova	Ovaries mg	Ova	Ovaries mg	Ova
FSH 2 ICSH 8	—	28	— 0/3	36	7 1/12	12	— 0/3	36	— 0/3
	FSH 8 ICSH 32	51	10 3/3	60	35 12/12	19	4 3/3	77	25 2/3
	FSH 8	43	6 3/3	83	49 3/3	21	10 2/3	39	16 5/6
	ICSH 32	48	5 3/3	50	28 18/18	26	— 0/3	43	7 2/3

* ICSH MED 12.5 μg used with the 25 μg FSH; MED 1 μg with all others.

In order more specifically to define the requirements for the supplement, experiments were conducted to determine whether this proportion and dose of FSH and ICSH (8 RU+32 RU) was optimal. Each component of the mixture was therefore examined separately, at the dose level contained in the mixture just described (Table 16). It was found that FSH alone at the 8 RU level was effective as a supplement under the conditions of this experiment. ICSH was then tried by itself at the same dose at which it had been present in the combined supplement (32 RU) and it too caused ovulation. In some instances, however, the number of animals ovulating and the number of ova shed were less than after the combination or after FSH alone; in fact there was one experiment in which not a single animal ovulated when ICSH only was used as a supplement at the 32 RU level.

Subsequently the efficacy of ICSH as an ovulatory supplement, following preparation of follicles by 2 RU FSH+8 RU ICSH, was analyzed more thoroughly at dose levels ranging from 2 to 40 RU. It was found that doses of 16 to 40 RU resulted in ovulation (Table 17). However, when the follicles were prepared by 4 RU of the same purified FSH given alone, and therefore containing only 4% intrinsic ICSH, even the highest supplementary dose of ICSH (32 RU) was not entirely effective (only 2 of 4 rats ovulated). When the FSH preparation used to develop the follicles contained 10% intrinsic ICSH, ovulation occurred following ICSH as a supplement at all levels: 8, 16 or 32 RU.

TABLE 17. GRADED DOSES OF ICSH AS THE OVULATORY SUPPLEMENT, AFTER FOLLICULAR DEVELOPMENT BY DIFFERENT TREATMENTS

Preparatory total dose, subcutaneous, days 1–4	Supplementary dose ICSH (MED 1 μg), day 4, subcutaneous, RU									
	0		8		16–20		32		40	
RU	Ov. mg	Ova	Ov. mg	Ova	Ov. mg	Ova	Ov. mg	Ova	Ov. mg	Ova
FSH 2 MED 4 μg 4% ICSH	36	7	46	15	43	33	48	37	52	17
ICSH 8 MED 1 μg		1/12		2/7		10/10		10/10		8/8
FSH 4 MED 4 μg	35	—	38	—	34	—	45	22		
4% ICSH		0/8		0/4		0/4		2/4		
FSH 4 MED 25 μg	39		53	*	56	*	60	*		
10% ICSH		0/10		2/4		3/4		4/4		

* Not counted; distended oviducts.

TABLE 18. GRADED DOSES OF CHORIONIC GONADOTROPIN (HCG) AS THE OVULATORY SUPPLEMENT, AFTER FOLLICLE DEVELOPMENT BY DIFFERENT TREATMENTS

Preparatory total dose, subcutaneous, days 1–4	Supplementary dose HCG, day 4, subcutaneous, IU									
	0		4		8		16		32	
RU	Ov. mg	Ova	Ov. mg	Ova	Ov. mg	Ova	Ov. mg	Ova	Ov. mg	Ova
FSH 2 MED 4 μg 4% ICSH	36	7	27	—	46	25	64	*	58	*
ICSH 8 MED 1 μg		1/12		0/1		5/6		4/4		4/4
FSH 4 MED 4 μg	35	—			47	—	55	6	60	44
4% ICSH		0/8				0/4		3/4		3/4
FSH 4 MED 25 μg	39	—	49	44	57	37	100	52		
10% ICSH		0/10		1/7		4/4		4/4		

* Not counted; distended oviducts.

Another luteinizing substance, human chorionic gonadotropin (HCG), was tested as a supplement at levels from 2 to 32 IU (Table 18, RU = IU). Doses of 8 or more IU HCG were found to be effective as ovulatory supplements following combinations of 2 RU FSH + 8 RU ICSH. The results were the same when 10% intrinsic ICSH was present in the FSH preparation, but following FSH containing 4% ICSH higher doses of HCG were required, 32 IU being optimal (Table 18).

The importance of the presence of more than 4% ICSH with the FSH during stimulation of follicular growth was exemplified further by experiments

TABLE 19. GRADED DOSES OF ICSH AS THE OVULATORY SUPPLEMENT, AFTER FOLLICULAR DEVELOPMENT BY PURIFIED FSH, WITH OR WITHOUT THE ADDITION OF 10% ICSH

Preparatory total dose, subcutaneous, days 1–4		Supplementary dose ICSH (MED 1 μg), day 4, subcutaneous, RU							
		0		8		16		32	
	RU	Ov. mg	Ova	Ov. mg	Ova	Ov. mg	Ova	Ov. mg	Ova
FSH MED 4 μg 4% ICSH	4	35	— 0/8	38	— 0/4	34	— 0/4	43	22 5/10
FSH MED 4 μg 4% ICSH ICSH MED 1 μg	4 0.4	45	— 0/12	57	* 4/6	63	* 6/6	37	* 6/6

* Not counted; distended oviducts.

TABLE 20. GRADED DOSES OF HCG AS THE OVULATORY SUPPLEMENT, AFTER FOLLICULAR DEVELOPMENT BY PURIFIED FSH, WITH OR WITHOUT THE ADDITION OF 10% ICSH

Preparatory total dose, subcutaneous, days 1–4		Supplementary dose HCG, day 4, subcutaneous, IU							
		0		8		16		32	
	RU	Ov. mg	Ova	Ov. mg	Ova	Ov. mg	Ova	Ov. mg	Ova
FSH MED 4 μg 4% ICSH	4	35	— 0/8	47	— 0/4	55	6 3/4	60	44 3/4
FSH MED 4 μg 4% ICSH ICSH MED 1 μg	4 0.4	45	0/12	77	* 6/6	60	* 6/6	69	* 6/6

* Not counted; distended oviducts.

in which 10% ICSH was added to the purified FSH during the preparatory treatment. ICSH was then effective as the ovulatory supplement in a greater number of animals, and at lower dose levels, than when following the FSH alone (Table 19). These results were confirmed with HCG (Table 20).

FSH was similarly evaluated as an ovulatory supplement at different dose levels, following different preparatory treatments. FSH had previously been shown to be effective as a supplement at the 8 RU level following follicular development by 2 RU FSH+8 RU ICSH. This held true for several FSH preparations of increasing purity (Table 16). As shown in Table 21, 4 RU of

TABLE 21. GRADED DOSES OF FSH AS THE OVULATORY SUPPLEMENT, AFTER FOLLICULAR DEVELOPMENT BY DIFFERENT TREATMENTS

Preparatory total dose, subcutaneous, days 1–4		Supplementary dose of the respective FSH, day 4, subcutaneous, RU					
		0		4		8	
	RU	Ovaries mg	Ova	Ovaries mg	Ova	Ovaries mg	Ova
FSH MED 4 μg 4% ICSH	2	36	7	46	34	54	28
ICSH MED 1 μg	8		1/12		2/3		15/15
FSH MED 4 μg 4% ICSH	4	35	— 0/8			54	6 12/34
FSH MED 25 μg 10% ICSH	4	39	— 0/10	75	* 6/6	61	27 28/34

* Not counted; distended oviducts.

purified FSH (MED 4 μg, 4% ICSH contamination) was still effective as a supplement after preparation of follicles by 2 RU FSH+8 RU ICSH. However, 8 RU FSH was less effective as a supplement when the follicles had been prepared by 4 RU of this FSH alone. The preparation used in determining the standard conditions, containing 10% intrinsic ICSH, was equally effective as an ovulatory supplement at 4 RU or at 8 RU, following follicular development by 4 RU of this preparation.

This apparent non-specificity of the gonadotropic supplementary stimulus to ovulation leaves several questions unanswered. That time is not the factor has been shown by failure of ovulation after the preparatory treatment alone, even though the rats were autopsied simultaneously with those which had received a supplementary injection in the interim. The occasional release of a few ova, reported here upon preparatory treatment by high unitages of FSH and ICSH, was accompanied by excessive luteinization of the majority of the follicles with enclosure of their ova. Sporadic instances of ovulation without supplementary treatment have also been observed during routine assay of gonadotropins, especially those of human pituitary origin, and here again the answer may lie in the high proportion of ICSH present. Ovulation in hypophysectomized rats after injection for four days of human pituitary has been reported by Bahn *et al.* (1) and by Velardo with sheep FSH and ICSH (28).

That the injection *per se* is not the stimulus has been shown by the inadequacy of lower doses of FSH, ICSH or HCG than those illustrated in the tables. A common factor might be sought in the possible contamination of all these products by minute amounts of substances such as posterior lobe hormones.* The existence of a separate "ovulatory hormone" has also been postulated (5). It is difficult, though not impossible, to conceive that another factor of sufficient biological potency could accompany FSH and ICSH in their present state of purification.

SUMMARY AND CONCLUSIONS

What has been learned thus far in experimental induction of ovulation in rat and monkey may be summarized as follows. Ovulation has been induced in normal immature and adult *Macaca mulatta* with sheep pituitary fractions high in FSH, and by 40% ethanol extracts of monkey anterior pituitary, with and without supplements of sheep ICSH or of HCG. Although the sheep preparations which caused ovulation in the monkey were designated as "FSH" and were prepared by methods which yielded potent FSH, which by physico-chemical criteria consisted of homogeneous protein, they were nevertheless not homogeneous biologically, and still contained small amounts of ICSH.

These experiments were also subject to the criticism that normal recipients were used and the pituitary undoubtedly contributed to the response. This criticism has been obviated in the studies conducted in hypophysectomized rats. Sheep FSH prepared similarly to that used in monkeys, as well as further purified FSH preparations of greater potency, in which ICSH contamination had been further reduced, have been examined carefully for their adequacy in induction of ovulation in the hypophysectomized rat. FSH preparations of potency comparable to those used in the monkey, with MED 25 μg and containing 10% ICSH were effective both in promoting growth of follicles and, terminally at higher doses, in giving the final impetus to ovulation. FSH preparations of greater potency, MED 4 to 1.7 μg, which

* Subsequent experiments have indicated that neither Pitressin, in doses of 0.5 or 0.05 dog pressor units, nor Pitocin, in doses of 0.5 or 0.05 guinea-pig uterine units, is effective as an ovulatory supplement after follicular development by the FSH preparation used in establishing standard conditions for ovulation. (The two products were supplied by Parke, Davis & Co.)

contained 4 to 1.5% ICSH contamination, were more variable in promoting ovulation and were improved by an increase of ICSH content to 10% during the preparatory phase of follicular growth.

A much higher content of ICSH than 10% did not interfere with the effectiveness of the FSH preparations either during the preparatory or supplementary phases. Combinations of FSH with 4-fold as much ICSH were active, optimally at doses of 2 RU FSH+8 RU ICSH. After stimulation of follicles by such combinations ovulation could be induced not only by the combination but also by either component given alone as the supplement. Purified FSH was somewhat more effective as a supplement and could be used at lower doses than ICSH (or HCG). It was clear, however, that FSH, though effective as a supplement, was sufficiently purified to require additional ICSH, more than 4%, during preparation of follicles.

It should be noted that the sheep preparations, at stages of purification after the 40% ethanol starting material, contained negligible amounts of other pituitary tropic hormones (growth, thyrotropic, adrenocorticotropic and lactogenic hormones) so that it appears improbable that the other pituitary tropic hormones are involved in either the preparatory or the supplementary impetus to ovulation. Perhaps it will be impossible to clarify further the proportion of the pituitary gonadotropic factors necessary for ovulation until FSH and ICSH have been prepared in pure form.

REFERENCES

1. BAHN, R. C., N. LORENZ, W. A. BENNETT and A. ALBERT, Gonadotropins of the pituitary gland and urine of the adult human male, *Proc. Soc. Exptl. Biol. and Med.* **82**, 777–782, 1953.
2. CARTER, F., M. E. SIMPSON and H. M. EVANS, Conditions necessary for the induction of ovulation in hypophysectomized rats, *Anat. Record* (*Proceedings*) **130**, 283, 1958.
3. ELLIS, S., A scheme for the separation of pituitary proteins, *J. Biol. Chem.* **233**, 63–68, 1958.
4. EVANS, H. M., M. E. SIMPSON, S. TOLKSDORF and H. JENSEN, Biological studies of the gonadotropic principles in sheep pituitary substance, *Endocrinology* **25**, 529–546, 1939.
5. EVERETT, J. W., The time of release of ovulating hormone from the rat hypophysis, *Endocrinology* **59**, 580–585, 1956.
6. FRAENKEL-CONRAT, H. L., M. E. SIMPSON and H. M. EVANS, Purification of follicle-stimulating hormone (FSH) of the anterior pituitary, *Proc. Soc. Exptl. Biol. and Med.* **45**, 627–630, 1940.
7. FRAENKEL-CONRAT, H. L., M. E. SIMPSON and H. M. EVANS, Purification of follicle-stimulating hormone of the anterior pituitary, *Anales de la Facultad de Medicina, Montevideo* **25**, 159–168, 1940.
8. GEMZELL, C. A., E. DICZFALUSY and K. G. TILLINGER, Clinical effect of human pituitary follicle-stimulating hormone (FSH), *J. Clin. Endocrinol. and Metab.* **18**, 1333–1348, 1958.

8a. GEMZELL, C. A., E. DICZFALUSY and K. G. TILLINGER, Ciba Foundation Colloquium on Human Pituitary Hormones, Buenos Aires, Argentina, Aug. 6–8, 1959.

9. HAMMOND, J., Jr., Induced ovulation and heat in anoestrous sheep, *J. Endocrinol.* **4**, 169–180, 1945.
10. HISAW, F. L., Development of the Graafian follicle and ovulation, *Physiol. Rev.* **27**, 95–119, 1947.

11. JENSEN, H., M. E. SIMPSON, S. TOLKSDORF and H. M. EVANS, Chemical fractionation of the gonadotropic factors present in sheep pituitary, *Endocrinology* **25**, 57–62, 1939.
12. KNOBIL, E., J. L. KOSTYO and R. O. GREEP, Production of ovulation in the hypophysectomized Rhesus monkey, *Endocrinology* **65**, 487–493, 1959.
13. LEONORA, J., W. H. MCSHAN and R. K. MEYER, Separation of LH fractions from sheep pituitary glands by use of ion exchange resins, *Endocrinology* **63**, 867, 1958.
14. LI, C. H., M. E. SIMPSON and H. M. EVANS, Interstitial cell-stimulating hormone. II. Method of preparation and some physico-chemical studies, *Endocrinology* **27**, 803–808, 1940.
15. LI, C. H., M. E. SIMPSON and H. M. EVANS, Isolation of pituitary follicle-stimulating hormone (FSH), *Science* **109**, 445–446, 1949.
16. MEYER, R. K. *et al.*, Conference on Human Pituitary Gonadotrophins (Sponsored by the Endocrinology Study Section, National Institutes of Health) Gatlinburg, Tennessee, December 3–5, 1959.
17. RAACKE, I. D., A. J. LOSTROH and C. H. LI, Zone electrophoresis on starch of preparations of follicle-stimulating hormone from sheep pituitary glands, *Arch. Biochem. Biophys.* **77**, 138–146, 1958.
18. ROSEMBERG, E. *et al.*, Conference on Human Pituitary Gonadotrophins (Sponsored by the Endocrinology Study Sections, National Institutes of Health) Gatlinburg, Tennessee, December 3–5, 1959.
19. ROWLANDS, I. W. and P. C. WILLIAMS, Comparative activity of the gonadotrophin in horse pituitary glands and in pregnant mare's serum, *J. Endocrinol.* **2**, 380–394, 1941.
20. ROWLANDS, I. W. and P. C. WILLIAMS, Production of ovulation in hypophysectomized rats, *J. Endocrinol.* **3**, 310–315, 1943.
21. SIMPSON, M. E. *et al.*, Conference on Human Pituitary Gonadotrophins (Sponsored by the Endocrinology Study Section, National Institutes of Health) Gatlinburg, Tennessee, December 3–5, 1959.
22. SIMPSON, M. E. and G. VAN WAGENEN, Experimental induction of ovulation in the macaque monkey, *Fertility and Sterility* **9**, 386–399, 1958.
23. SQUIRE, P. G. and C. H. LI, Purification and properties of an interstitial cell-stimulating hormone from sheep pituitaries, *Science* **127**, 32, 1958.
24. SQUIRE, P. G. and C. H. LI, Purification and properties of interstitial cell-stimulating hormone from sheep pituitary glands, *J. Biol. Chem.* **234**, 520–525, 1959.
25. STEELMAN, S. L. and A. SEGALOFF, *Abstracts*, The Endocrine Society, 39th meeting, New York, May 1957, p. 158.
26. VAN WAGENEN, G. and M. E. SIMPSON, Induction of multiple ovulation in the Rhesus monkey (*Macaca mulatta*), *Endocrinology* **61**, 316–318, 1957.
27. VAN WAGENEN, G. and M. E. SIMPSON, Experimentally induced ovulation in the Rhesus monkey (*Macaca mulatta*), *Revue Suisse de Zoologie* **64**, 807–819, 1957.
28. VELARDO, J. T., Induction of ovulation in immature hypophysectomized rats, *Science* **131**, 357–359, 1960.
29. WILLIAMS, P. C., Studies of the biological action of serum gonadotrophin. 2. Ovarian response after hypophysectomy and oestrogen treatment, *J. Endocrinol.* **4**, 131–136, 1945.
30. WOODS, M. C. and M. E. SIMPSON, Chromatography of sheep pituitary gonadotropins on DEAE-cellulose, *Federation Proc.* **18**, 687, 1959.
31. WOODS, M. C. and M. E. SIMPSON, Purification of sheep pituitary follicle-stimulating hormone (FSH) by ion exchange chromatography on diethylaminoethyl (DEAE)-cellulose, *Endocrinology* **66**, 575–584, 1960.

DISCUSSION

Dr. Ernest Knobil: I would much prefer to stand in mute admiration of Dr. Simpson's impressive studies, but since she has mentioned some of our work dealing with ovulation in the hypophysectomized rhesus monkey, I will accept this opportunity to take the floor.

As Dr. Simpson indicated, we were able to induce ovulation in hypophysectomized monkeys by the subcutaneous administration of porcine FSH followed by the simultaneous administration of this FSH preparation and HCG (*Endocrinology* **65**, 487, 1959). We most certainly concur with Dr. Simpson that non-primate FSH preparations are highly active in the monkey and that their administration, in small quantities, all too easily leads to the production of cystic follicles.

Our few attempts to induce ovulation in hypophysectomized monkeys with LH preparations other than HCG (non-primate pituitary LH) were uniformly unsuccessful. These findings, the difficulties encountered by other workers in the induction of ovulation in normal monkeys with non-primate pituitary LH preparations, coupled with our experiences with the species specificity of growth hormone, prompted us to determine whether a similar specificity could account for the apparent ineffectiveness of non-primate LH preparations in primates.

Because of the complexities in the ovulatory mechanism and other matters described by Dr. Simpson we decided to test the effects of these LH preparations in the male hypophysectomized monkey rather than in the female. We estimated their stimulatory effect on androgen secretion by the interstitial cells of Leydig by measuring the secondary effects on the epithelium of the seminal vesicles and on the seminiferous tubules of the testes.

It was also felt that considerations of species specificity would be equally applicable to both sexes. With the apologia for the interjection of the testis into an ovarian conference I should like to summarize some of our experiments.

Male monkeys which had been hypophysectomized for 2 months to 3½ years were used. Testicular and seminal vesicle biopsies were performed approximately two weeks before the treatment period. The tissues were stained with hematoxylin and eosin. In addition, frozen sections of a portion of the testicular biopsy material were prepared and stained with Sudan black B. The various hormone preparations were administered twice daily by subcutaneous injection in 1 ml of 12% gelatin. This regimen was continued for 14 days in all instances. On the day following the last injection the contralateral testis and seminal vesicle were biopsied and the tissues prepared as before. The hormone preparations used with their daily doses were as follows: HCG (500 Units), Equine LH–Armour (10 mg equivalent of Armour standard), Ovine LH–NIH (10 mg equivalent of Armour standard), and a human pituitary gonadotropin concentrate kindly provided by Dr. S. L. Steelman. The latter was given at a dose of 10 mg per day but its relative potency has not been established.

All of these treatments resulted, within a few days, in edema and pigmentation of the scrotum as well as variable degrees of testicular descent. The biopsies revealed distinct stimulation of the secretory epithelium of the seminal vesicle and enlargement of the seminiferous tubules. The equine and human preparations which contained large quantities of FSH as determined by rat assay occasioned, in addition, marked mitotic activity in the spermatogenic elements of the tubules.

Gonadotropin treatment, while producing but modest and inconsistent hypertrophy and hyperplasia of Leydig cells, resulted in a most striking sudanophilia of the interstitial tissue. Figures 8 and 9 illustrate the response of a hypophysectomized monkey to ovine LH.

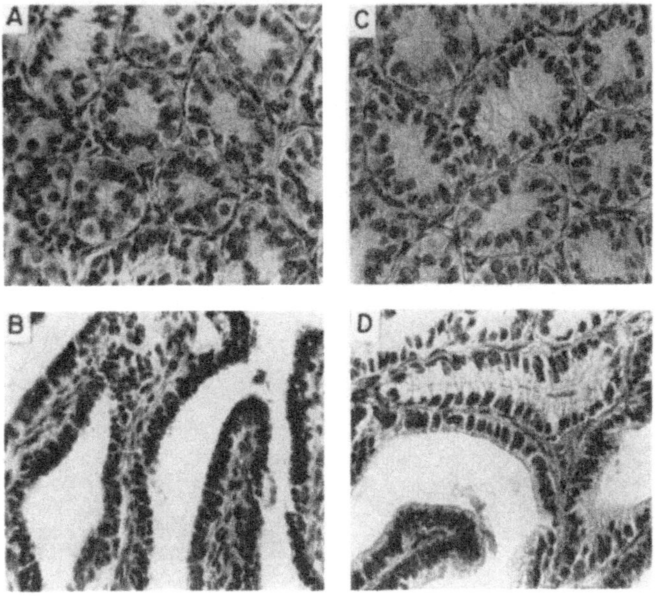

FIG. 8. Monkey 182 (4 kg BW). Hypophysectomized 2 months previously. A, Control testis; B, Control seminal vesicle; C, Appearance of testis following treatment with ovine LH (10 mg per day for 14 days); D, Seminal vesicle following treatment. Note increase in cell height and accumulation of cytoplasm characteristic of androgen stimulation. H and E.

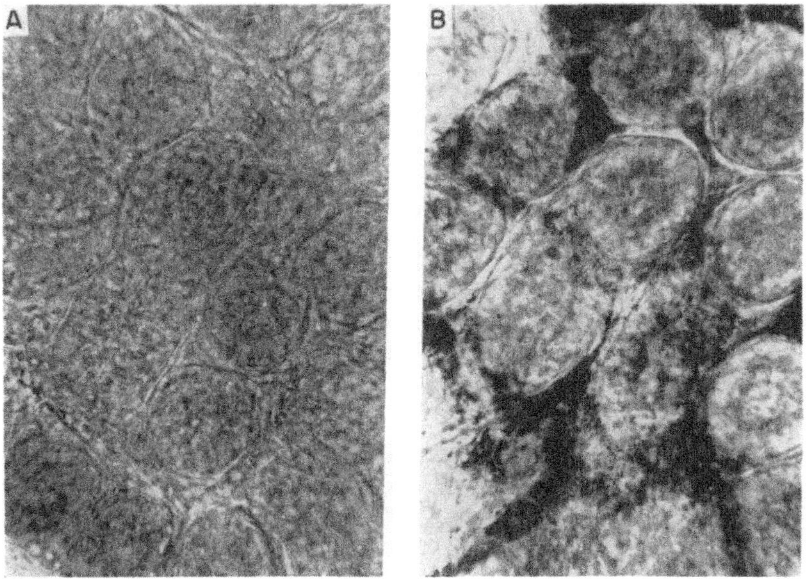

FIG. 9. Frozen sections of testicular tissue stained with Sudan black B. A, Hypophysectomized control; B, Following treatment as in FIG. 8 (monkey 182).

We conclude from these observations that LH preparations of non-primate origin are capable of stimulating the interstitial cells of the hypophysectomized male monkey with resultant increases in androgen secretion. While preliminary evidence indicates that quantitative differences may exist in the potencies of various LH preparations in the monkey, an absolute species specificity analogous to that described for growth hormone cannot be attributed to FSH and LH, at least as far as the monkey is concerned. The difficulties encountered in experimental ovulation in primates must reside, as Dr. Simpson has so clearly indicated, in problems concerned with the dosages and ratios of the hormones used as well as the timing of their administration.

FOLLICULAR DEVELOPMENT, OVULAR MATURATION AND OVULATION IN OVARIAN TISSUE TRANSPLANTED TO THE EYE

R. W. Noyes, T. H. Clewe and A. M. Yamate
Department of Obstetrics and Gynecology
Stanford University School of Medicine, Palo Alto, California

Previous studies on ovarian tissue transplanted into the anterior chamber of the eye have been mainly concerned with the ovary as an endocrine organ. Although both ovulation and follicular hemorrhage have been reported (7, 13), little attention has been paid to the maturation of ova in the anterior chamber of the eye. Our interest has been to obtain mature fertile ova from primordial follicles after the ovary has been removed from the body. Similar attempts, using tissue culture methods (4, 8, 14) have failed, and ova removed from the ovarian follicles do not mature normally *in vivo* (9) or *in vitro* (11), though certain nuclear changes simulate meiosis (2).

Follicles are maturing and undergoing atresia concomitantly in the mammalian ovary, and there is no way to distinguish a growing from an atretic follicle by inspecting the ovary at any particular time of the cycle. In order to correlate the growth rate of a follicle with the maturity of its contained ovum, it is essential that the follicle be observed continuously. We have taken advantage of the remarkable tolerance of the anterior chamber of the eye for both interspecies and intraspecies transplants to study follicular growth and ovulation.

MATERIALS AND METHODS

Whole fetal ovaries, halves of immature ovaries and fractions of adult ovaries without corpora lutea were transplanted, using Goodman's technique (5), to the anterior chamber of the eyes of 1296 albino rats of the Sprague-Dawley strain. In most cases the donor animals were 25 days old, since it was found that about that period of time was required for the ovaries of newborn rats to develop a degree of follicle growth sufficient to insure adequate response to the gonadotropic hormones. The host animals included males and females, also 25 days old, both intact and gonadectomized.

In a typical experiment, half an ovary from a black pigmented donor rat was placed in the anterior chamber of the eye of an albino male recipient rat, and the graft was observed daily with the aid of an 18-power dissecting microscope equipped with an eyepiece micrometer. On the fourth day after the operation the host was castrated and injected with 15 I.U. of pregnant mare's serum gonadotropin (PMS). Fifty-six hours later, 25 I.U. of human chorionic gonadotropin (HCG) was injected, this sequence having been found to cause superovulation in immature rats (12).

The maturity of ova from the above transplants was evaluated histologically and biologically. The ovarian grafts were recovered by killing the host and dissecting the ovarian tissue away from the iris. The follicles were pierced with a sharp blade and the ova were extruded into saline. Some of the ova were fixed and stained whole under a coverslip, others were transferred into the ovarian bursas of recently mated adult female rats of the Sprague-Dawley strain. If such transferred ova were mature they became fertilized, implanted and developed into normal young in the foster mother. Since the donor ova came from a strain of black rats, the donor had black iris pigment, whereas the young native to the foster mother had no iris pigment.

In some experiments the ovarian grafts were fixed and serially sectioned, and the volume of the larger follicles was calculated. Two diameters were measured at right angles to each other with the eyepiece micrometer and the third diameter was estimated from the number of sections in which the follicle appeared ($V = 1/6\pi d^3$).

In a few instances, donor ovarian tissue was taken from rabbits, or from other rodent species (*Microtus californicus* (1), *Peromyscus maniculatus*, *Mus musculus*), and from young adult women at the time of operation. Ten guinea-pigs and 6 rabbits were used as recipients, and cortisone, x-ray, and desensitization of embryos with cellular suspensions from future donor species, all were tried in order to reduce recipient antigenicity (10).

MORPHOLOGIC OBSERVATIONS

Of 1296 transplants of rat ovarian tissue into the eyes of rats, 1084 (84%) became vascularized within 4 days of the time of transfer. Ovulation did not occur spontaneously, but was observed in about 6% of grafts following gonadotropin injections. Ovulation usually occurred 14 to 18 hr after the second injection, and was more common in the eyes of castrated males than of ovariectomized females. Although usually 6 to 8 large follicles developed, no more than 2 ova were ovulated at one time. Ovulation occurred as early as the seventh day after transplantation and could be induced again eleven days later, but the critical intervals were not determined. In some cases the ovulated ova were grossly and microscopically indistinguishable from normal ova, but in others the cumulus cells were densely packed (as around an immature ovum) and the vitellus showed degenerative changes suggesting atresia.

The initial growth and maturation of follicular ova in ovarian tissue transplanted from black donor rats to albino hosts was indistinguishable from that observed in albino-to-albino transfers. However, after fourteen days the tissue from the blacks became unresponsive to gonadotropins and began to degenerate. The albino-to-albino transplants lasted indefinitely; several animals being observed for as long as one hundred and eighty days without regression of the transplants.

The interspecific transplants often became vascularized, and one crop of follicles sometimes developed. However, neither ovulation nor ovum maturation was observed. The average period of viability of such grafts was 10 days. The details of these interspecific experiments are recorded elsewhere (3, 10).

Figures 1 and 2 are low and high power photomicrographs of ovarian tissue from a 25-day-old rat. After four days in the eye, all of the original antrum-containing follicles degenerated, and the few surviving primordial follicles were located along the interface between the ovary and the iris (FIG. 3). The earliest of the *new* antrum-containing follicles appeared on the fourth day (FIG. 4). Fifty-six hours after castration and gonadotropin injection of the host, the new follicles had enlarged greatly (FIG. 5) and the ova had begun to separate from the mural granulosa. The nuclei in most of the ova remained in the immature or germinal vesicle stage (see FIG. 2), although occasional ova formed the first meiotic spindle (FIG. 6). Fourteen hours following the injection of HCG, the follicles enlarged still further, and an occasional follicle ovulated (FIG. 7). Ova in the maturing follicles usually completed meiosis by this time and they were separated completely from the mural granulosa. Mitotic activity in the cumulus cells was abundant (FIG. 8).

Corpora lutea were formed 22 hr after the administration of HCG (FIG. 9), and ova that had not been ovulated were found compressed among the lutein cells (FIG. 10). The relationship of the transplant to the iris and to the cornea is shown in FIG. 9. In this particular section the connection between the iris and the ovary is narrow, but usually the transplant was attached to a wide area of the iris.

Figure 11 is a photograph of a transplant taken through the cornea at the same magnification that was routinely used with the dissecting microscope. A freshly ovulated ovum, still surrounded by cumulus oophorus, is visible.

Plate I

FIG. 1. Ovary from a 25-day-old rat. (× 20)

FIG. 2. An early antrum follicle from FIG. 1. Volume = 65 × 10^6 μ^3. (× 90)

FIG. 3. Half an ovary from a 25-day-old donor rat, 4 days after transfer to the anterior chamber of the eye of a 25-day-old recipient rat of a different strain. (× 20)

FIG. 4. An early antrum follicle from Fig. 3. Volume = 4.6 × 10^6 μ^3. (× 90)

FIG. 5. Rat ovarian transplant 56 hr after injection of the recipient rat with 15 I.U. pregnant mare's serum gonadotropin. (× 20)

FIG. 6. Developing follicle from FIG. 5. Volume 110 × 10^6 μ^3. The ovum is unusual in that it has formed the first meiotic spindle. (× 90)

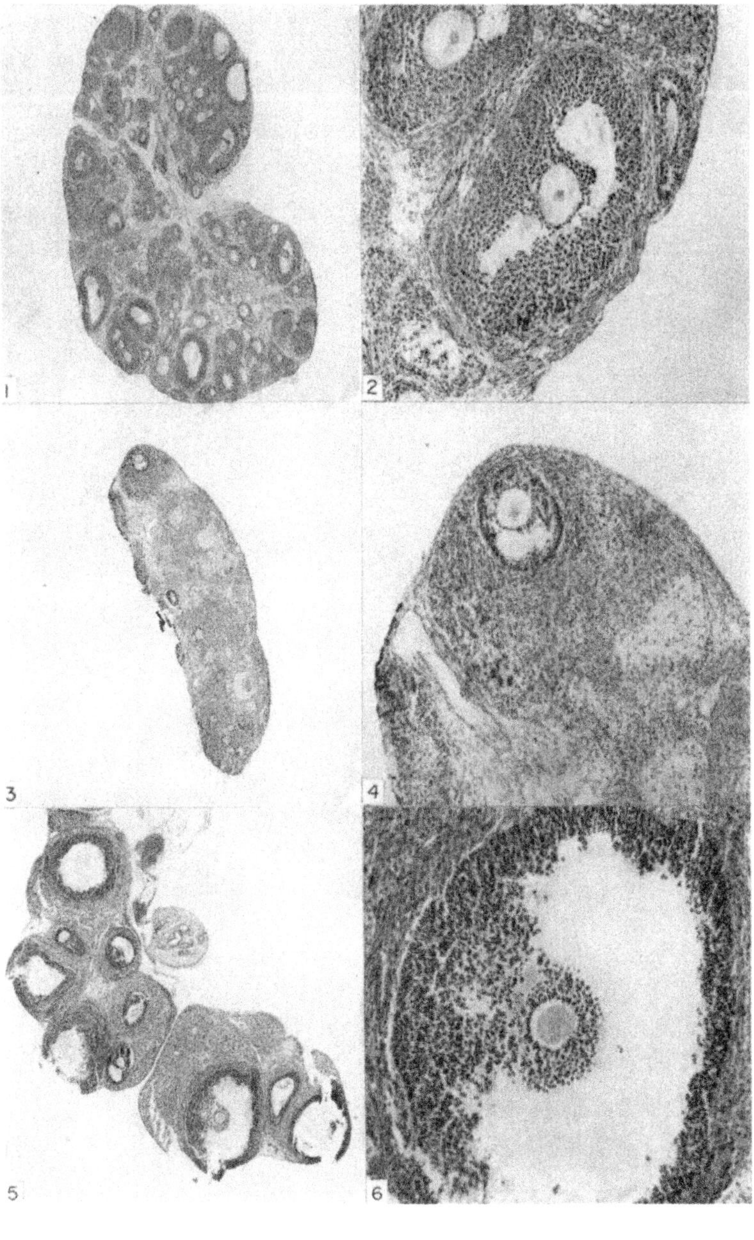

PLATE I

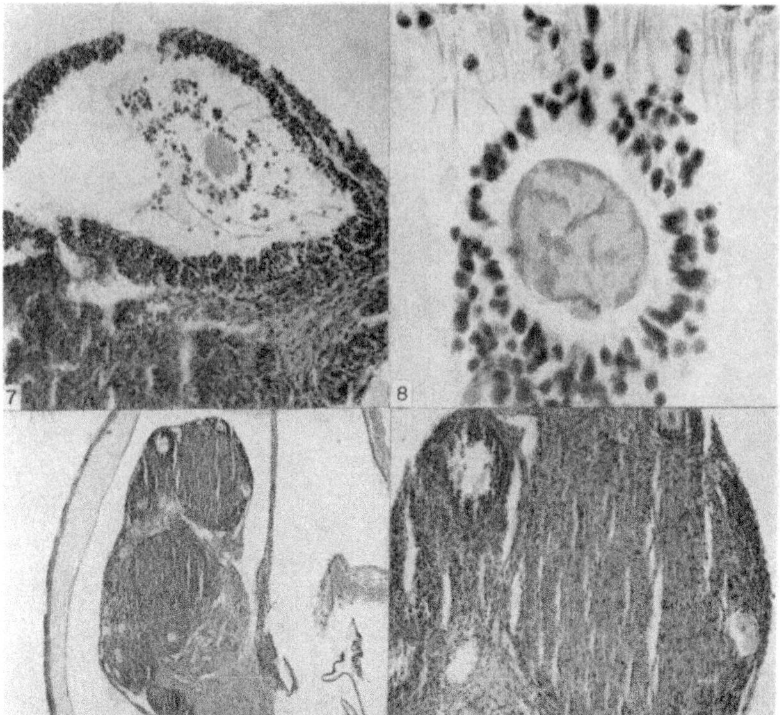

Plate II

Figure 12 shows a mature follicular ovum that has been stained *in toto* under a coverslip. The crescentic first polar body has recently been abstricted from the horseshoe-shaped telophase spindle.

THE RATE OF FORMATION OF MATURING FOLLICLES

Daily sketches were made of 36 ovarian transplants between the fourth and seventh days following transplantation. The host animals to 30 of these transplants were subjected to PMS and HCG injections, and 6 were untreated controls. The rate of appearance of the follicles growing in treated animals did not differ from the controls. This suggests that the intrinsic pituitary gonadotropin level of the immature castrate male recipient is high enough to stimulate all follicles that are mature enough to respond.

Sixty-five follicles appeared (diameter 0.25 mm) in the 36 transplants on the fourth, 60 on the fifth, 32 on the sixth, and 28 on the seventh postoperative day. The number of follicles that appear each day diminishes rapidly after the first 2 days, and this cannot be prevented by supplementary gonadotropin injections. These direct observations are in agreement with the theory that the original stimulus for follicular maturation is independent of gonadotropic hormone stimulation.

In order to compare the performance of transplants with that of ovaries *in situ*, 25-day-old female rats were injected with gonadotropin on the same schedule that has been outlined above. Serial sections of these normal control ovaries showed that the average number of follicles that "appear" each day is five times that observed in the transplants. Probably the smaller original size of the transplant, plus the massive follicular degeneration that occurs before its new blood supply develops is sufficient to account for this difference. It is not likely that antigenic influences would be manifest so soon after transplantation.

Plate II

FIG. 7. A developing follicle from an ovarian transplant 70 hr after injecting the recipient with PMS and 14 hr following the injection of 30 international units of human chorionic gonadotropin. Volume = $90 \times 10^6\ \mu^3$. The opening in the follicle is possibly the point of ovulation. (× 90)

FIG. 8. An ovum 14 hr following HCG injection, showing the first polar body. Mitosis of a cumulus cell can be seen to the upper right. (× 370)

FIG. 9. An ovarian transplant 78 hr following PMS and 22 hr following HCG, showing early corpora lutea. The cornea is on the left and the attachment of the iris to the graft is shown to the right. (× 20)

FIG. 10. An early corpus luteum from FIG. 9, showing a squeezed atretic ovum to the right. (× 20)

FIG. 11. An ovarian transplant as seen through the dissecting microscope, 14 hr following HCG, and showing, to the left, an ovulated ovum in front of the iris. (× 20)

FIG. 12. A follicular rat ovum that has been fixed and stained *in toto* under a coverslip. The first polar body is being abstricted from the horseshoe-shaped late telophase spindle. (× 1300)

VOLUME CHANGES IN MATURING FOLLICLES

The diameter of a given follicle, as measured in the anterior chamber of the eye using an eyepiece micrometer, was estimated to be accurate to within about ±0.25 mm. The volumes of 157 follicles in 36 transplants were recorded daily from the fourth through the seventh postoperative days. In 24 of the transplants, both PMS and HCG were given to the recipient animal; in 6,

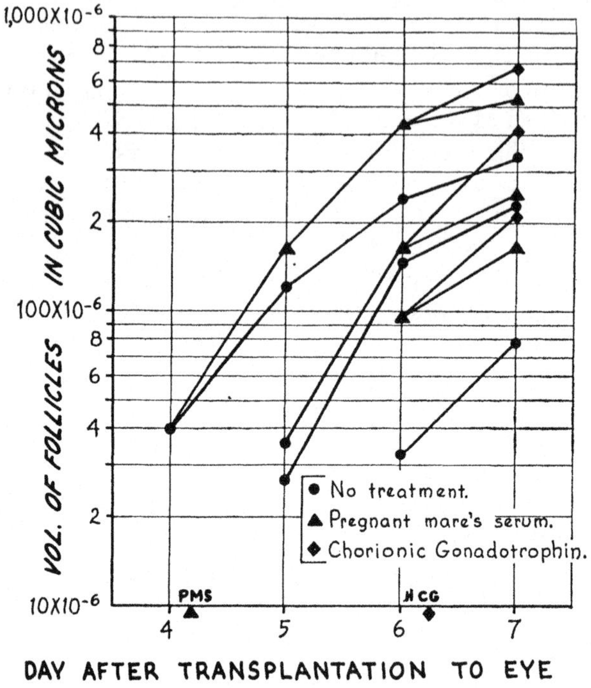

FIG. 13. Growth of ovarian follicles in the anterior chamber of the eye as affected by pregnant mare's serum and human chorionic gonadotropin injections. Each point represents the average volume of all of the grossly visible follicles in many transplants. The measurements were made on living follicles. The points that pertain to a group of follicles that first appeared on the same day are connected by lines. The time of injection and dosage of PMS and HCG are given in the text.

only PMS was given; and in 6 no gonadotropin was given. The average volume for each group of follicles that appeared on a given day in each of the three groups of animals was plotted against time (FIG. 13). The average volume of 65 follicles that appeared on the fourth day was $40 \times 10^6\ \mu^3$, and one day later, following castration and PMS administration, the average volume had increased to $165 \times 10^6\ \mu^3$. When the recipients were castrated, but no PMS was given, the average volume was slightly less, $120 \times 10^6\ \mu^3$, and although they continued to grow, the follicles in uninjected animals grew more slowly than those in the treated animals.

When HCG is given there is a further increase in the follicular growth rate. The curve of growth is very similar for each group of follicles irrespective of the day on which they appeared. In the group of animals treated with PMS, the average volume of follicles that first appeared on the sixth day is much larger than that in the preceding groups. This artifact is caused by the sudden emergence into view of older follicles that had been growing deeply on the

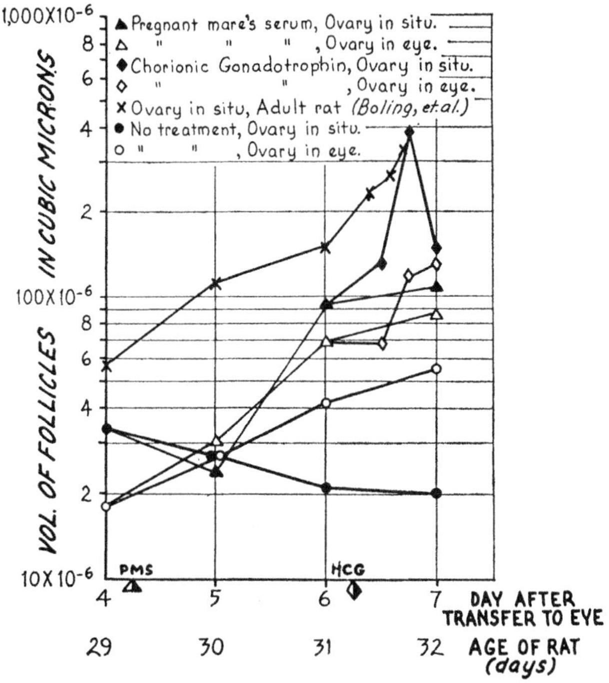

FIG. 14. The effect of gonadotropin injections on the volumes of ovarian follicles in eye transplants and in normal immature ovaries *in situ*. Each point represents the average volume of many follicles from different ovaries. The measurements were made on fixed, sectioned tissue. The time of injection and dosage of PMS and HCG are given in the text.

interface between the iris and the ovary. Although they appear on the sixth day many of these follicles are actually older, and thus larger, than the more superficial follicles. These observations were not continued long enough to include the declining growth of follicles as they become atretic, or the curves for those that formed corpora lutea.

Similar data were plotted from the average volumes of the larger follicles in the serially sectioned transplants (FIG. 14). Again, three groups of transplants were studied (castration only, PMS only, and PMS plus HCG), and a parallel series of three groups of normal immature rat ovaries *in situ* was studied for comparison.

The average follicular volume in the normal untreated ovary does not increase between the twenty-ninth and the thirty-second day of age, but there is a steady rise in the follicular volume each day the ovarian transplant remains in the eye of the castrate male recipient. None of the follicles in untreated animals matures completely, although there is a tendency for ova in some atretic follicles to undergo early meiotic nuclear activity. The volume of both *in situ* and transplanted ovaries increases rapidly following PMS treatment, and injection of HCG causes still further growth after a short lag period. In the *in situ* ovaries, ovulation and regression follow the final dramatic growth spurt.

Follicles in the eye transplants grow more slowly, and do not attain the large preovulatory volumes that follicles in normal ovaries do. However, the rate of nuclear maturation of the ova appears to be the same whether the ovary is in the eye or in its normal location.

The curve of follicular growth obtained in the normal ovary of adult female rats by Boling *et al.* (1) is very similar to the curve for superovulated ovaries *in situ* although the time sequences cannot be directly compared. No doubt the lack of a final growth spurt in transplanted ovarian follicles is related in some way to their low rate of ovulation. At these early stages there is no evidence that intraocular pressure is increased, or that moderate increases in extrinsic pressure would interfere with follicular growth or ovulation. In the sectioned transplants blood vessels are smaller and less numerous than in the normal immature ovary. Perhaps the failure of preovulatory growth and ovulation can be explained on the basis of inadequate blood supply.

Shrinkage resulting from fixation of the tissue accounts for the smaller over-all follicular volumes in the sectioned material compared with the living transplants, but other than this, the data from the two series are quite comparable. More than 100 ova were stained *in toto* to correlate the growth-rate of the follicle with the maturation of the contained ovum. The results were exactly the same as those for the serially sectioned ova. In each group of ova recovered from ovarian transplants, however, a few immature vesicular ova from the smaller follicles of an earlier generation were seen. Although these unripe ova were obviously unlike the maturing ova when they were fixed and stained, they were not easy to distinguish in the living state.

THE FERTILITY OF FOLLICULAR OVA FROM OVARIAN TRANSPLANTS

From 470 transplants, 1154 ova were obtained by lancing large follicles under saline, an average of 2.5 ova per transplant. More than twice this number of large follicles was counted under the dissecting microscope and in the sectioned material, so it is obvious that our recovery technic was imperfect.

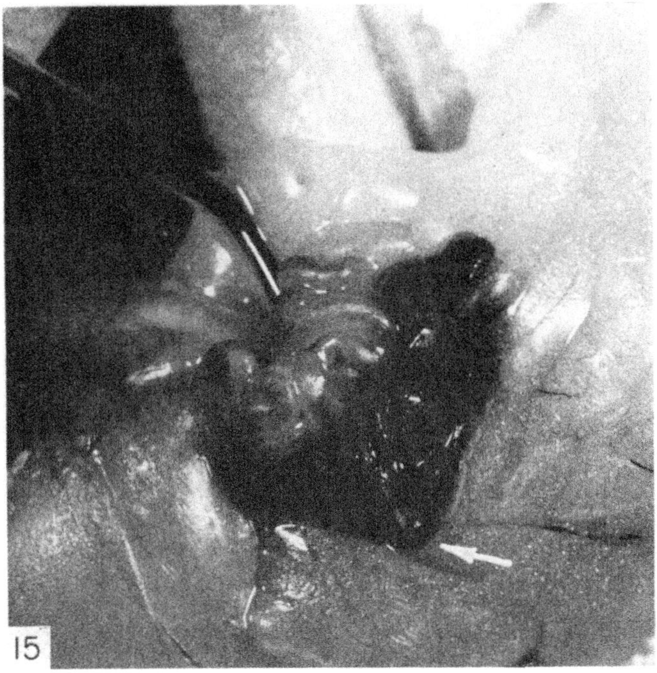

Fig. 15. Method for transferring follicular ova into the ovarian bursa. The tip of the pipet (see arrow) is visible behind the bursal membrane.

Approximately 6 follicular ova were pipetted into each of 184 ovarian bursas of previously mated albino recipient animals. The method for injecting ova is illustrated in FIG. 15.

In a previous experiment (1), when 130 developing follicular ova were removed from the ovaries of normal adult animals six hours or less before the expected time of ovulation, and were then transferred into the bursas of 19 recipient animals, 44 (34%) of the ova were fertilized and developed to term embryos.

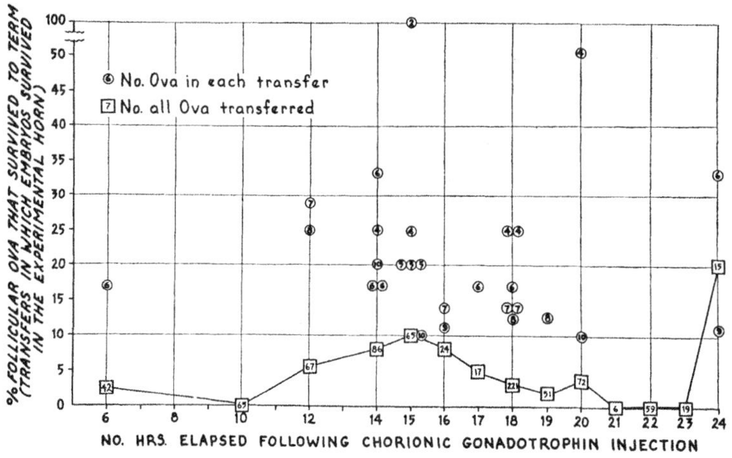

FIG. 16. The fertility of follicular rat ova taken from ovaries transplanted to the eyes of recipient rats of a different strain. The data are from Table 1. The figures within the circles are the numbers of ova in each transfer in which one or more of the transferred ova developed to term. The figures in the squares represent the number of all ova transferred into recipient bursas at a given hour following chorionic gonadotropin injection.

Our present experience with the fertility of follicular ova obtained from eye transplants is not nearly this encouraging (Table 1). When 809 maturing ova from eye transplants were transferred to 131 bursas, only 36 (4.5%) developed into term embryos.

The optimal stage of follicular development was between the fourteenth and sixteenth hours following the administration of HCG (FIG. 16), but even at this time only 10% of transferred ova survived. The results of individual experiments were quite variable, and the apparent high fertility of ova occurring 24 hr after HCG was probably a chance occurrence. This was a very rigorous test for fertility, with many chances for ova to be lost and for inadequate conditions for fertilization to be present. However, the conditions in these eye transplant experiments were similar to those with normal follicular ova, yet only one-tenth as many of the ova from the eye transplants were fertile as compared with the preovulatory ova from ovarian follicles *in situ*.

TABLE 1. FOLLICULAR OVA TRANSFERRED INTO THE OVARIAN BURSAS OF RECIPIENT HOST RATS

	No. hr elapsed after chorionic gonadotropin injection														Totals
	6	10	12	14	15	16	17	18	19	20	21	22	23	24	
Transfers in which follicular ova survived to term in the experimental *uterine horn*															
Transfers	1	0	2	5	6	2	1	6	1	2	0	0	0	2	28
Ova	6	0	15	32	31	16	6	36	8	12	0	0	0	15	177
Ova surviving	**1**	**0**	**4**	**7**	**7**	**2**	**1**	**7**	**1**	**3**	**0**	**0**	**0**	**3**	**36**
Transfers in which only control embryos survived in the experimental uterine horn															
Transfers	8	10	6	14	8	1	2	24	5	7	1	16	3	0	105
Ova	36	65	52	54	34	8	11	185	43	60	6	59	19	0	632
Subtotals	**9 42**	**10 65**	**8 67**	**19 86**	**14 65**	**3 24**	**3 17**	**30 221**	**6 51**	**9 72**	**1 6**	**16 59**	**3 19**	**2 15**	**133 809**
Transfers in which the recipient was pregnant, but no embryo survived in the experimental uterine horn															
Transfers	7	6	4	0	3	2	0	4	1	0	1	0	0	1	29
Ova	47	42	32	0	20	20	0	25	5	0	10	0	0	6	207
Transfers in which the recipient failed to continue pregnancy															
Transfers	5	5	1	2	5	0	0	1	0	1	0	1	0	1	22
Ova	23	46	6	9	31	0	0	9	0	7	0	2	0	5	138
Totals															
Transfers	**21**	**21**	**13**	**21**	**22**	**5**	**3**	**35**	**7**	**10**	**2**	**17**	**3**	**4**	**184**
Ova	**112**	**153**	**105**	**95**	**116**	**44**	**17**	**255**	**56**	**79**	**16**	**61**	**19**	**26**	**1154**
Ova surviving	**1**	**0**	**4**	**7**	**7**	**2**	**1**	**7**	**1**	**3**	**0**	**0**	**0**	**3**	**36**

SUMMARY AND CONCLUSIONS

Transfers of immature rat ovarian tissue to the anterior chamber of the eyes of immature male recipient rats of a different strain produced vascularized, growing grafts in 84% of trials. Most of the antrum-containing follicles of these grafts degenerate, but new ones grow from surviving primordial follicles within 4 days following transplantation. One to 4 new follicles begin to grow each day, and an average of 6 mature within 4 days. The number of follicles that appear is independent of extrinsic gonadotropin injections, but is dependent on the intrinsic rise of gonadotropin level following castration of the host animal.

When treated with pregnant mare's serum gonadotropin, the follicles increase in volume at about the same rate that has been reported for follicles in the mature ovary *in situ*, while in untreated grafts, follicular growth lags. Following the injection of human chorionic gonadotropin, the follicles in transplants do not grow so rapidly or become so large as those developing in ovaries *in situ*, and ovulation is rare. However, meiotic changes in the ovum's nucleus, and cumulus maturation of these ova, seem to progress at the normal rate despite their smaller volume. Only 4.5% of ova removed from follicles that seemed to be maturing proved to be fertile. This is only one-tenth the fertility rate expected from previous experiments on follicular ova obtained from mature ovaries *in situ*. Ovulation occurred in 6% of the grafted ovaries.

Interspecies transplants of ovarian tissue from rabbit to rat, from rat to rabbit, and from human to rat, rabbit or guinea pig, all failed to produce normal ova despite extensive and varied treatments aimed at reducing the antigenic response of the host.

From an immunologic point of view it is interesting that in these acute experiments, ova can be brought to maturity despite the fact that these intraspecies grafts invariably degenerate a short time later. It is felt that inadequate blood supply, rather than antigenicity, may be the cause for the failure of rapid growth following the injection of chorionic gonadotropin. Slow growth may in turn be responsible for the failure of ovulation, and still more remotely may decrease the fertility of these ova. Further advances in solving this problem will depend on better immunologic control in the recipient host, so that transplants may grow long enough to attain a normal blood supply before ovum maturation is attempted.

Acknowledgments—This investigation was supported in part by PHS Research Grant RG 4470 from the National Institutes of Health, Public Health Service, and in part by the generosity of Mrs. Lilian Howell.

REFERENCES

1. BOLING, J. L. *et al.*, Growth of the Graafian follicle and the time of ovulation in the albino rat, *Anat. Rec.* **79**, 313, 1941.
2. CHANG, M. C., Maturation of rabbit oocytes in culture and their maturation, activation, fertilization and subsequent development in fallopian tubes, *J. Exper. Zool.* **82**, 85, 1939.
3. CLEWE, T. H., A. M. YAMATE and R. W. NOYES, Maturation of ova in mammalian ovaries in the anterior chamber of the eye, *Internat. J. Fertil.* **3**, 187, 1958.
4. GAILLARD, P. J., Growth and differentiation of explanted tissues. *Internat. Rev. Cytol.* **2**, 331, 1953.
5. GOODMAN, L., Observations on transplanted immature ovaries in the eyes of adult male and female rats, *Anat. Rec.* **59**, 223, 1934.
6. GREENE, H. S. N., Use of mouse eye in transplantation experiments, *Cancer Research* **7**, 491, 1947.
7. LANE, C. E. and J. E. MARKEE, Response of ovarian intra-ocular transplants to gonado-trophins, *Growth* **5**, 61, 1941.
8. MARTINOVITCH, P. N., Effect of subnormal temperature on differentiation and survival of cultivated *in vitro* embryonic and infantile rat and mouse ovaries, *Proc. Roy. Soc. London* **B 128**, 138, 1939.
9. NOYES, R. W., Fertilization of follicular ova, *Fertil. & Steril.* **3**, 1, 1952.
10. NOYES, R. W., A. M. YAMATE and T. H. CLEWE, Ovarian transplants to the anterior chamber of the eye, *Fertil. & Steril.* **9**, 99, 1958.
11. PINCUS, G., Comparative behavior of mammalian eggs *in vivo* and *in vitro*. IV. Development of fertilized and artificially activated rabbit eggs, *J. Exper. Zool.* **82**, 85, 1939.
12. ROWLANDS, I. W., Production of ovulation in the immature rat, *J. Endocrinol.* **3**, 384, 1944.
13. WARD, J. E., J. L. GARDNER and B. L. NEWTON, Anterior ocular ovarian grafts in the rabbit, *Am. J. Obst. & Gynec.* **66**, 1200, 1953.
14. WOLFF, E., Sur la différenciation sexuelle des gonades de souris explantées *in vitro*, *Compt. Rend.* **234**, 1712, 1952.

DISCUSSION

Chairman: Roy O. Greep

Dr. John Hammond, Jr.: I have one idea that I should like to put to you because it follows what was said about ovulation.

Dr. Noyes seems to disregard the effect of the intra-ocular pressure, and it seems to me that that might be of some considerable importance. Ovulation depends upon the formation of the ovulation cone and that cone formation, I suppose, depends upon the occlusion of the vessels. And that point, that occlusion, depends upon the pressure gradient across the wall of the follicle.

Now, I have heard the follicle picturesquely described as a blister on the surface of the ovary, and I think that is more than a figure of speech. We think of the liquor as secretion of the cells. It is in part, particularly in the early stages when you have a lot of cells and cement substance around the oocyte, a viscous sort of fluid; but, in the later stages of the follicle, you get rapid accumulation of fluid, of tertiary liquor.

Some Italians (R. Catavaglios and R. Cilotti, *J. Endocrinol* **15**, 273, 1957) analyzed the liquor and showed that it contains most of the blood proteins; the largest molecules are present in reduced amounts, but it seems more or less to be a transudate from the thecal vessels, and yet collecting amongst the epithelium of the granulosa. This is very much like the formation of a blister. You burn yourself, and a fluid is liberated from the blood vessels of the dermis, yet in like manner, the fluid accumulates in the epithelium of the epidermis. If the liquor is a transudate, its formation depends upon the hydrostatic pressure in the blood vessels.

The intra-ocular pressure in the human eye is about 30 mm of mercury, and the ordinary capillary hydrostatic pressure is of the order of 30 mm of mercury. I don't know what it is in the ovary but it does not seem to be surprising that when you inject pregnancy urine, the follicle doesn't grow so rapidly as it does in its normal position because there is obviously much greater pressure opposing the filtration of the liquor.

Dr. Noyes also said that the two phenomena of the maturation of the eggs and of ovulation were not necessarily due to the same causes. But I wonder if the stimulus to ovulate which the follicle gets may not produce the maturation of the oocyte and liberate it from the follicle wall, and induce the secretion of the tertiary-liquor, all by the same mechanism. Whether, in fact, the stimulus to ovulate may produce an incipient process of degeneration in the granulosa cells, and that this, on the one hand, liberates the ovum from the wall of the follicle, and at the same time it may also, perhaps, free the ovum from an inhibition of cleavage and allow it to go through the reduction division. Perhaps the degenerating cells release a substance which increases the permeability of the thecal vessel walls, and this results in the sudden increase in pressure and accumulation of fluid, inside the follicle.

I think one might, perhaps, understand the way in which the pituitary works in inducing ovulation, if one could reconstruct the way in which the process has evolved. For that, I can see two main clues, and perhaps there are many others. One is this: It seems very improbable that FSH and LH should have appeared simultaneously as hormones regulating the process of ovulation. Secondly, one has the probability that the steroid hormones started as gonadal organizer substances. Working from this, I would like to put forward an idea. Initially, I suppose that the ovary was regulated purely by nutrition. I suppose the gonad was a late-developing part of the body. It only developed fully when feeding conditions and nutritive conditions were good. When it did, the germ cells developed and were surrounded by the satellite cells; and when the oocytes were full-grown they went automatically, as cells have a habit of doing, through the next stage, which is that of cell division. In this case, of course, this is the reduction division.

Then there came the necessity of restricting the season of reproduction. Food is plentiful in autumn, but it is a poor time for young animals to have to start their development. I suppose this seasonal restriction was imposed, first of all, by the granulosa cells, inhibiting the germinal meiosis, and secondly, that the granulosa came under the influence of the pituitary through the regulation of the thecal-organizing substance.

I imagine that the first gonadotropin was something like PMS, with both FSH and LH activities, and that the response of the thecal cell depended on its maturity. I here partly follow, with modification, the ideas of Gadrenstroom and de Jongh (*Research in Holland.* Elsevier, Amsterdam, 1946). When the thecal cell was young it responded to the FSH part of the molecule, and the FSH caused thecal estrogen secretion which maintained the granulosa cells. As the thecal cell became older it responded to the LH part of the molecule, and secreted androgen that produced the effect of destroying the granulosa, thus removing the inhibition to meiosis and at the same time freeing the egg.

When estrogen becomes a hormone as well as an organizer, its output has to increase as the follicle ripens—when one supposes the theca becomes reactive to LH. One may imagine, then, the evolution of LH as a separate hormone, synergizing with FSH for estrogen secretion; and also the evolution of interstitial cells, derived from the theca and stimulated by LH, in which estrogen can be produced at a site remote from the follicle—and so can act as a hormone without also having an effect on the follicle where it might antagonize the presumed thecal androgen production, which organizes ovulation by destroying the granulosa. Later still, the granulosa will not be destroyed, but stimulated to luteinize when vascularized.

Finally, a question I would like to put to Dr. Noyes. How do you know that the follicles haven't been stimulated and maturation changes initiated by discharge from the host pituitary before you give chorionic gonadotropin?

THE ROLE OF STEROIDS IN THE CONTROL OF MAMMALIAN OVULATION*

GREGORY PINCUS and ANNE P. MERRILL
The Worcester Foundation for Experimental Biology
Shrewsbury, Massachusetts

WE have previously described methods for determining the effects of various compounds on copulation-induced ovulation in the rabbit (1, 2, 3). Our standard procedure is to administer the test substance to a post-partum female rabbit and then mate her to a male of known fertility 18 to 24 hr later. On the day following the mating the occurrence of ovulation is ascertained by examining the ovaries for rupture points at laparotomy. The occurrence of pregnancy in such mated rabbits may easily be determined by palpation of uteri for implantations at the tenth to fourteenth day after mating. In order to obtain a preliminary idea of the effectiveness of any given compound, our usual procedure is to administer a dose of 10 mg per animal to each of five post-partum females. In view of the fact that approximately 90% of untreated post-partum rabbits ovulate under these conditions, the absence of ovulation in all of the five test animals is highly significant; if one out of five ovulates the effect is considered marginally significant.

In FIGS. 1 through 12 are presented the structural formulae of those steroids which have given some indication of acting as ovulation inhibitors when administered to groups of five post-partum rabbits. At the dosage underlined with a solid line, all animals failed to ovulate; at the dosages underlined with a broken line, marginally significant frequency of inhibition occurred.

Among the estrogens (ring A unsaturated) and their derivatives, nine compounds gave indication of activity (FIGS. 1 and 2). Consistent evidence of inhibition following subcutaneous injection at various dosages is given by estrone (IV, FIG. 1) and 17α-ethyl-17β-estradiol (II, FIG. 1). Estradiol (I, FIG. 1) itself, which we expected to be quite a potent inhibitor and which was thus tested at relatively low dosages, gave a marginally significant effect at 0.1 mg per rabbit by mouth but not at 0.5 mg per rabbit. All of the other compounds listed in FIGS. 1 and 2 appear to be of rather low potency.

* Investigations described in this paper have been conducted with grants-in-aid from G. D. Searle & Company and the Population Council, Inc.

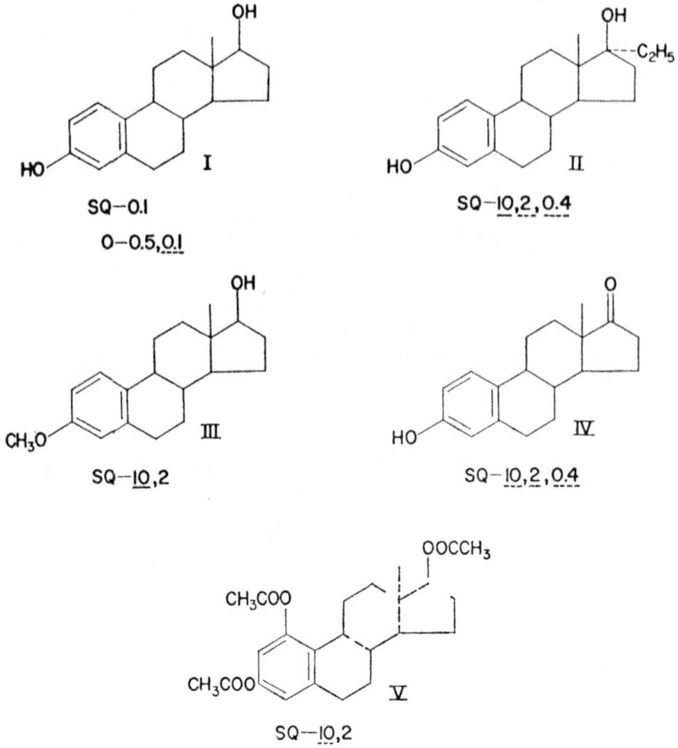

FIG. 1. Estrogens and derivatives. (Dosage in milligrams. SQ = subcutaneous injection; O = by gavage.)

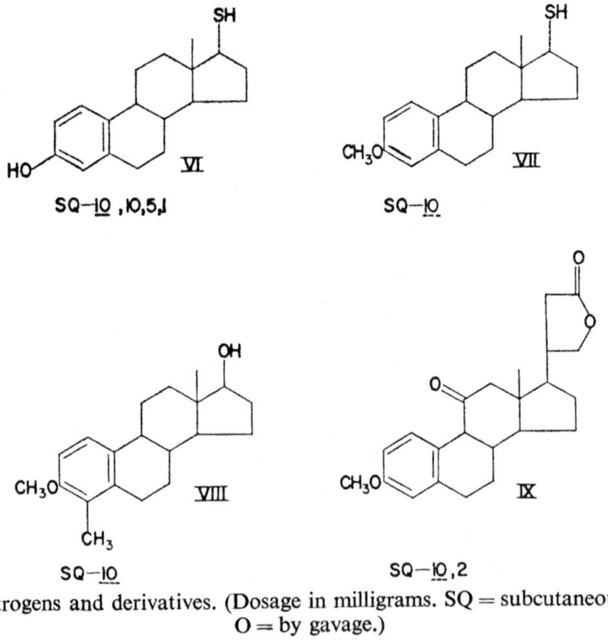

FIG. 2. Estrogens and derivatives. (Dosage in milligrams. SQ = subcutaneous injection; O = by gavage.)

Seven compounds classifiable as androgens and their derivatives (FIG. 3) are clearly of low or marginal potency.

Among a large number of progesterone derivatives and analogs tested, we list in FIG. 4 two epoxides (XVII and XVIII) which gave marginal indications of activity, two 16-substituted compounds of which one (XX) is clearly of

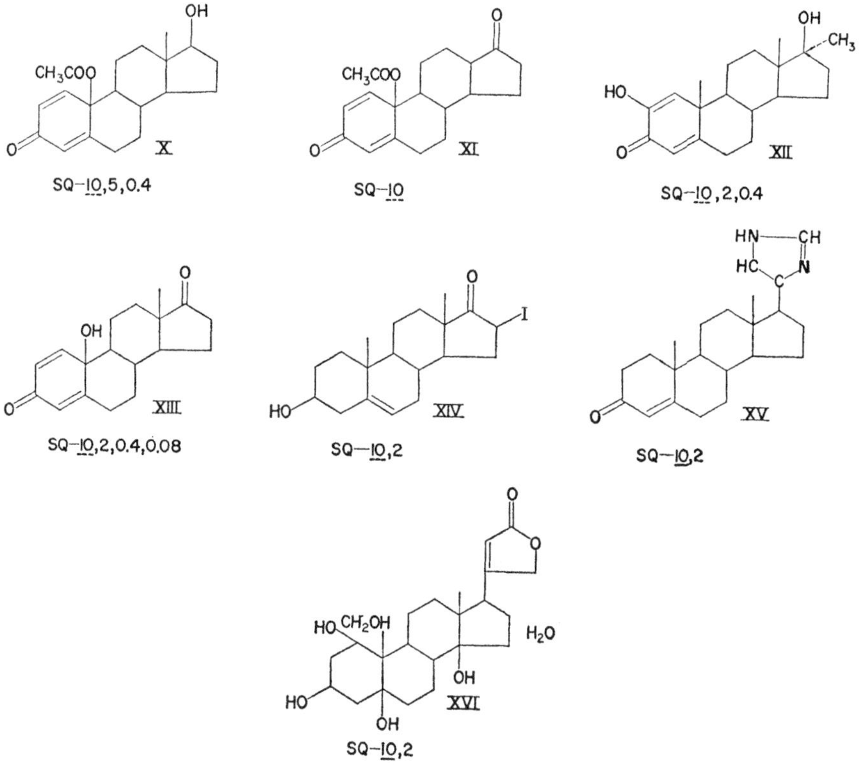

FIG. 3. Androgens and derivatives. (Dosage in milligrams. SQ = subcutaneous injection; O = by gavage.)

low potency and the other (XIX) is inconsistently active by injection and of low potency by mouth, and 11-keto-Δ^6-progesterone (XXI) which is of moderate potency by injection. In FIG. 5, among the 21-substituted progesterone derivatives only 21-fluoroprogesterone (XXVI) shows consistent activity to a dosage as low as 0.4 mg per rabbit. Among a group classified as miscellaneous progesterone derivatives (FIG. 6) only one, XXIX, is consistently inhibitory by the subcutaneous route. It appears to be inactive on oral administration.

The reported high progestational activity of certain derivatives of 17-hydroxyprogesterone (4, 5) led us to test a number of them (FIGS. 7 and 8).

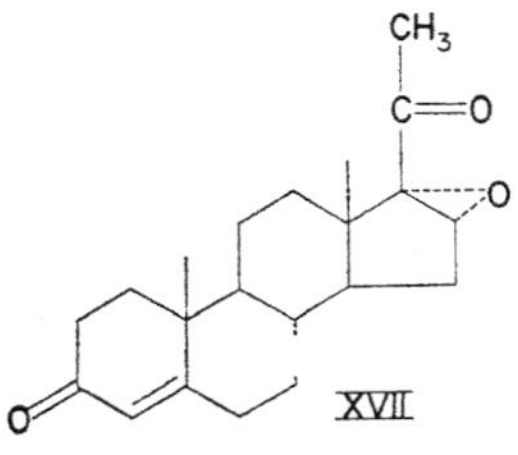
XVII

SQ–2,0.4

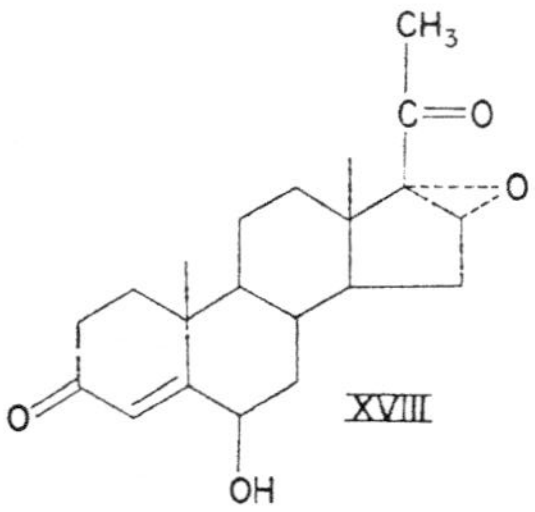
XVIII

SQ–10,2

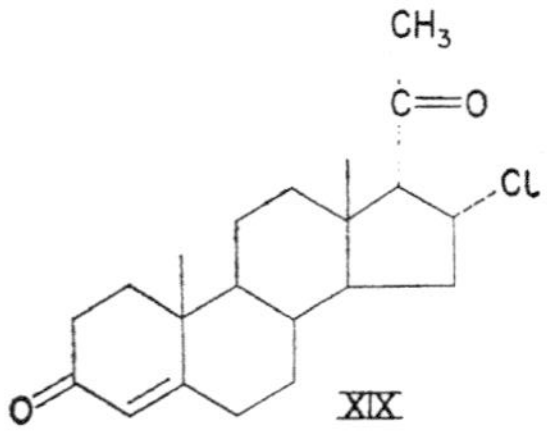
XIX

SQ–2, 0.08
O–10,2,0.4,0.08,0.004

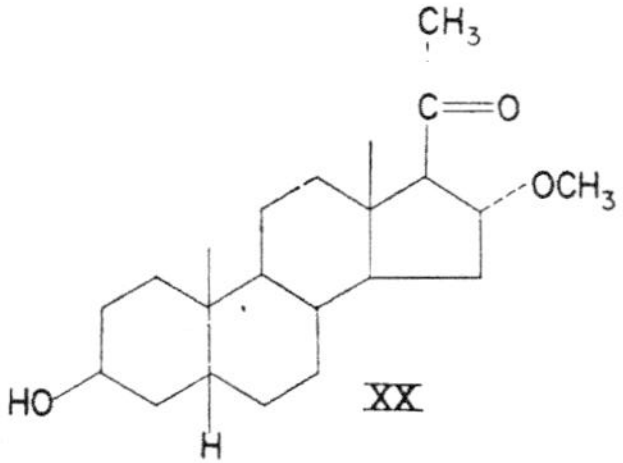
XX

SQ–10,5,2

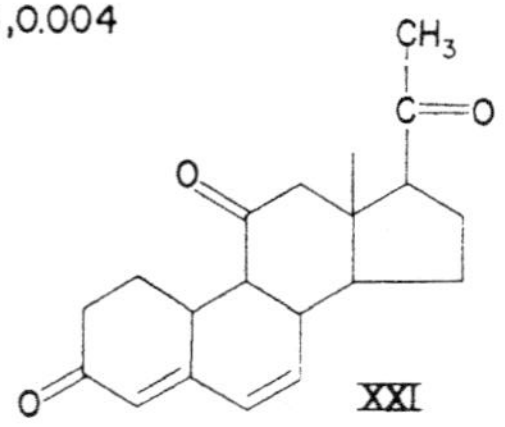
XXI

SQ–10,2,0.4

FIG. 4. Progesterone derivatives: epoxides, 16- and 11-substituted. (Dosage in milligrams. SQ = subcutaneous injection; O = gavage.)

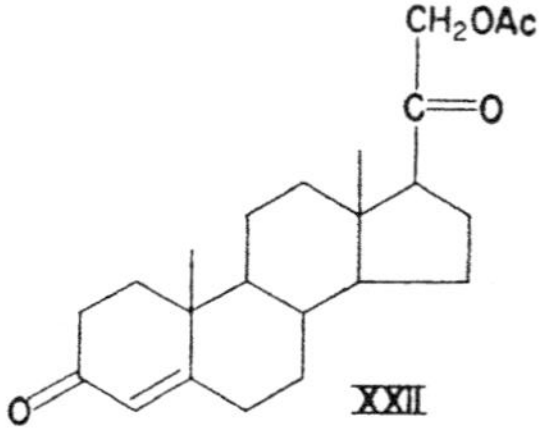
XXII

SQ–2, 0.4

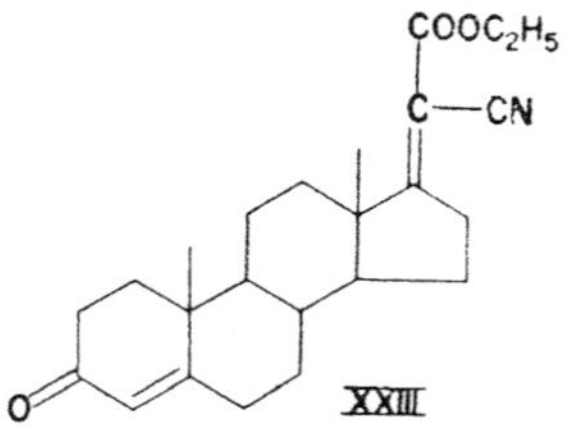
XXIII

SQ–2
O–10

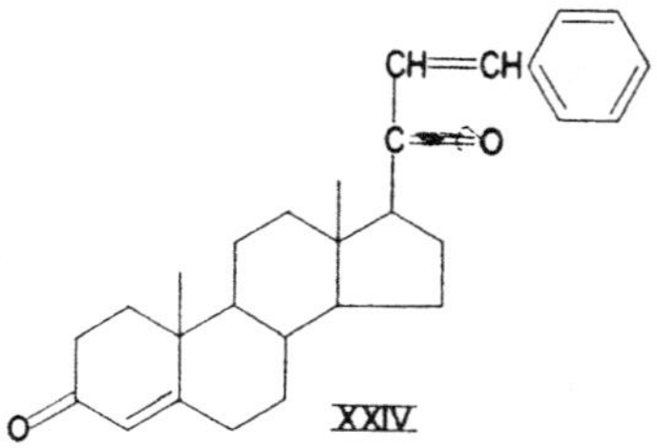
XXIV

SQ–10,5

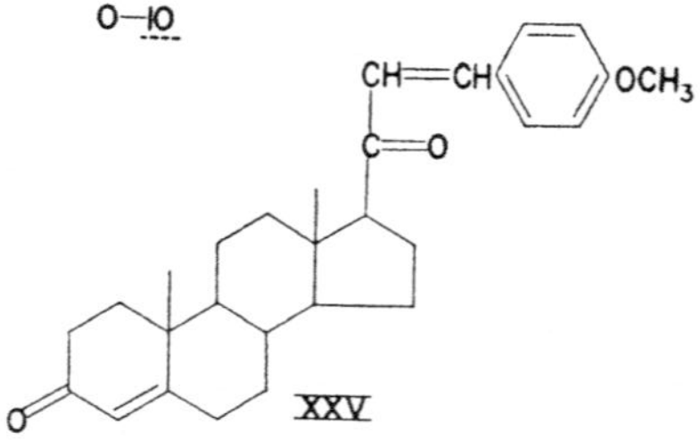
XXV

SQ–10,5

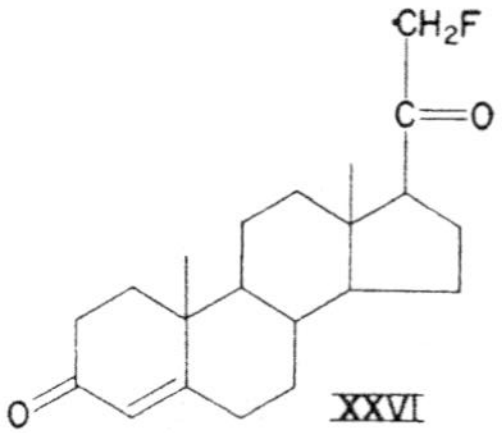
XXVI

SQ–10, 2, 0.4, 0.016

FIG. 5. 21-Substituted progesterone derivatives. (Dosage in milligrams. SQ = subcutaneous injection; O = by gavage.)

Previously we had found 17-hydroxyprogesterone itself to be inactive as an ovulation inhibitor in the rabbit (1) and, as can be seen in FIG. 7, four compounds with a free 17α-hydroxyl group proved to be marginally active (numbers XXXII to XXXV). Acetylation of the 17α-hydroxyl alone (XXXVI) confers consistent and rather high inhibitory activity by the subcutaneous

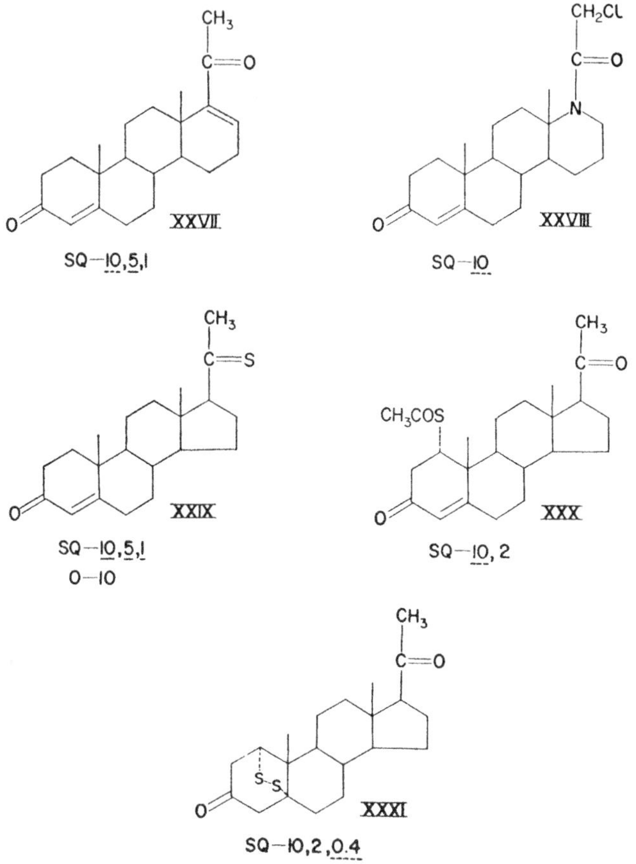

FIG. 6. Miscellaneous progesterone derivatives. (Dosage in milligrams. SQ = subcutaneous injection; O = by gavage.)

route. This parallels the emergence of progestational activity with 17-esterification (6). It should be noted that oral activity is not pronounced. Various derivatives of 17-acetoxyprogesterone are listed in FIG. 8. Two (XXXVII and XXXVIII) give evidence of minimal activity, and the two most thoroughly tested (XL and XLI) are highly potent by the subcutaneous route and somewhat less active when administered orally.

In FIGS. 9 through 12 are listed active compounds classified as 19-nor-steroids. These are basically derivatives of 19-nortestosterone. The potent

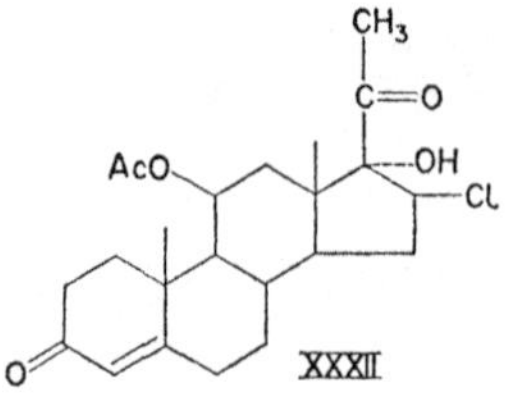

XXXII

SQ–20,5

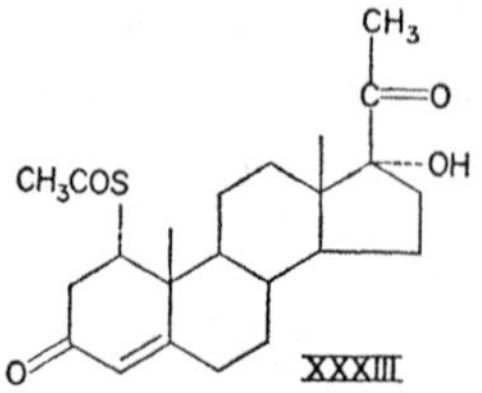

XXXIII

SQ–10,2

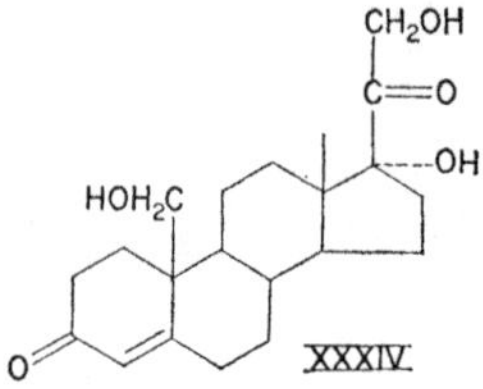

XXXIV

SQ–10

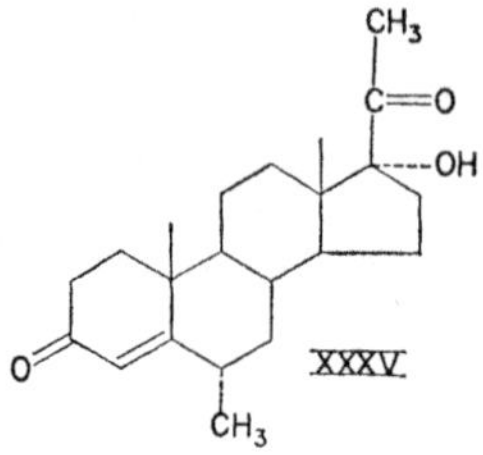

XXXV

SQ–10,2
O–20

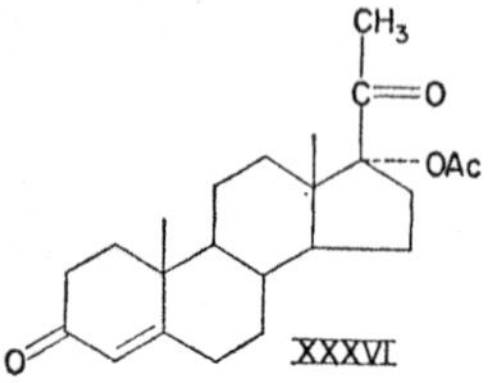

XXXVI

SQ–2,0.4,0.08,0.016
O–10,2

FIG. 7. Derivatives of 17-hydroxyprogesterone. (Dosage in milligrams. SQ = subcutaneous injection; O = by gavage.)

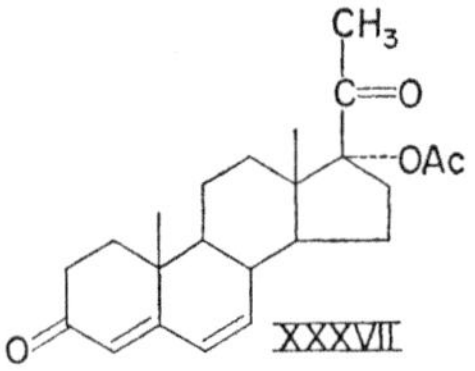

XXXVII

SQ–10,2, 0.4

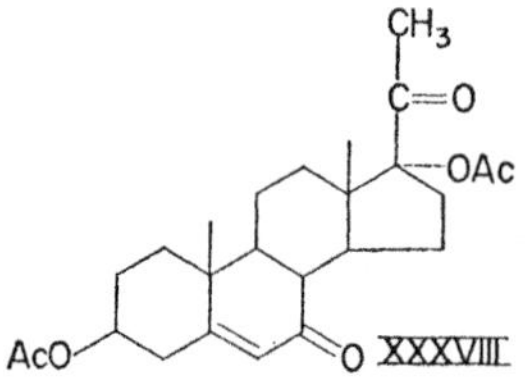

XXXVIII

SQ–10

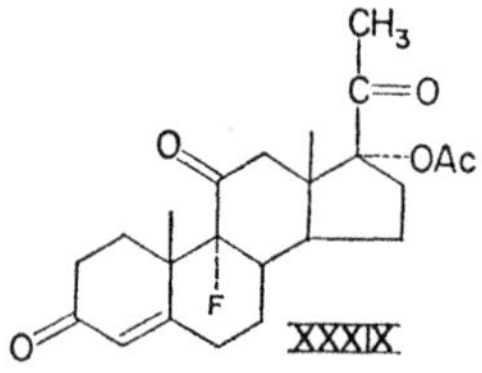

XXXIX

SQ–10

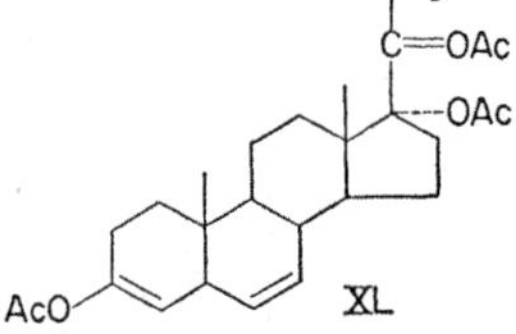

XL

SQ–10 ,0.4,0.08,0.016
O–2,0.4,0.08

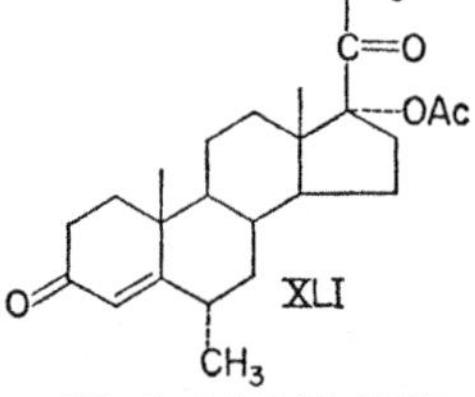

XLI

SQ–2,0.4,0.08,0.016
O–10,2,0.4, 0.016

FIG. 8. Derivatives of 17-hydroxyprogesterone. (Dosage in milligrams. SQ = subcutaneous injection; O = by gavage.)

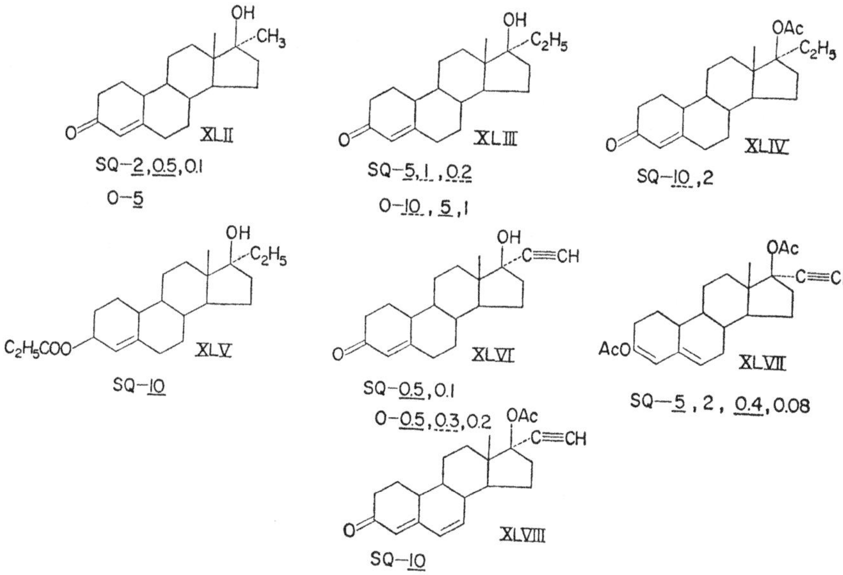

FIG. 9. 17α-Methyl, ethyl and ethinyl derivatives of 19-nortestosterone. (Dosage in milligrams. SQ = subcutaneous injection; O = by gavage.)

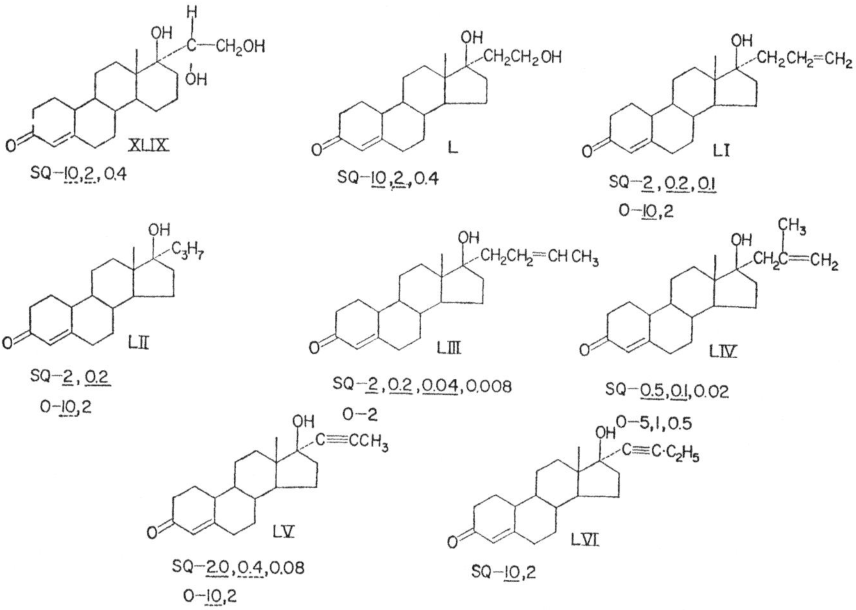

FIG. 10. Higher 17α-derivatives of 19-nortestosterone. (Dosage in milligrams. SQ = subcutaneous injections; O = by gavage.)

oral progestational activity of 17α-ethinyl-19-nortestosterone (XLVI) was first reported by Hertz *et al.* (7). We reported *in extenso* (2, 3, 4) on the progestational, ovulation-inhibiting, deciduomagenic and other properties of four 17α-alkyl-19-norsteroids (XLVI, XLII, XLIII and LXII), as well as on their effects on ovulation and various menstrual cycle phenomena in women (2, 8, 9, 10). Of the compounds listed in FIG. 9, all save XLIV are potent ovulation inhibitors. Among the higher alkyl derivatives of 19-nortestosterone (FIG. 10), significant ovulation inhibition at fairly low dosages is exhibited on subcutaneous injection, but all the compounds of high potency by this route are much less active by the oral route (cf. LI, LIII,

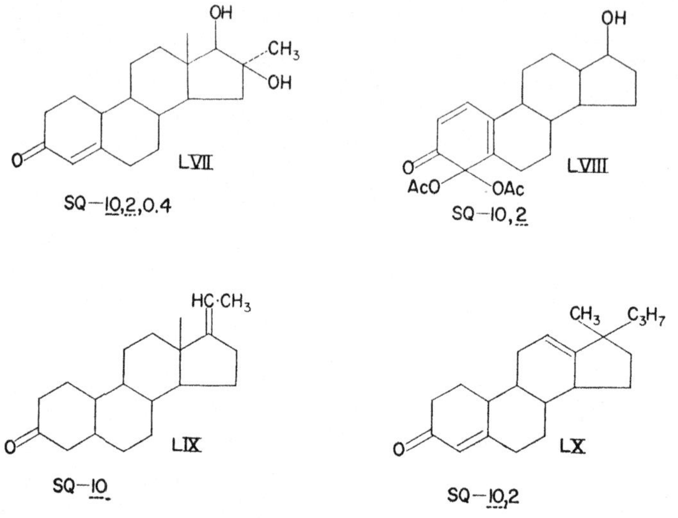

FIG. 11. Miscellaneous 19-norsteroids. (Dosage in milligrams. SQ = subcutaneous injection; O = by gavage.)

LIV and LV). Certain miscellaneous 19-norsteroids listed in FIG. 11 are either marginally active or of low potency. Finally, the shifting of the ring A double bond from the 4, 5 to the 5, 10 position may reduce the ovulation-inhibiting activity by subcutaneous administration (cf. LXII and XLVI; LXIII and XLIII; LXIV and LII), but highly potent activity is exhibited by the one compound (LXII) tested orally.

We have presented in the foregoing figures a list of sixty-four steroid compounds indicated as ovulation inhibitors in the rabbit. One hundred and twenty-three additional steroid compounds have been submitted to this test, with negative results. In Table 1 we list the numbers tested in various classifications and the percentages of active compounds. It is clear that the largest proportion of active compounds is in the group of 19-norsteroids, with the 17-hydroxyprogesterone derivatives ranking next. These percentage figures probably represent in part the deliberate selection of potentially active substances, but it should be noted that in those groups where the proportion of active compounds is lowest the potency of those deemed active is relatively low.

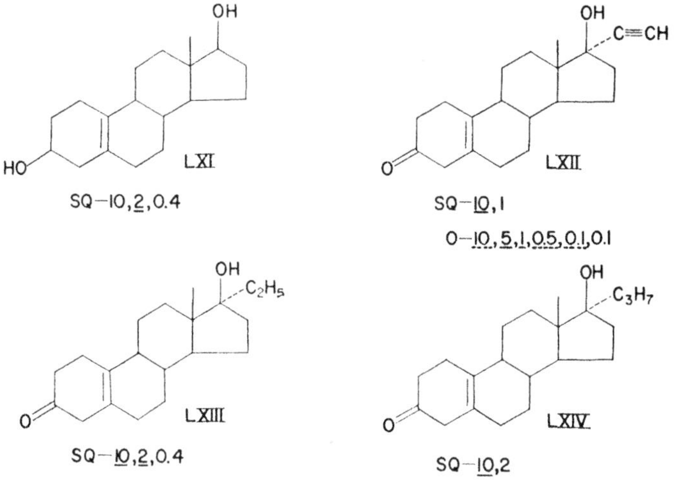

FIG. 12. $\Delta^{5,10}$-19-Norsteroids. (Dosage in milligrams. SQ = subcutaneous injections; O = by gavage.)

TABLE 1. THE NUMBERS IN VARIOUS CLASSES OF STEROID COMPOUNDS TESTED AS OVULATION INHIBITORS

Type of compound	Number demonstrating activity	Number inactive	% active
Estrogens and derivatives	9	34	21
Androgens and derivatives	7	28	20
Progesterone derivatives	15	42	26
17-OH-progesterone derivatives	10	9	52
19-Norsteroids	23	10	70

One feature of our findings which requires further remark is the discrepancy between activity by mouth and by injection exhibited particularly by some of the more potent substances. This is illustrated in Table 2 where we present the calculated minimal effective doses of five compounds which have been sufficiently tested by both routes both as ovulation inhibitors and as progestins. The data on oral : subcutaneous progestational potency ratios are from the paper by Miyake and Pincus (4). The parallelism in relative oral effectiveness is evident. The fact that XLVI is somewhat and LXII very much more potent by mouth suggests that these may be transformed to more potent ovulation inhibitors following oral ingestion. In this connection it should be noted that, in addition to finding them more potent as oral than as parenteral progestins, Saunders and Drill (11) were unable to find evidence

TABLE 2. THE RELATIVE EFFECTIVENESS OF CERTAIN STEROIDS BY PARENTERAL AND ORAL ROUTES AS OVULATION INHIBITORS AND AS PROGESTINS

Compound number	Minimal effective ovulation-inhibiting dose		$\frac{SQ}{O}$	Oral/subcutaneous ratio as progestins†
	SQ*	O*		
XXXVI	0.05	5	0.01	0.1
XLI	0.05	0.4	0.13	0.2
XLIII	0.2	2	0.10	0.6
XLVI	0.3	0.25	1.2	1.4
LXII	5	0.2	25	5.4

* SQ = by subcutaneous injection; O = by gavage.
† From Miyake and Pincus (4).

of direct effect on the endometrium with intrauterine implants. Their transformation to active progestins somewhere outside the uterus is indicated by this evidence as well as by our data on the oral : subcutaneous ratio.

If this *in vivo* conversion to a potent progestin be accepted, then it may be asked if the unknown conversion product is also responsible for the ovulation inhibition. The fact is that a number of highly potent progestins are also rather potent ovulation inhibitors on injection (e.g. LIII, XLI and related compounds). Presumably their reduced activity by mouth is due to some inactivation process in the gut or in the liver. We have considered the possibility that norethynodrel (LXII) and norethindrone (XLVI) are converted to estrogenic compounds which in turn are the active ovulation inhibitors. The rather unremarkable record of the estrogens as ovulation inhibitors in our tests (see FIG. 1) has led us to discount this possibility. We have, in fact, tested the 3-methyl ether of ethinyl estradiol subcutaneously at dosages of 10, 5, 1 and 0.1 mg and have had no significant inhibition of ovulation. However, 17α-ethinyl estradiol itself is the probable estrogenic metabolite, and we have not as yet tested this compound as an ovulation inhibitor in the rabbit.

Before concluding this presentation, I should like to exhibit data which we have obtained on the ovaries of rats receiving norethynodrel. These are presented in Tables 3 and 4, in which the numbers of corpora lutea, of various follicle types, and of primordial ova per unit area are given for control and for norethynodrel-injected rats. The rats were injected daily for fourteen days and sacrificed at the fifteenth day. In both groups of animals there was consistent reduction over the control values only in the number of corpora lutea.

The significantly lower number of normal follicles without antra in the 30-day-old rat series is certainly not seen in the 90-day-old rat series. The reduction in corpus luteum number may be due to a reduction in the number of follicles ovulating or to a facilitation of corpus luteum resorption, or, indeed, to a retention of corpora lutea present at the time the injections were begun. A direct examination of the oviducts for ova could perhaps resolve these possibilities.

TABLE 3. THE STATE OF THE OVARIES IN THIRTY-DAY-OLD RATS RECEIVING NORETHYNODREL BY DAILY INJECTION IN A FIFTEEN-DAY PERIOD

Treatment	Total dosage (mg)	No. of animals	Number per unit area					
			Corpora lutea	Follicles with antra		Follicles without antra		Primordial ova
				Atretic	Normal	Atretic	Normal	
None	—	20	2.0±0.30	5.1±0.93	1.4±0.40	8.7±1.42	7.1±1.13	8.8±1.45
Norethynodrel	2.8	18	0.7±0.31	4.9±0.67	1.4±0.33	7.5±1.39	7.5±0.96	12.5±2.17
Norethynodrel	14.0	17	<u>0.2±0.14</u>	6.2±0.71	0.6±0.26	11.5±1.52	<u>2.7±0.63</u>	9.5±1.39

Underlined values differ significantly from control values.

TABLE 4. THE STATE OF THE OVARIES IN NINETY-DAY-OLD RATS RECEIVING NORETHYNODREL BY DAILY INJECTION IN A FIFTEEN-DAY PERIOD

Treatment	Total dosage (mg)	No. of animals	Number per unit area					
			Corpora lutea	Follicles with antra		Follicles without antra		Primordial ova
				Atretic	Normal	Atretic	Normal	
None	—	20	6.6±0.46	6.0±0.84	0.6±0.21	8.4±1.25	2.2±0.48	5.7±0.97
Norethynodrel	2.8	18	4.4±0.69	5.6±0.44	0.2±0.35	8.7±1.12	2.1±0.57	12.1±3.71
Norethynodrel	14.0	16	<u>3.9±0.49</u>	5.6±1.00	0.8±0.35	7.9±0.75	2.7±0.57	7.7±1.27

Underlined values differ significantly from control values.

In conclusion, I should like to summarize as follows: (*a*) a good number of steroid substances give evidence of acting as ovulation inhibitors in the rabbit; (*b*) except, however, for certain progestational steroids, most of these substances are of low or dubious activity; (*c*) among the compounds of relatively high potency by subcutaneous injection, there are several in which activity by mouth is apparently absent (e.g. XXIX, LIV) or much less than by the parenteral route (e.g. XLI, LV); (*d*) one compound, norethynodrel, is highly active on oral administration (in fact it is the most active ovulation inhibitor) but of quite low potency by injection; norethindrone is similarly somewhat more active by mouth than by injection. It is interesting to note that thus far the most consistent oral ovulation inhibitors in women are these two compounds, whereas others (e.g. XLI and LIV) are by themselves not very effective oral agents in women (12, 13).

REFERENCES

1. Pincus, G. and M. C. Chang, *Acta Physiol. Latino-americana* **3**, 177, 1953.
2. Pincus, G., *Proc. 5th Internat. Conf. Planned Parenthood*, p. 176, 1955.
3. Pincus, G., M. C. Chang, M. X. Zarrow, E. S. E. Hafez and A. Merrill, *Endocrinology* **59**, 695, 1956.
4. Miyake, T. and G. Pincus, *Endocrinology* **63**, 816, 1958.
5. Saunders, F. J. and R. L. Elton, in *Endocrinology of Reproduction* (Edited by C. W. Lloyd), p. 227. Academic Press, New York, 1959.
6. Junkmann, K., *Arch. Exptl. Pathol. Pharmakol.* **223**, 244, 1954.
7. Hertz, R., W. Tullner and E. Raffelt, *Endocrinology* **54**, 228, 1954.
8. Rock, J., G. Pincus and C. R. Garcia, *Science* **124**, 891, 1956.
9. Rock, J., C. R. Garcia and G. Pincus, *Recent Progress in Hormone Research* **13**, 323, 1957.
10. Garcia, C. R., G. Pincus and J. Rock, *Am. J. Obstet. & Gynec.* **75**, 82, 1958.
11. Saunders, F. J. and V. A. Drill, *Ann. N.Y. Acad. Sci.* **71**, 516, 1958.
12. Pincus, G., *Vitamins and Hormones* **17**, 307, 1959.
13. Rock, J. and C. R. Garcia (this volume).

DISCUSSIONS

Chairman: Dr. Roy O. Greep

Dr. Frederick L. Hisaw: The experiments reported by Dr. Simpson on the induction of ovulation in monkeys (*Macaca mulatta*) and rats deal with two mammalian species that differ widely in sensitivity to exogenous pituitary gonadotropins, and particularly in responsiveness to the luteinizing hormone (LH). An unfractionated pituitary extract that contains both FSH and LH, when given subcutaneously to monkeys in moderate doses, produces primary growth of follicles, most of which may be cystic and show little or no luteinization of the granulosa. If, following follicular development, the same preparation is injected intravenously, luteinization usually occurs and occasionally a follicle may rupture, but when this happens it always involves a follicle of approximately normal size that has not become cystic. In contrast with this, a similar preparation invariably causes luteinization in rats when administered subcutaneously in effective doses for a period longer than 3 or 4 days.

Therefore, as Dr. Simpson has emphasized, an analysis of follicular development and ovulation as induced by pituitary gonadotropins must depend in large measure on the purity of FSH and LH preparations, the length of treatment, the relation of the two hormones in the reactions, and the responsiveness of the experimental animal. It seems that LH can be obtained free of FSH but it is disappointing that so far no one has succeeded in isolating FSH in sufficient purity that it will not produce luteinization when given in large doses. This, of course, could mean an incomplete separation of the two hormones but the possibility should be considered that the weak luteinizing action of purified FSH may be due to an amino-acid sequence held in common with LH as has been found for the melanophore-stimulating hormone (MSH) and adrenocorticotropin (ACTH).

It may not be an unimportant observation that the conditions most favorable for follicular development when induced by gonadotropins are also at the same time most favorable for stimulating estrogen secretion. Both FSH and LH are notoriously ineffective when given alone in dosages that are very effective when the two hormones act concurrently. A notable difference between the two situations is that in the former estrogen is not secreted and in the latter it is. The follicular growth produced by large doses of FSH is probably facilitated by the weak LH action that is invariably present, and also estrogen is secreted.

The association of estrogen secretion with follicular growth seems to apply equally well to ovarian responses induced by the chorionic luteotropin, HCG. This hormone is capable of causing the secretion of both estrogen and progesterone provided follicles and corpora lutea (particularly the latter) are present when it is administered. It also can substitute for LH when FSH is given. However, it cannot promote follicular growth, at reasonable dosage, in the involuted ovaries of hypophysectomized rats or in the ovaries of juvenile monkeys, and in neither instance is estrogen secreted. The probable importance of estrogen is suggested by the fact that the ovaries of hypophysectomized rats will respond to HCG when the treatment is preceded by a series of injections of estrogen. Also, estrogen will facilitate the action of FSH.

Another placental hormone, PMS, is of interest in this connection in that it can mimic both FSH and LH, particularly the former, and, of course, estrogen secretion is associated with its effects. It is an excellent hormone for producing follicular growth and is useful in experimental ovulation. However, both it and HCG are, in reality, hormones of gestation that are designed for the specific physiological needs of the species in which they are found and are useful in studies of ovulation only in so far as their pharmacological actions assist in the elucidation of the physiology of FSH and LH.

It may not be of direct practical importance for the problem in hand, but I do think it adds interest to keep in mind that the interactions of pituitary and ovarian hormones in the regulation of follicular development and ovulation, as found in vertebrate animals, represent the culmination in the evolution of a long series of adaptations. The present evidence indicates that in the vertebrates the hormonal situation is basically the same in all reproductive cycles up to and including ovulation. The principal hormones seem to be FSH, LH and estrogen. This means of course that the cycle in all vertebrates is physiologically homologous with the follicular phase of a mammalian estrous cycle. Also, it seems quite possible that the steroid hormone of the Graafian follicle in all instances is estradiol-17β. This is supported by the isolation of estradiol-17β from ovaries of such distantly related vertebrates as the mammal, bird, lung fish and dogfish. It is also of added interest that estradiol-17β has been found in the ovaries of certain invertebrates, i.e. a starfish, sea urchin and pecten. It is also a possibility that progesterone is an ubiquitous steroid. A steroidal substance has been obtained from the ovaries of invertebrates, by using methods applicable to mammalian tissues, which has been tentatively identified as progesterone on the basis of column chromatography, paper chromatography and positive Hooker–Forbes reactions.

The general presence of these steroids raises the question of their importance and function in the physiology of the follicle itself. When reduced to its simplest form, it is conceivable that estrogens and progesterone along with various other steroids and sterols were deposited in the ovum by the surrounding nurse cells or granulosa, with which ova are commonly associated, long before they assumed hormonal functions. It is not even necessary to assume that these compounds were synthesized and secreted by the nurse cells. There is some evidence that they are present in plants and consequently might have been obtained ready formed as is true of most vitamins. However, regardless of origin, the most important point is the probability that the nurse cells of the follicle from the inception of the practice of passing materials along to the ovum were metabolically acquainted with steroid compounds and also it is a further assumption that the initial endocrine functions were concerned only with physiological processes in the follicle. The acquisition of the status of bodily hormones was probably a specialization that came later.

The only endocrine features that seem to be common throughout the life of a follicle in both vertebrates and invertebrates are the presence of steroid hormones and the fact that the follicle normally ruptures. Therefore, the solution of the problem of ovulation may be found by investigating the basic physiological processes that go on in the follicle. There have been very few analytical efforts in this direction. Most research has been concerned with the regulatory mechanisms that affect follicular physiology. Those factors which originate outside the ovary are for the most part timing devices to guarantee that ovulation occurs at the most favorable moment and season for fertilization and survival of the embryo. It is of course a familiar fact that environmental factors such as light, temperature, humidity, food, etc., can influence the secretion of gonadotropins by the pituitary and it is now quite evident that these effects are mediated by the nervous system.

It is of course a familiar and interesting observation that ovarian development and ovulation generally is attuned to environmental influences such as light, temperature, humidity and food. These influences in vertebrates are mediated by the pituitary but it is obvious that ovulation was a well-established phenomenon long before a pituitary was invented. Therefore, the physiology of the follicle itself should hold the solution of the problem and steroid action may be the answer.

The research reported by Dr. Pincus deals with the most important practical problem that confronts the human race today. The destiny of mankind most certainly depends more on control of the world's population than it does on the curious international competition now raging over such comparatively trivial things as who is to enjoy the dubious distinction of being the first to get a peek at the sea's bottom or the moon's backside. Even so, finding a method for the inhibition of ovulation is in reality a problem in endocrine engineering which relies on basic information rather than contributing to it. However, these studies have raised many important questions regarding essential molecular morphology of an effective steroid inhibitor and the nature of the inhibitory process.

CHAIRMAN GREEP: Dr. Folley, would you like to comment on any of these three papers?

DR. S. JOHN FOLLEY: At this rather early stage of the proceedings I do not think that any comment of an all-embracing nature has occurred to me, except for one point in connection with what Dr. Hammond has just said about the follicular fluid. We know that, in addition to the proteins, salts and so forth mentioned by him, follicular fluid also contains other substances, in particular at least two mucopolysaccharides. I have often wondered if there is some connection between the fact that the gonadotropins are glycoproteins and the fact that the cells lining the follicles, at least some of them, are cells which secrete mucopolysaccharides. I am afraid I cannot offer any more specific suggestions about this at the present time, but it would seem to me to be a point which is worth some consideration. More pertinent, perhaps, is the fact that these mucopolysaccharides undergo depolymerization just before ovulation, with a concomitant rise in the colloid osmotic pressure of the follicular fluid (Zacharias and Jensen, *Acta Endocrinol.* **27**, 343, 356, 1958), and one cannot help wondering whether estrogen produced by the follicular cells plays any role in this as it seems to do in the liquefaction of the cervical mucus at estrus. I throw this out to the meeting as something which might be thought about and perhaps we might have some ideas about it.

CHAIRMAN GREEP: Is there any one who would like to comment, or is there any one who would like to pose a question to any of our speakers of the afternoon?

DR. WARREN O. NELSON: I wonder, Gregory, harking back to your remarks about inhibition of ovulation in the rat whether it would not be appropriate to take into account the fact that the 19 nor-compounds behave very much, under some circumstances, as estrogens do. If they are given to adult rats corpora lutea are maintained. Your objective was, of course, to examine the inhibitory activity of these compounds which, indeed, are very effective gonadotropin inhibitors, but I wonder if the presence of corpora lutea in animals, treated for fifteen days, would not reflect the fact that corpora lutea were present at the time treatment was begun and were caused to persist by treatment.

DR. GREGORY PINCUS: That is a probable explanation in the 90-day-olds, and perhaps in the 30-day-old animals, although you would know, perhaps, better than I, whether you would get ovulation in a 30-day-rat.

There is one possibility that we are examining and that is the possibility that there is in the young rat perhaps some initial stimulation by steroid; I don't think it is true, though, because the ovaries, as you well know, even after two weeks' treatment, are smaller than those of the controls and though there are corpora lutea, they are less in number.

Also we have run the animals for a longer period of time, and eventually we see no corpora lutea. So I was merely being over-conservative in saying that there may have been an ovulation. Actually, we have no proof.

In the mouse, we have looked for ova, and it is quite clear that the ova are not produced. Maybe I should have made that remark in my presentation. Otherwise, I quite agree with you that these are just as potent gonadotropin inhibitors in the rat and mouse, by the standards that we have been able to set up, as they are in the rabbit and the human.

DR. ERNEST KNOBIL: May I ask Dr. Hisaw whether he has failed to find estrogen in any of these invertebrate animals he has investigated?

DR. FREDERICK L. HISAW: So far we have studied ovarian material from only three species of invertebrates: a starfish (*Pisaster ochraceous*), a sea-urchin (*Strongylocentrotus franciscanus*) and a pecten (*Pecten hericins*). Estradiol-17β and progesterone were present in all three, as determined by techniques commonly employed in the isolation and identification of these steroids in mammalian tissue. Lots of 10 to 14 kg of ripe ovaries were extracted. The amounts of these steroids on a tissue-weight basis were very small and we were interested primarily at this time in identification rather than quantitation. However, the estrogen content in pecten ovaries was found to be much greater than in the ovaries of either the starfish or sea-urchin.

DR. JANET MCARTHUR: I would like to ask Dr. Simpson what sort of extrapolation she would make from these studies to her applied work on the FSH and ICSH content of the monkey pituitary during different stages of the menstrual cycle.

DR. MIRIAM E. SIMPSON: I do not think we are in a position to answer your question. I made the point for the rat, that we have not so far been able to show a relationship between the pituitary hormone content at different stages of the cycle and the ability to induce ovulation. The preparations of rat pituitary used were crude preparations.

Such studies have not been conducted with monkey pituitaries removed at different stages of the menstrual cycle.

DR. JANET MCARTHUR: In your monkey studies, the FSH went up as well as the LH in the cycle?

DR. MIRIAM E. SIMPSON: There are several things that would indicate that the presence of ICSH is necessary for ovulation. The stimulation from FSH preparation may in part be attributable to a masked ICSH in FSH preparations. ICSH cannot be recognized at as low doses in the presence of FSH as when given alone.

When very high doses of ICSH were injected during preparation of follicles premature thecal luteinization with enclosure of eggs occurred.

CHAIRMAN GREEP: The ovulatory process may really start with the growth of the follicle. Perhaps the processes producing ovulation have to follow a given sequence right from the very beginning. Do you see what I am driving at?

DR. MIRIAM E. SIMPSON: They have to go on in a normal sequence.

CHAIRMAN GREEP: This, we haven't unravelled as yet, but your data indicate to me that if you had a pure FSH, you might not be able to ovulate the follicle when it was fully grown, because certain of the processes had lagged behind, and could not then catch up.

DR. MIRIAM E. SIMPSON: Although it is commonly assumed that some ICSH must be present with FSH before full maturity of the follicles and estrous response can be elicited, nevertheless the exact amount of ICSH needed is not known accurately. I think we are agreed that a follicle needs a vascular envelopment for development, and this is supplied by the theca.

CHAIRMAN GREEP: It seems that the importance of balance is not just at the time of ovulation, but long before that. You have to have the proper preparation all the way along, in order to get really effective ovulation.

DR. SOMERS H. STURGIS: I would like to ask Dr. Pincus a question. I gather that the steroids were given just after mating so that you had 10 hr in which they had to work, presumably to prevent ovulation. This would seem to me to be a very short time for these compounds to work, particularly those that were given by the oral route. It suggests some mode of action other than through pituitary inhibition. What about the possibility of some direct action on the follicles themselves? We don't know very much about the activity of an ovarian steroid as estrogen or progesterone on the ovary itself, yet in the hypophysectomized rat, estrogen certainly does maintain and perhaps even stimulate the growth of follicles and granulosa. Last fall, Vasicka reported at the American College of Surgeons some evidence for the direct action of Enovid on human ovaries. In ovarian biopsies, he felt that he could show an increase in follicle atresia following Enovid medication.

In this regard, do you want to say something about the possibility of some direct action of these steroids on the ovarian follicles, or do you believe that the effect that you have shown us on inhibition of ovulation can and must take place through the pituitary, even when giving oral preparations after mating with only ten hours for effective action before ovulation will occur?

DR. GREGORY PINCUS: Dr. Chang and I originally found that with progesterone, we could practically invariably ovulate the animal receiving an inhibiting dose, by giving gonadotropins intravenously. Whether this would be true of all the compounds we have tested, I don't know. I know it is true in some cases. As to the possibility of a direct influence on the ovary, this ties in with Dr. Hisaw's and Dr. Hammond's discussion; it is something that fascinates me very much.

If we had been lucky enough to find a steroid which causes ovulation, the course of reproductive physiology might have changed markedly. I think that there may be such a substance.

If there is something which can stimulate ovulation, there are certainly plenty of things you should be able to do to reverse such stimulation. We know that steroids can act as antagonists to each other in many situations. We have tried to find some evidence for direct action of steroids upon the ovaries in studies with the mouse. What we did was to use PMS and HCG to ovulate the mice, administer the steroid, and then see if ova were produced.

The most potent ovulation inhibitors proved to be reserpin and chlorpromazine. So we probably weren't by-passing the pituitary of the animals but affecting an endogenous factor that acts with the administered gonadotropins. Certain of the steroids also were active in inhibiting ovulation.

The last point I want to make is in reference to Dr. Hisaw's remarks. As far as the genesis of hormonal steroids is concerned, in every species of mammals studied so far, the process is identical. The major precursor is cholesterol; this is transformed to Δ^5-pregnenolone, which is the parent of all the steroid hormones.

One of the possibilities very much overlooked is that some of these steroids are mitosis-stimulating and others mitosis-inhibiting. What relationship this would have to egg development and maturation has never been studied. With modern techniques, one ought to be able to isolate and grow eggs to see whether there are inhibiting and stimulating steroids.

CHAIRMAN GREEP: Is there a biologist in the house? I would like to have someone comment on the work of Witschi and Chang.

DR. SHELDON SEGAL: I am reminded of three recent studies that bear on today's discussion. The first is by Meyer and Bradbury (*Endocrinology* **66**, 121–128, 1960), demonstrating a direct effect of estrogen on growing ovaries. Using both immature and hypophysectomized rats, they found that estrogen priming (stilbestrol) enhanced the ovarian response to gonadotropin. This principle may be of significance with respect to some aspects of the work reported by Dr. Noyes and Dr. Simpson. In each case, the failure of the ovary to respond to stimulation could be correlated with an absence of estrogen. In the experiments of Dr. Noyes, the ovarian implants were made in castrate hosts. Would the addition of estrogen improve the performance of the ovarian implants? Dr. Simpson reports that FSH preparations most purified and free of ICSH contamination ($<4\%$) are least effective as a supplement in causing ovulation. Do these results correlate with the effect of the preparations on causing ovarian estrogen production?

The two other studies I would like to mention deal with *in vitro* ovulation using frog ovaries. Witschi and Chang (*Endocrinology* **61**, 514–519, 1957) found that exposure of primed segments of frog ovaries to cortisone *in vitro* favored egg-release. Bergers and Li (*Endocrinology* **66**, 255–259, 1960) reported that *in vitro* ovulation by this test is induced by progesterone. ICSH and GH, from mammalian sources, induced ovulation also under the conditions of the experiment. Neither study included a report of the activity of estrogen in this *in vitro* test. It would be of interest to learn about this in view of the evidence for the direct effect of estrogen on the mammalian ovary.

DR. VILLEE: I would like to ask Dr. Simpson whether she had tried to add estrogens in the course of the preparation of the follicles.

DR. MIRIAM E. SIMPSON: Estrogens have not been injected. Furthermore, there was not sufficient time to present the estrogenic properties of each of the follicle-stimulating preparations injected. The purified follicle-stimulating preparations were very different in regard to their ovulating capacity and eventually we will present the correlation between the capacity of FSH preparations to induce ovulation and to cause estrous uterine response.

DR. ROBERT W. NOYES: It always appeared to me that a follicle may make enough estrogen to prepare the endometrium on its own. Occasionally, in post-menopausal women, a pregnancy may occur two or three years after the last period, and you wonder if a single follicle was able to make enough estrogen and progesterone to support implantation and pregnancy.

NALBANDOV: In connection with Bradbury's work, it seems significant to me that the doses of estrogen or stilbestrol required to produce these effects on the ovary are extremely high. I believe that a minimum of 1 mg of the steroid per day must be given. This fact suggests that this is not a physiological mechanism and raises the question whether the effect is produced by the hormone itself or by a metabolite of these substances.

DR. SHELDON SEGAL: One can't decide that issue until he does a subsequent step of making local implantations of estrogen crystals or small pieces of estrogen in one ovary, in relation to the next step. We will have to wait for those results before deciding whether it is a physiological thing or not.

DR. GREGORY PINCUS: I would like to say one thing in regard to that. He may not be using the right estrogen.

Maybe it is natural. If you study ovarian vein blood and study the estrogens in there, you would be surprised. They are not the usual estrogens, but they may be of importance physiologically.

DR. W. R. BRENEMAN: Perhaps I should let Dr. Segal speak on the following point since I believe that the non-mammalian vertebrates provide information relative to the effect of steroid hormones on the gonads. For example, in the amphibia distinct primary and secondary cords usually are present in both testes and ovaries and Burns demonstrated in the 1930's that sex hormones were able to regulate the development of the cords. Genetic males could be transformed into females with estrone. Unfortunately, this result does not follow in all amphibia as Witschi demonstrated in frogs.

The experiments of Burns provide evidence for the direct effect of sex hormones on the development of the primary and secondary cords of the developing gonad.

Changes in the nature of the follicular contents have been referred to in the discussion. It is interesting that Van Oordt and his co-workers have observed comparable changes with the seminiferous tubules. The administration of anterior pituitary hormones transforms the viscous contents of the tubules to a watery consistency and there is a simultaneous disappearance of mucopolysaccharide. However, I suppose caution should be exercised in considering this to be homologous with changes in the ovarian follicle.

Finally, it may be of interest to report in connection with Dr. Simpson's results some observations of Dr. R. R. Humphrey on axolotls. He tried to ovulate these animals with Armour LH with which we provided him. This experiment was unsuccessful. Armour FSH, on the other hand, did a beautiful job in ovulating the axolotls.

DR. M. C. CHANG: I should like to comment here about Dr. Noyes' paper in connection with the point raised by Dr. Pincus, whether the presence of estrogen in the follicle would inhibit or facilitate maturation of the egg. In 1955 (*J. Exp. Zool.* **128**, 379; *Science* **121**, 867) I did some work on the cultivation and transplantation of follicular eggs in the rabbit. It was found that eggs recovered from follicles of the unmated rabbit could mature, that is, there was disappearance of the nuclear membrane, formation of the first maturation spindle, extrusion of the first polar body and formation of the second maturation spindle, either in culture or in the fallopian tubes. It seems to me that there is perhaps a factor in the follicle which inhibits the maturation of the egg. Whether it is estrogen, I do not know. Some of these eggs can be fertilized, but most of them failed to develop into normal young after fertilization. It seems to me that whether an egg with second maturation spindle observed outside the follicle is really matured in the follicle or matured *in vitro* is uncertain and whether or not they are really normal is also difficult to say. By application of potassium fluoride, Nadamitsu (*J. Sci. Hiroshima Univ.* **17**, 47, 1957) observed the ovulation of rat ovaries *in vitro* and claimed that the eggs are normal because of the presence of the second maturation chromosomes. I wonder whether these eggs ovulated *in vitro* or in the anterior chamber of eye are really normal.

DR. GREGORY PINCUS: The experimenter has done more than that. He has actually taken eggs and added gonadotropin *in vitro*, and decided that unless the gonadotropin is present, the eggs do not go through the first maturation division. Unfortunately, I don't think that he is statistically minded, so we cannot find out more details.

All you need to do with rabbit eggs is take them out of the follicles, put them in culture, and it can be a variety of types of cultures, and they will go through the first maturation division.

The second division doesn't occur, ordinarily, unless the egg is fertilized or parthenogenetically activated.

It is the first maturation division which occurs in the ovaries in practically all species.

DR. ROBERT W. NOYES: These early follicular eggs cannot be fertilized because of the immaturity of the cumulus, corona and probably zona pellucida. Although certain features of nuclear maturation and meiosis take place in such ova removed to *in vitro* conditions, the cumulus and corona do not mature, and spermatozoa do not penetrate these coats if the cultured ova are transferred into a recipient oviduct.

CHAIRMAN GREEP: Does any one know about the hyperemia test?

DR. CHARLES A. BARRACLOUGH: Would the development beyond the secondary follicle occur with a smaller amount of FSH, given to the estrogen-primed animal?

DR. MIRIAM SIMPSON: As estrogens will cause follicular growth in hypophysectomized rats I think it is quite possible the follicular growth resulting from the combination of FSH and estrogen might be greater than that which results from either alone.

DR. FREDERICK L. HISAW: I should like to suggest that probably the frog's ovary could be used to test certain ideas that have been mentioned regarding ovulation. One advantage offered is that ovarian fragments can be induced to ovulate quite easily *in vitro*. Also, sufficient material for a rather large series of experiments can be obtained from a single ovary. Several investigators have reported results of experiments of this sort and the chief difficulty encountered seems to be variability in responsiveness of ovaries from different animals. This is at least partly due to such things as the time of year the frogs are collected and the conditions under which they are kept. Best results can be expected when the animals are taken directly from hibernation under natural conditions. Also, the responsiveness of the ovaries can be greatly increased by administering a subovulatory dose of frog pituitary tissue or by hypophysectomizing the animal a day or so before the ovaries are removed. It may also be added that physiological solutions used should be low or even lacking in calcium.

THE PITUITARY STALK AND OVULATION

G. W. HARRIS

Department of Neuroendocrinology, Institute of Psychiatry
Maudsley Hospital, London S.E.5, England

THE ripening of an ovarian follicle and its rupture, with discharge of an ovum, is dependent on the secretion of the anterior pituitary gland. Administration of purified follicle-stimulating hormone (FSH) results in follicular enlargement, but such follicles are unable to reach full size or secrete estrogen unless some luteinizing hormone (LH) is also present (39). Ovulation is most effectively produced by administration of FSH with a small amount of LH (ratio about 10 : 1).

FOLLICULAR GROWTH

Until recently the central neural factors responsible for regulating the pituitary secretion of FSH had received little attention. Studies of such factors require the use of animals with quiescent ovaries; either immature animals or adult animals with a well-marked anestrous period.

(i) *The Hypothalamus and Development of Puberty*

It was at first thought that the onset of puberty was due to an ageing or maturation process in the endocrine glands concerned. However, Foà (34) showed that ageing of ovarian tissue could not be concerned since the ovaries of immature animals transplanted to mature animals show changes typical of the adult organ; likewise ovaries from a mature animal transplanted to the prepubertal become quiescent and undergo atrophy. After it was realized that the anterior pituitary gland was responsible for ovarian activity, it was found that this gland contained active gonadotropic hormone before the onset of maturity and that the implantation of anterior lobes of immature animals into other immature animals might induce gonadal activity. Further, Harris and Jacobsohn (48) found that pituitary tissue obtained from *new-born* rats grafted under the hypothalamus of hypophysectomized adult female rats became vascularized by the hypophysial portal vessels, and was capable of supporting full adult reproductive functions. Thus the functional activity of the ovary and anterior pituitary gland in the immature animal does not depend on an intrinsic property of the tissue but on the "environment" in which it is situated.

In considering the sequence of events underlying the onset of puberty, account must be taken of the endocrine status of the immature animal. It is likely that the adenohypophysis and gonads are active, secreting glands in prepubertal forms. The data for this statement have been reviewed in detail by Donovan and Harris (20) and may be summarized as follows:

(*a*) The immature gonad secretes sex hormones, since prepubertal castration in the rat results in regression of the seminal vesicles and penis (15), an increase in pituitary content of gonadotropin (52) and the development of castration cells in the pituitary gland (17).

(*b*) The immature pituitary gland secretes gonadotropic hormones since hypophysectomy in infantile rats results in regression of both ovarian (84) and testicular (83) development.

(*c*) A feed-back action of gonadal hormones on pituitary function is indicated by the fact that castration of one of a pair of infantile rats united in parabiosis leads to precocious puberty in the other (61, 62); this can be prevented by the administration of low doses of gonadal hormone to the castrate partner (13). It is probable that a temporary fall in blood concentration of ovarian hormones, resulting in increased gonadotropin secretion, underlies the precocious puberty seen to follow auto-transplantation of infantile ovaries (74, 40).

It seems then that before puberty the anterior pituitary gland and gonads are functionally active but, although capable of maintaining adult reproductive function at this time, their activity is restricted to a low level. The fact that a feed-back mechanism of gonadal hormones is present in the immature form implies the existence of some control mechanism regulating gonadal activity at this level.

In 1956 Donovan and van der Werff ten Bosch (21) reported that vaginal canalization in the rat, which serves as an index of ovarian maturation, occurred significantly earlier in animals with lesions in the anterior hypothalamus than in control animals. In a recent report (23) these workers give an account of a study based on over 200 animals divided into the following groups—normals, blank-operated and those with various hypothalamic or preoptic lesions. It was found that lesions placed in the anterior region of the hypothalamus in animals 10–15 days of age will, on the average, advance puberty by 5–7 days. In one experiment 34 blank-operated animals had a mean pubertal age of 43.3 days, whilst 13 rats with hypothalamic lesions had a mean pubertal age of 38.1 days. Lesions in the preoptic region did not hasten the onset of puberty. It is of interest that some of the sexually precocious rats displayed cycles of prolonged estrus, and their ovaries contained no corpora lutea, though others had normal vaginal cycles and were fertile. The effective lesions were found to be situated basally in the hypothalamus immediately behind the optic chiasma. Such lesions did not result in hyperphagia and obesity and did not significantly affect the weight of the adrenal glands. Bogdanove and Schoen (9) have recently obtained confirmatory results to the above in the rat. In attempting an explanation of these findings Donovan and van der Werff ten Bosch (23) suggest that anterior hypothalamic lesions damage or destroy some neural mechanism sensitive to the feed-back action of gonadal hormones. It seems clear in adult animals that this feed-back action is exerted on the hypothalamus, and that this structure in turn exerts a restraining influence over gonadotropin secretion by the pituitary gland. A reduced sensitivity of the hypothalamus to gonadal hormone may be one of the changes occurring in the development of sexual maturity, since Hohlweg and Dohrn (57) found that in infantile rats the cytological changes in the pituitary after gonadectomy could be prevented by gonadal hormone in doses approximately one-hundredth of that required in the adult.

In comparing the experimental findings with the clinical data on cases in which hypothalamic lesions have been found associated with precocious puberty in children (85, 3), two facts are outstanding. Firstly, various lesions (especially hamartomata—a type of congenital abnormality) may result in a greater advancement of puberty in the human than the experimental lesions do in the rat. It is possible, however, that lesions placed in the hypothalamus of fetal rats might yield results more equivalent to those seen in the human in this respect. Secondly, the site of the hypothalamic lesions in clinical cases of pubertas praecox may be well circumscribed and localized, and are often found to be in the posterior part of the tuber cinereum or in the region of the mammillary bodies. Ganong (37) has recently mentioned the results of unpublished experiments by Gellert and Ganong in which lesions just in front of the mammillary bodies of rats have been found to be the most effective in accelerating the onset of puberty. He states that "Lesions in the thalamus and the cerebral cortex also accelerate the onset of vaginal opening to a slight degree, suggesting a non-specific 'stress' effect. . . . However, it should be emphasized that this acceleration is slight when compared to the marked acceleration produced by posterior hypothalamic lesions."

It is possible that the central nervous system exerts a restraining influence on prepubertal gonadal activity in a wide variety of biological forms. Wells and Wells (86) have found, in the octopus, that blinding by optic nerve section or optic lobe removal, that lesions placed in the subpedunculate/dorsal basal region of the posterior part of the supraesophageal lobes of the brain, or that interference with the nerve supply to the optic glands, all result in enlargement of the optic glands and gonads. The ovary may enlarge from 1/500th to as much as 1/5th of the total body weight, and may visibly distort the body of the operated animal. Such females may lay viable eggs and brood in a normal manner. Wells and Wells suggest that a neural reflex arc, consisting of the optic nerves–optic lobes–supraesophageal lobes of the brain–and the nerve supply to the optic glands, normally exerts an inhibitory influence on the secretory activity of the optic glands. Lesions in the reflex arc thus allow a release effect on the optic glands, the secretory product of which in turn stimulates the gonads. They compare this suggested mechanism with that in insects in which, after the last moult, the corpus allatum becomes a source of gonadotropic hormone under the control of an inhibitory center in the supraesophageal ganglion and an opposing excitatory center in the subesophageal ganglion.

(ii) *The Hypothalamus and Follicular Ripening following Anestrus*

The physiological factors responsible for regulating FSH secretion at the beginning of the breeding season have received little attention. It is well known that various environmental factors, such as conditions of lighting, are of major importance in determining the onset of reproductive activity following a period of sexual quiescence. Rowan (78) was the first to demonstrate that artificial illumination during the hours of darkness in winter causes enlargement of the gonads and sperm production in the junco finch. These findings were extended to mammals by Baker and Ranson (field mouse, 2) and Bissonnette (ferret, 7). Other mammals whose reproductive rhythm has been found sensitive to changes in light exposure include the rat, hedgehog, cat, mink, goat and sheep.

The ferret shows a well-marked breeding season from March to July or August and in the estrous state exhibits a prodigious vulval swelling. On account of these facts it has been used in experimental work to analyze the light-estrus reflex. The following facts have been established:

(*a*) Extra illumination with light of wave lengths 6500–3650 Å (red-near ultra-violet) accelerates the onset of estrus in winter (68).
(*b*) The acceleration of estrus may be correlated with the intensity of the extra illumination (67).
(*c*) Long periods of light alternating with short periods of darkness are more effective than continuous illumination (42).
(*d*) Hypophysectomized ferrets do not respond to extra illumination (55).
(*e*) Section of the optic nerves or blinding by other means (8, 16, 79) frees the onset of estrus from photic influence.

It thus seems clear that the influence of light is mediated through the retina and optic nerves to stimulate the release of FSH from the adenohypophysis. The anatomical pathway intervening between the optic nerve fibers and anterior pituitary cells is not clear. Data adduced by Clark, McKeown and Zuckerman (16) and Jefferson (58) indicated that the pathway does not involve the optic tracts in the region of the lateral geniculate body. In order to see whether the central nervous pathway involved the pituitary stalk, Donovan and Harris (18) cut the stalk in a series of female ferrets. They found that animals in which regeneration of the blood vessels of the stalk (the hypophysial portal vessels) had been prevented by placement of a waxed

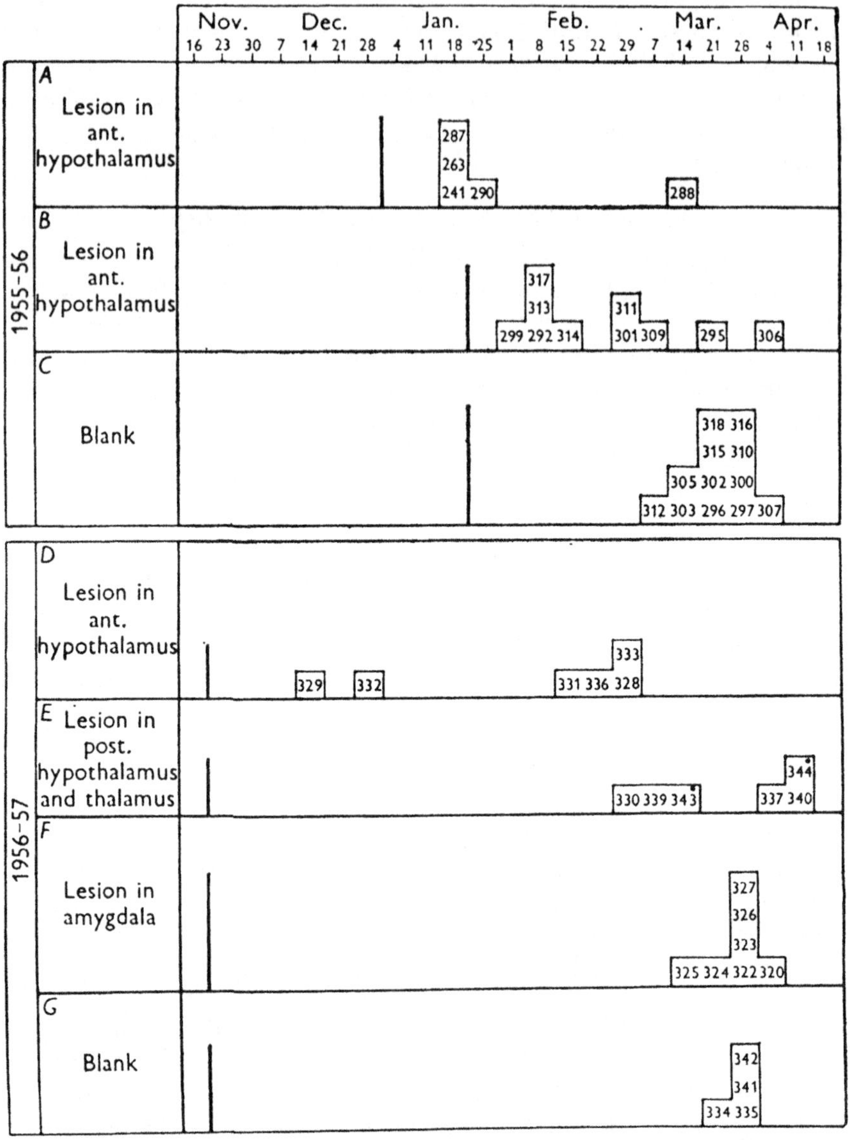

FIG. 1. Diagram to illustrate the effect of various operations on the brain on the onset of estrus in the ferret. In this figure the height of the block indicates the number of animals which began to show vulval swelling each week. The numerals within the block identify individual animals. The animals marked by an asterisk possessed lesions confined to the thalamus. The solid vertical bars indicate the time of operation. (From Donovan and van der Werff ten Bosch, 24.)

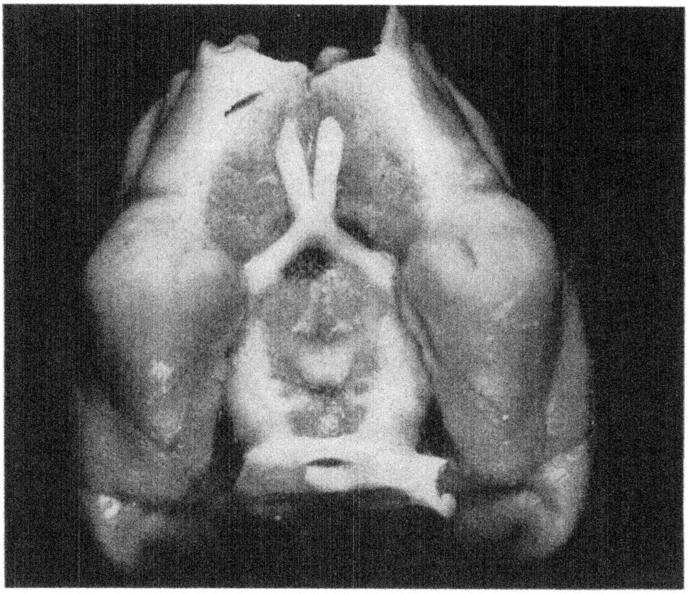

FIG. 2. View of ventral surface of brain of ferret. Note the dark damaged area posterior to the optic chiasma and extending forward over the left optic tract. (From Donovan and van der Werff ten Bosch, 24.)

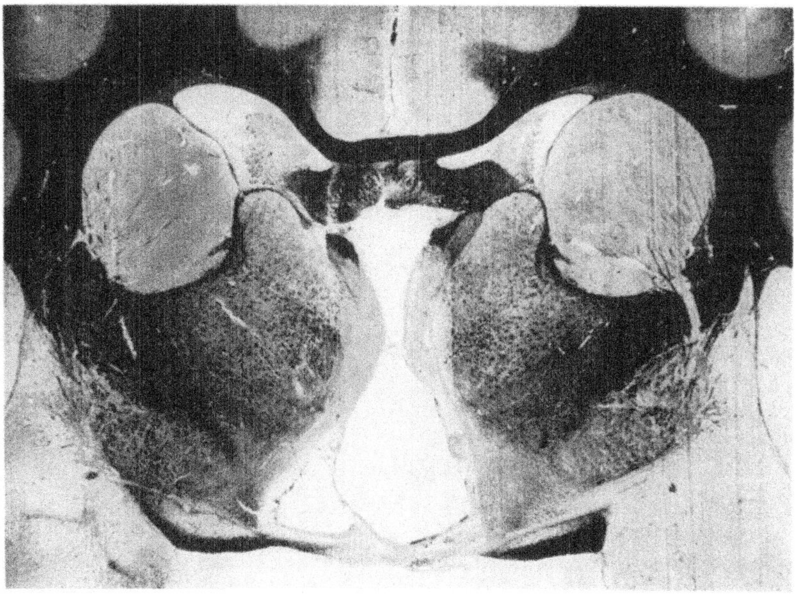

FIG. 3. Transverse section through the anterior hypothalamus of the brain shown in FIG. 2, showing the region in the midline destroyed by the lesion. (Loyez stain, 25 μ.) From Donovan and van der Werff ten Bosch, 24.)

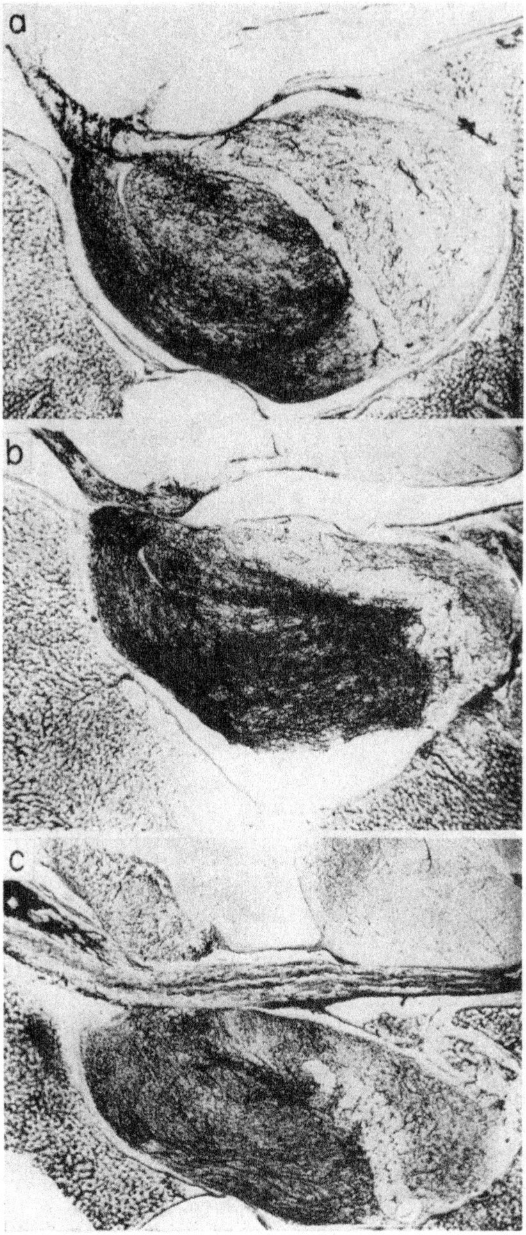

FIG. 5. Photomicrographs of midline sagittal sections through the hypothalamus, pituitary gland and base of skull of three rabbits. (*a*) Normal animal. Note the portal vessels passing from the median eminence to the pars distalis. (*b*) Stalk-sectioned animal. Regeneration has occurred across the site of stalk section. The neural lobe is atrophic. (*c*) Stalk-sectioned animal with waxed paper plate placed to intervene between the hypothalamus and pituitary gland. Neural lobe atrophic. In all cases the vascular system was perfused with India ink after death. (From Fortier, Harris and McDonald, 35.)

paper plate between the cut ends of the stalk, remained anestrus. Ferrets in which the stalk had been cut, but in which vascular regeneration had occurred across the site of the injury, became estrus on exposure to prolonged illumination. The results of their study indicate that the final connecting link from brain to pituitary gland involves the hypophysial portal vessels [Thomson and Zuckerman (80) have drawn different conclusions].

To investigate the possibility that reflex nerve tracts between the chiasmal region of the optic pathway and the upper end of the pituitary stalk (median eminence of the tuber cinereum) were involved in the increased secretion of FSH occurring in the spring, Donovan and van der Werff ten Bosch (22, 24) placed lesions in this part of the hypothalamus of the female ferret during winter. Electrolytic lesions were placed with the aid of a stereotaxic machine, with the animals anesthetized with Nembutal (pentobarbitone sodium). Since the plan of the experiment was to see whether such lesions delayed or prevented the onset of the breeding season in the spring it was surprising to find that about 75% of the animals with anterior hypothalamic lesions became estrous early; that is, at a time of the year when normal animals, blank-operated animals and those with lesions in the posterior hypothalamus and thalamus, or amygdala, were still in the winter anestrum (FIG. 1). Many of the animals that showed early estrus were placed with males, and produced litters which they reared successfully. Serial sections through the brains showed that the effective lesions were situated basally in the anterior part of the hypothalamus, between the optic chiasma and pituitary stalk, extending upward to the level of the paraventricular nuclei (FIGS. 2 and 3). The optic chiasma, suprachiasmatic nuclei and fornices were usually involved. In only one animal was the pituitary stalk partly damaged. Ineffective lesions involved the mammillary bodies, medial nuclei of the thalamus and habenular complex, and amygdaloid area. In view of the fact that the hypothalamic lesions might have exerted a stimulating effect by pressure on surrounding structures, Donovan and van der Werff ten Bosch (24) electrically stimulated various regions in the anterior hypothalamus. These experiments were carried out with implanted electrodes and stimulation continued for periods of weeks or months during winter. There was no indication of any release of gonadotropin by stimulation.

The specificity of the above results has been questioned by Herbert and Zuckerman (53, 54) who claim that estrus in ferrets is advanced by lesions placed in the thalamus or adjacent areas and by blank operations. The reason for this discrepancy is, at the moment, not clear.

General Conclusions

The most likely explanation of the finding that hypothalamic lesions result in FSH secretion, follicular ripening and estrus, in both the immature, or the mature anestrous, animal, is to be found in terms of a neural mechanism situated in the anterior hypothalamus which exerts a tonic inhibitory effect over the release of FSH. Such a mechanism may be supposed to be sensitive

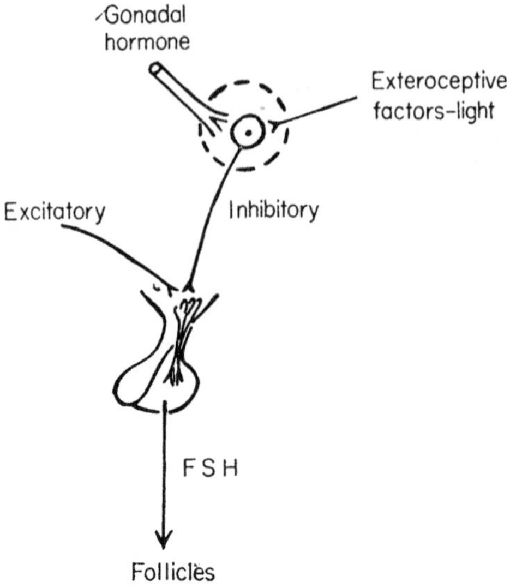

FIG. 4. Diagram to illustrate the influence of the hypothalamus on FSH secretion. Since pituitary stalk section may result in atrophy of the reproductive organs, whereas anterior hypothalamic lesions lead to premature release of FSH and block the feed-back action of ovarian steroids, it is necessary to postulate both excitatory and inhibitory neural effects.

to the effects of both environmental stimuli (light) and the blood concentration of gonadal hormones (FIG. 4). The present evidence may be summarized:

(1) Light. Increased illumination hastens the onset of puberty in infantile rats (63, 30, 59). The onset of puberty varies in many forms with the time of year of birth. An increasing or decreasing day length, or period of artificial illumination, is a potent factor in determining the onset of the breeding season in many forms.

(2) Ovarian Hormones. The immature animal appears especially sensitive to the feed-back action of ovarian hormones (57). The work of Flerkó has been important in establishing the paraventricular region of the hypothalamus as an important site of action for the feed-back mechanism in adult animals. Flerkó (31) found that lesions in the region of the hypothalamic paraventricular nuclei prevented the gonadal atrophy induced by estrogen administration, and Flerkó and Illei (32) found that similar lesions interfere with the inhibition of gonadotropin secretion produced by testosterone propionate. By autotransplanting small fragments of ovarian tissue into the hypothalamus Flerkó and

Szentágothai (33) demonstrated that the hormones released from the graft depressed gonadotropin secretion if in the region of the paraventricular nuclei.

(3) Anterior Hypothalamic Lesions. Such lesions result in a discharge of FSH that would not occur in the immature or mature anestrous female (see above). Since pituitary stalk section results in atrophy of the reproductive organs it is necessary to suppose that the inhibitory action of the anterior hypothalamus over FSH release is normally in balance with an excitatory effect exerted by some other hypothalamic area, both acting through the "final common path" of the hypophysial stalk.

FOLLICULAR RUPTURE—OVULATION

Non-spontaneous Ovulation

Ovulation occurs spontaneously in most mammals, but in some forms requires the sensory stimuli normally supplied by the presence of a male and coitus for its occurrence. These latter forms include many birds, the rabbit, ferret, cat, ground squirrel, short tailed shrew and mink, and possibly (see Eckstein and Zuckerman, 25) the hare, weasel, Asiatic vole (*Microtus guentheri*), certain marsupials (i.e. *Didelphus azarae*) and a tropical fruitbat (*Pteropus giganteus*). Marshall (66) and Heape (51) first reported that ovulation follows copulation in the ferret and rabbit, respectively. Early studies showed that ovulation in the rabbit was *not* due (1) to absorption of semen from the female reproductive tract, (2) to release of a hormone from the vaginal wall, (3) to a direct nervous reflex acting on the ovaries [ovulation occurred in transplanted ovaries—Asdell (1), Friedman (36)], and the idea became current that a neuro-humoral reflex arc was involved: that sensory nerve pathways caused activation of the anterior pituitary gland and the released gonadotropic hormone brought about follicular rupture. This view received support when it was found that hypophysectomy within one hour of coitus prevented ovulation from occurring some nine hours later, though hypophysectomy later than this was followed by ovulation (28).

Sensory Stimuli

The sensory stimuli involved appear to be varied. Since artificial stimulation of the vulva or vagina may result in ovulation, the sensory receptors in these regions would seem of importance. However, local anesthesia of the vulva and vagina (29), or denervation of these structures by removal of the sacral region of the spinal cord (even when supplemented by complete abdominal sympathectomy, hysterectomy and extirpation of the proximal half of the vagina (11)) does not prevent ovulation following coitus. Brooks (11) also studied the effect of bilateral destruction of the labyrinths and auditory apparatus, enucleation of the eyes and the olfactory lobes, and removal of the cerebral cortex. He found that none of these structures was essential for post-coital ovulation in the rabbit, and concludes ". . . that ovulation occurs as a result of intense sexual or emotional excitement rather than as a result of a reflex initiated by stimulation of any specific group of sensory endings". It seems likely, then, that under normal conditions of coitus afferent impulses from many different receptors converge in the diencephalon and in some way excite anterior pituitary activity.

Electrical Stimulation of Central Nervous System

The first positive evidence that reflex nerve tracts do activate LH release came from the experiments of Marshall and Verney (69). These workers showed that electrical stimuli applied through the lumbar spinal cord or through the head of rabbits resulted in ovulation and pseudopregnancy in a large proportion of animals. The stimulation used was strong and diffuse, resulting in generalized convulsions, so that no localization was possible. It seemed likely, however, that the site of action was some region in the central nervous system. The results of experiments in which localized stimuli were applied to different sites in the diencephalon were soon forthcoming. Harris (43), using a stereotaxic machine, stimulated the hypothalamus or pituitary gland of ether-anesthetized rabbits. It was found that stimulation of the tuber cinereum, posterior hypothalamus or pituitary gland directly might result in ovulation or the formation of cystic or hemorrhagic follicles. Similar results were reported by Haterius and Derbyshire (50) who found that electrical stimuli applied to the preoptic region evoked ovulation. Some ten years after these reports two groups of workers observed that electrical stimuli, too weak to excite LH discharge and ovulation if applied directly to the pituitary gland, might be fully effective if applied to the tuber cinereum. Markee, Sawyer and Hollinshead (65) anesthetized rabbits with ether and stimulated the pituitary at operation by a pharyngeal or temporal route, and the hypothalamus via the superior orbital fissure. It was found that stimulation of the pituitary did not result in ovulation unless there were signs of spread of the stimulus, whereas stimulation of the hypothalamus at a lower voltage resulted in ovulation in three out of four animals. Harris (44) used the remote control method of stimulation which permits the use of unanesthetized animals and the repetition of an experiment in any one animal. The method consisted essentially of implanting a coil of wire (about 2000 turns) beneath the scalp. The ends of the coil were connected to electrodes, one of which was inserted through a trephine hole in the skull so that the stimulating tip was placed in some part of the hypothalamus or pituitary gland. After recovery from the operation, electrical stimulation was applied by placing the animal in an electro-magnetic field. Forty-two experiments on seventeen rabbits showed that stimuli applied to various regions of the tuber cinereum might elicit a full ovulatory response, even when applied for as short a time as three minutes, whereas stimuli applied to the pituitary stalk (below the level of the median eminence) or to the pars distalis of the gland, for periods of up to 7½ hours, were not followed by any ovarian response. Both Markee, Sawyer and Hollinshead (65) and Harris (44) suggested that the failure of the anterior pituitary to respond to electrical stimulation might be due to the fact that the hypothalamus normally regulates the activity of this gland by a humoral mechanism rather than by a direct nerve supply. Such a suggestion had been tentatively put forward by various workers previously (56, 43, 12) in an attempt to explain the absence of a well-marked nerve supply to the pars distalis.

Anatomical Pathway from Hypothalamus to Pituitary

The anatomical pathway by which the hypothalamus influences the adenohypophysis has been discussed many times (for recent and detailed reviews, see 46, 5, 20). Data relating to the various suggested pathways may be summarized, for the present purpose, as follows:

(1) *Direct nerve supply*

(*a*) Cervical sympathetic supply carried to the gland via the carotid plexus. But, ovulation still follows sterile coitus in the partially or completely sympathectomized rabbit (49, 10).

(*b*) Parasympathetic supply carried to the gland via the greater superficial petrosal nerves. However, ovulation still follows coitus after bilateral avulsion of the facial nerve and geniculate ganglion, or after destruction of the petrosal nerves at the geniculate ganglion (41, 82).

(*c*) A nerve supply passing to the gland via the pituitary stalk. However, prolonged electrical stimulation of the pituitary stalk at a level below the median eminence does not evoke ovulation (44). Section of the pituitary stalk in the rabbit (35) may be followed by a normal ovulation reflex if vascular regeneration has occurred across the cut. All available evidence indicates that hypothalamic nerve fibers do not regenerate across the site of pituitary stalk section.

Histological studies, although unable to prove a negative finding, give very strong indication that the pars distalis of the anterior pituitary receives a very scanty nerve supply, if any at all (77, 38, 87).

(2) *Vascular path*

(*a*) General systemic circulation. There are no data that the hypothalamus regulates the anterior pituitary release of FSH or LH through the general circulation. Unlike the ovary, testis, adrenal cortex and thyroid, the pituitary gland does not maintain normal internal secretory activity if transplanted to a distant site in the body. General ovarian and follicular atrophy have been repeatedly observed in well-controlled studies of pituitary transplants.

(*b*) Hypophysial portal circulation. This system of vessels, first described by Popa and Fielding (75, 76) in man, has now been extensively studied.

A *primary plexus* of vessels, formed by a multitude of capillary loops or twisted skeins of capillaries, is situated in the median eminence of the tuber cinereum. This plexus drains into wide vascular trunks which pass down the pituitary stalk and break up to distribute blood into the sinusoids of the anterior pituitary. The system is supplied with blood by small arterial twigs, from the internal carotid arteries or Circle of Willis, which penetrate the pars tuberalis and median eminence. The portal vessels form a constant link between the median eminence and anterior pituitary in all vertebrates investigated from amphibians to man. Analogous vessels are found in cyclostomes and fishes. Microscopic examination in living amphibians, rats, dogs and mice has established the direction of blood flow as being from the tuber cinereum to the pituitary. From the anatomical point of view these vessels form the only direct and constant system linking the central nervous system and adenohypophysis.

Experimental data confirm the importance of the hypophysial portal vessels for normal anterior pituitary function:

(*a*) As mentioned above, Markee, Sawyer and Hollinshead (65) and Harris (44) found electrical stimulation of the tuber cinereum effective in evoking ovulation in the rabbit, though similar stimuli applied to the pituitary gland did not cause ovulation. These data are compatible with the view that the hypothalamus controls the adenohypophysis by humoral means.

(*b*) Pituitary stalk section is followed by very varied results so far as anterior pituitary activity is concerned. The extensive literature on this topic has been recently reviewed (20). It was found first in rats (45) and later in other forms—the duck (4), ferret (18), rabbit (35) and *Triturus cristatus* (71)—that the return of normal, or near normal, levels of anterior pituitary function after operation occurs in those animals in which regeneration of the hypophysial portal vessels takes place across the site of stalk section. If regeneration is prevented by the placement of a barrier between the hypothalamus and pituitary, FSH and LH secretion ceases. The results of Fortier, Harris and McDonald (35) may be taken as an example. These workers cut the pituitary stalk in thirty-two rabbits. In twenty-two the stalk was severed and a paper plate left *in situ* between the cut ends. These animals all showed atrophic reproductive organs when killed. In ten rabbits the stalk was cut, a paper plate inserted between the cut ends but immediately removed (FIG. 5). Six of these animals showed marked portal vessel regeneration and had ovarian weights not significantly different from the normal (two of them accepted the male and ovulated in the normal way).

(*c*) Transplantation of the anterior pituitary gland to a site in the body remote from the sella turcica results in a marked loss of anterior pituitary function, though if the tissue is placed in the subarachnoid space beneath the median eminence it becomes vascularized by the hypophysial portal vessels and apparently normal anterior pituitary function returns (48, 73, 81).

It is clear then that a normal level of function of the anterior pituitary depends on its vascularization by the hypophysial portal vessels and that the central nervous system through the hypothalamus exerts an influence over the gland through the mediation of this vascular system. It is probable that nerve fibers from the hypothalamus liberate some humoral substance(s) into the capillaries of the primary plexus in the median eminence and that this substance is carried by the portal vessels to excite or inhibit the cells of the adenohypophysis.

Many important investigations have now been undertaken in an attempt to identify such humoral agents. Most of this work has however been concerned with the regulation of secretion of the adrenocorticotropic hormone (ACTH); a fact which has added to the difficulties of the problem, since the discharge of ACTH is evoked so easily by so many and varied stimuli. The identification of any particular substance as a physiological humoral agent involved in anterior pituitary control, and indeed the neurohumoral view as a whole, will only be established if it is possible to ". . . firstly identify a particular substance which exerts a direct action on anterior pituitary cells; secondly, to show this substance is present in the blood in the hypophysial portal vessels in greater amount than in systemic blood; thirdly, to show that the concentration of this substance in the blood of the hypophysial portal vessels varies according to electrical or reflex activation of hypothalamic nerve tracts; and fourthly, to demonstrate that the activity of the adenohypophysis is correlated with this varying concentration". (Harris, 47.) Data such as this are not yet available for any of the substances postulated for the role of a transmitter agent. Various reports have suggested that the substance involved in gonadotropin release may be (*a*) adrenergic in nature (64, see, however, 19), (*b*) intermedin (60), (*c*) oxytocic hormone (6, 72), (*d*) posterior pituitary polypeptides (70).

Work at the Institute of Psychiatry, London, has recently been undertaken to see the effect of infusing various brain extracts into the adenohypophysis of rabbits on the release of thyrotropic hormone (TSH) and LH (H. J. Campbell, G. Feuer, J. Garcia and G. W. Harris, unpublished). Careful consideration was first paid to two points—the anatomical limits of the region which might be expected to contain active material and the methods to be used for applying this material with minimal concurrent trauma to anterior pituitary tissue.

The median eminence of the tuber cinereum is the region of the infundibulum which contains the primary plexus of the portal vessels, surrounded by a wealth of nerve fibers (Fig. 6). Extracts of the median eminence might then be expected to contain a greater concentration of any humoral transmitter agent than surrounding structures. In the brain of the freshly-killed animal the median eminence may be identified from adjacent hypothalamic tissue as the pink and bulbous upper end of the pituitary stalk. If the brain is forcibly removed from the skull the median eminence often tears away from the hypothalamus and remains attached by the stalk to the sella turcica and its contents. After hypophysectomy or pituitary stalk section the portal vessels thrombose and the median eminence is clearly defined as a hard

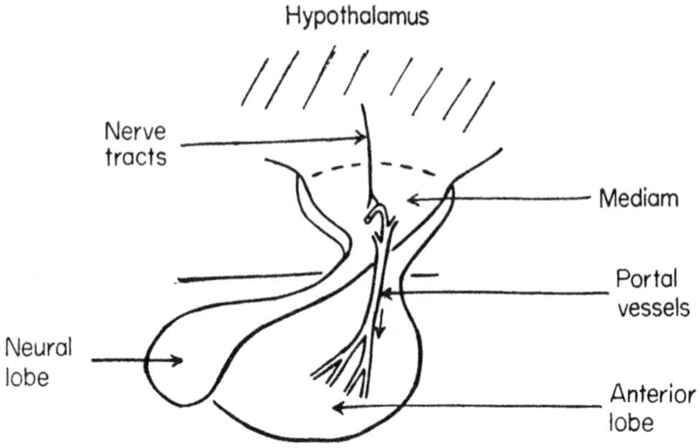

FIG. 6. To show the region—the median eminence—probably involved in the transfer of humoral agents from hypothalamic nerve tracts to the hypophysial portal vessels.

plum-colored nodule whose vessels have undergone retrograde thrombosis (FIG. 7). Since the median eminence is structurally part of the neurohypophysis (and forms about 12% of total neurohypophysial tissue—see Campbell and Harris, 14), many workers have investigated the effect of posterior pituitary extracts on anterior pituitary activity. *A priori* there would appear to be little to support this procedure, since—firstly, the median eminence : anterior pituitary complex is evolutionarily the basic unit, with the neural lobe arising as a secondary outgrowth from the median eminence in terrestrial forms (38); secondly, the median eminence in all probability contains nerve tracts with their fiber terminations and chemical constituents that are not present in the neural lobe; and thirdly, although the median eminence is constantly connected to the adenohypophysis by a rich vascular unit, the neural lobe is connected by scanty capillaries at most. Some authors have laid emphasis on the existence of these capillaries, but there is little data that they possess much functional significance and, indeed, in some mammals (whale, porpoise, sea-cow, armadillo, Indian elephant) and birds the two lobes of the pituitary are separated by an intervening fibrous septum. Thus although there is much data that the median eminence of the neurohypophysis is directly related to anterior pituitary function there are few reasons for believing the neural lobe of the neurohypophysis is so related.

Some reports in the literature have dealt with the effects of extracts of the hypothalamus (presumably including the median eminence) on anterior

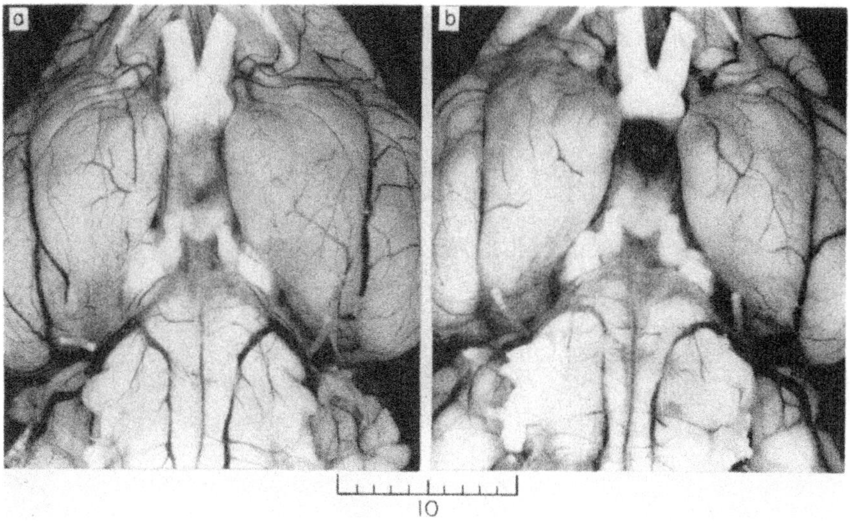

FIG. 7. To illustrate the anatomical extent of the median eminence as seen on the base of the rabbit brain. (*a*) Base of brain of normal rabbit; (*b*) base of brain of rabbit hypophysectomized 6 hr before death. Hypophysectomy severs the hypophysial portal vessels. The primary plexus of these vessels in the median eminence therefore undergoes retrograde thrombosis and the median eminence may then be clearly seen as a hardened, plum-colored nodule. Anterior to the median eminence is the optic chiasma, and posterior is the mammillary body, the posterior perforated substance and the emergence of the oculomotor nerves from the midbrain. Scale in mm.

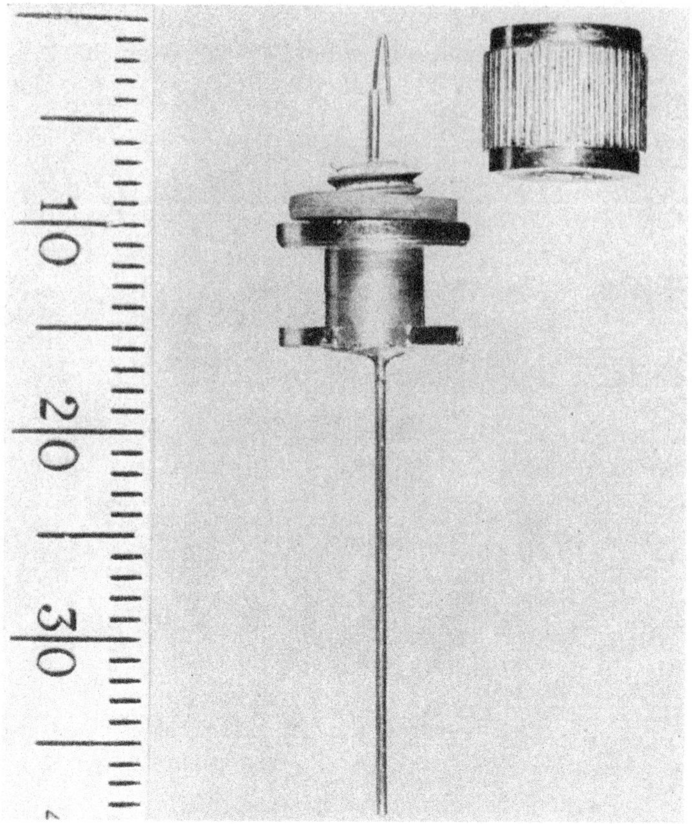

FIG. 8. Photograph of the cannula with inserted stilette (seen as bent wire protruding from upper end) and protective screw cap. Scale in mm.

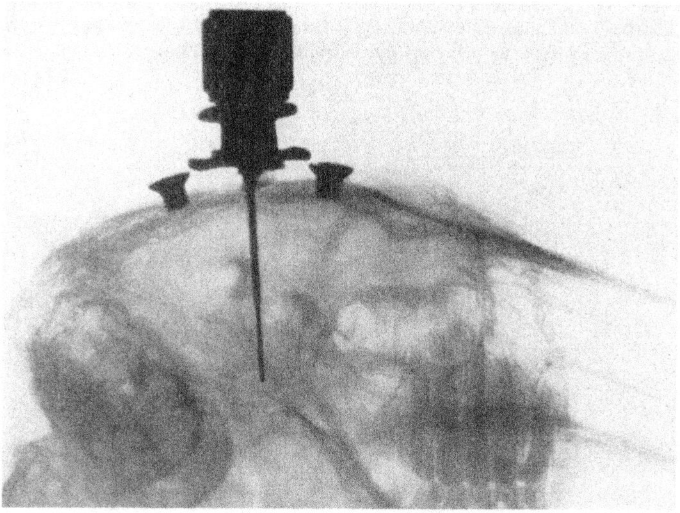

FIG. 9. X-ray photograph of cannula *in situ* in head of rabbit. The stainless steel, anchoring screws may be seen in the vault of the skull, though the mound of dental cement fixing the cannula to these screws is invisible by X-ray photography.

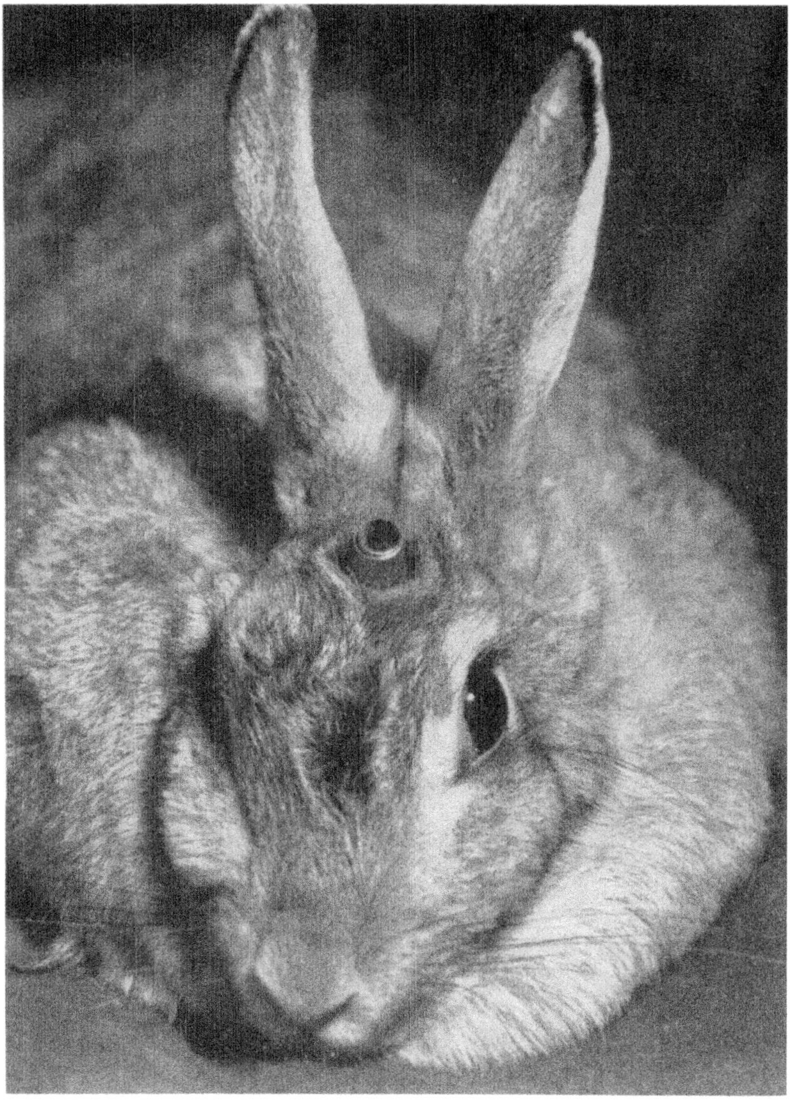

Fig. 10. Photograph of rabbit after recovery from the operation of cannula implantation. For infusion of extracts into the pituitary gland, the stainless steel screw cap and the stilette in the cannula are removed, and the upper end of the cannula connected by fine polythene tubing to a syringe operated by a Palmer slow injection apparatus, by which means infusion is made at a constant rate.

pituitary activity. If, for the reasons given above, the median eminence contains the greatest concentration of any agent, then this would be greatly diluted by taking a relatively large mass of surrounding hypothalamic tissue.

In the present work eight extracts of median eminence tissue have been studied. The first six of these were obtained from rabbits and the last two from cattle (steers). For each extract made from rabbit tissue four normal adult female rabbits, that had been isolated for several weeks, were anesthetized with ether, the skin of the head reflected and the head sawn through in the transverse plane so that the cut severed the midbrain. The forebrain in the front end of the skull was quickly removed from the bone, care being taken to cut the pituitary stalk with fine scissors so that no fragment of pars distalis tissue was removed with the stalk. The median eminence, the hypothalamus and samples of cerebral cortex were dissected and immediately frozen. The cattle material was obtained from a slaughter house, but in this case the animals (castrated) had been killed (by bleeding) $\frac{1}{2}$–2 hr previously. The same tissues were taken from each brain; material from about twelve brains being pooled for each cattle extract. Again the tissues were immediately frozen after dissection. The extracts were prepared by homogenizing the pooled samples in 0.5% acetic acid and centrifuging. The solutions were then neutralized and made isotonic by addition of appropriate amounts of solid sodium bicarbonate and sodium chloride, centrifuged for 15 min at 10,000 r.p.m. at 0°C, and the supernatant distributed into sealed ampoules and kept in the frozen state. The volume of the final extracts of the different brain samples was equivalent on the basis of wet tissue weight.

The technique finally chosen for infusing the extracts directly into the anterior pituitary in the conscious animal was a modification of that used by von Euler and Holmgren (26). In a preliminary operation cannulae consisting of fine platinum tubing (SWG 25) are inserted through a small trephine hole in the vault of the skull so that the tip of the cannula is located in the pars distalis of the pituitary. This is easily and simply performed with the use of a stereotaxic machine and X-ray control. A flange attached to the upper end of the tubing is then fixed to stainless steel screws inserted in the skull with dental cement, a fine wire stilette inserted in the cannula, the skin sutured around the cannula mounting and a protective cap screwed to the mounting (see FIGS. 8, 9, 10).

In early experiments attention was paid to the spread of infused dye, or radioactive I^{131}, when different rates of administration were used. An infusion rate of 0.06–0.07 ml/hr, for a 2-hr period, was finally chosen.

Since the majority of the animals in this work were being used to see the effect of the various infusions on both TSH and LH release, the experimental procedure was usually as follows. After recovery from the operation of implanting the cannula, the animals received 100 μc I^{131} subcutaneously.

Four days later half-hourly blood samples (0.5 ml each) were taken from the marginal vein of the ear for 6–8 hr, during which time the infusion of the various extracts or solutions was made either into the pituitary (at the above rate) or intravenously (at a rate of 2.1 ml/hr) for 2 hr. Two days later the animals were killed and the ovaries inspected under a binocular microscope. If any sign of follicular activation was observed, serial sections were made of the ovaries and histological studies carried out.

Since ovulation is said to occur "spontaneously" in the occasional female rabbit, it is necessary to know the frequency with which this happens in any particular colony. In thirty-one normal, isolated Chinchilla rabbits from the present stock, killed for various reasons, corpora lutea of various ages were found in the ovaries of three. In a previous study, in which various adrenalin and noradrenalin solutions were infused under ether anesthesia into the anterior pituitary gland, Donovan and Harris (19) found three out of thirty-eight isolated Chinchilla rabbits had ovulated. For control purposes then, one out of about eleven rabbits could be expected to show corpora lutea in the ovaries. But since freshly ruptured follicles are distinguishable from mature corpora lutea the experimental error would be less than indicated by these figures.

Infusion of median eminence extract in various doses into the pituitary gland resulted in ovulation in nine out of sixteen rabbits. In three cases, fresh cystic and hemorrhagic follicles were found in the ovaries, though no ruptured follicles were present.

Following infusion of extracts of the cerebral cortex, hypothalamus or solvent only, into the pituitary gland only one animal out of thirteen rabbits was found to have ovulated.

Infusion of median eminence extract intravenously, in doses greater than those given (ranging up to ×20) in the pituitary resulted, in ovulation in three out of seventeen rabbits.

The following conclusions may be tentatively put forward:

(1) Infusion of extracts of median eminence tissue directly into the anterior pituitary gland results in an increased blood level of LH, and so ovulation.

(2) It is unlikely that this result can be explained in terms of damage to anterior pituitary tissue, since control infusions of hypothalamic extract, cerebral cortical extract or solvent only did not produce a similar result.

(3) It is unlikely that the effect is due to gonadotropic material in the median eminence extract, since intravenous infusion did not evoke comparable results.

(4) It is probable that there is some substance in extracts of the median eminence which is active in causing discharge of LH from anterior pituitary cells.

Infusion of Median Eminence Extracts into Rats

Concurrently with the above study, Dr. M. Nikitovitch-Winer, working in this department, has been investigating the effect of intrapituitary infusions of median eminence, and other extracts in rats in which spontaneous ovulation has been blocked with nembutal. The procedure used is as follows.

Adult female rats (Wistar strain), whose vaginal cycles had been found to be regular for at least two weeks, were anesthetized early in the day of proestrus and a fine platinum or platinum–iridium cannula (SWG 27) was inserted in the right half of the pars distalis with a stereotaxic machine. In general principle the technique used was similar to that described above for the rabbit. Later on the same day, the spontaneous release of LH, and subsequent ovulation, was blocked by intraperitoneal injections of 30 mg/kg body weight "nembutal" (pentobarbitone sodium) at 11.00 a.m. and 2.00 p.m. (see Everett and Sawyer, 27). In the afternoon, usually between one and three o'clock, the brain extracts (from cattle) were infused either into the pituitary gland directly (at a rate of 0.005–0.006 ml/hr or 0.008–0.009 ml/hr for one to two hours) or intravenously (0.016–0.019 ml/hr) for the same period. The following morning, the animals were anesthetized, the pituitary glands infused with a dye solution at the same rate and for the same period as perfused on the previous day, and the ovaries and Fallopian tubes removed.

TABLE 1. INDUCTION OF OVULATION BY DIRECT INTRA-PITUITARY INFUSION OF MEDIAN EMINENCE EXTRACTS INTO "NEMBUTAL-BLOCKED" PROESTROUS FEMALE RATS

	No. of animals	Ovulation		Dose mg wet wt.
		Yes	No	
Nembutal intra-pituitary infusion median eminence extract	10	8	2*	0.88–2.3
Nembutal intra-pituitary infusion cortical extract	6	0	6	1.9–2.4
Nembutal intravenous infusion median eminence extract	8	1†	7	2.2–5.4
Nembutal + cannula	6	0	6	—
Nembutal	7	0	7	—

* 0.44 mg infusion.
† Fast infusion over a period of 1 min.

After killing the animal, the cranium was opened and the position of the tip of the cannula and the spread of the dye was observed. The ovaries were examined for fresh rupture points, and the ampullae of the oviducts searched for ova. The results obtained are shown in Table 1. It may be seen that median eminence extracts infused in the pituitary were effective in evoking ovulation (except in the case of the two animals that received the smallest dose), whereas control infusions of the cerebral cortex in the pituitary failed to excite the same response. Intravenous infusion of median eminence extract was likewise ineffective in causing ovulation except in one animal that was exceptional in that it was injected with the maximal dose (5.4 mg of extract) over a period of *one minute*. Thirteen animals in which no infusion was given failed to ovulate after nembutal treatment.

The preliminary results presented above dealing with the infusion of median eminence extracts into the pituitary glands of rabbits and rats are suggestive, but further work is necessary before any definite conclusions can be drawn.

Acknowledgments—The original work reported in this paper (by H. J. Campbell, G. Feuer, J. Garcia and G. W. Harris) was performed with the assistance of a grant from the United States Air Force (Contract No. AF61 (514)–953) and (by M. Nikitovitch-Winer) a postdoctoral Fellowship Award from United States National Institutes of Health (AF-8155-CI).

REFERENCES

1. ASDELL, S. A., Studies in the physiology of lactation, Dissertation, Cambridge University, England, 1926.
2. BAKER, J. R. and R. M. RANSON, *Proc. Roy. Soc. B* **110**, 313, 1932.
3. BAUER, H. G., *J. clin. Endocrinol.* **14**, 13, 1954.
4. BENOIT, J. and I. ASSENMACHER, *Arch. Anat. micr.* **42**, 334, 1953.
5. BENOIT, J. and I. ASSENMACHER, *J. Physiol. (Paris)* **47**, 427, 1955.
6. BENSON, G. K. and S. J. FOLLEY, *J. Endocrinol.* **16**, 189, 1957.
7. BISSONNETTE, T. H., *Proc. Roy. Soc. B* **110**, 322, 1932.
8. BISSONNETTE, T. H., *Res. Publ. Ass. nerv. ment. Dis.* **17**, 361, 1938.
9. BOGDANOVE, E. M. and H. C. SCHOEN, *Proc. Soc. exp. Biol., N.Y.* **100**, 664, 1959.
10. BROOKS, C. McC., *Amer. J. Physiol.* **113**, 18 P, 1935.
11. BROOKS, C. McC., *Amer. J. Physiol.* **120**, 544, 1937.
12. BROOKS, C. McC., *Amer. J. Physiol.* **121**, 157, 1938.
13. BYRNES, W. W. and R. K. MEYER, *Endocrinology* **48**, 133, 1951.
14. CAMPBELL, H. J. and G. W. HARRIS, *J. Physiol.* **136**, 333, 1957.
15. CLARK, H. M., *Anat. Rec.* **61**, 175, 1935.
16. CLARK, W. E. LE GROS, T. MCKEOWN and S. ZUCKERMAN, *Proc. Roy. Soc. B* **126**, 449, 1939.
17. DOHRN M. and W. HOHLWEG, *Proc. II Int. Congr., Sex Res.*, pp. 436–442, London, 1931.
18. DONOVAN, B. T. and G. W. HARRIS, *J. Physiol.* **131**, 102, 1956.
19. DONOVAN, B. T. and G. W. HARRIS, *J. Physiol.* **132**, 577, 1956.
20. DONOVAN, B. T. and G. W. HARRIS, in *Marshall's Physiology of Reproduction*, Vol. **I**, Part 2 (Edited by A. S. Parkes) (in press). Longmans, Green & Co., London, 1960.
21. DONOVAN, B. T. and J. J. VAN DER WERFF TEN BOSCH, *Nature, Lond.* **178**, 745, 1956.
22. DONOVAN, B. T. and J. J. VAN DER WERFF TEN BOSCH, *J. Physiol.* **132**, 57P, 1956.
23. DONOVAN, B. T. and J. J. VAN DER WERFF TEN BOSCH, *J. Physiol.* **147**, 78, 1959.
24. DONOVAN, B. T. and J. J. VAN DER WERFF TEN BOSCH, *J. Physiol.* **147**, 93, 1959.
25. ECKSTEIN, P. and S. ZUCKERMAN, in *Marshall's Physiology of Reproduction*, 3rd Ed., Vol. **I**, Part 1 (Edited by A. S. Parkes), p. 257, Longmans, Green & Co., London, 1956.

26. von Euler, C. and B. Holmgren, *J. Physiol.* **131**, 125, 1956.
27. Everett, J. W. and C. H. Sawyer, *Endocrinology* **47**, 198, 1950.
28. Fee, A. R. and A. S. Parkes, *J. Physiol.* **67**, 383, 1929.
29. Fee, A. R. and A. S. Parkes, *J. Physiol.* **70**, 385, 1930.
30. Fiske, V. M., *Endocrinology* **29**, 187, 1941.
31. Flerkó, B., *Acta Morphol. Hung.* **4**, 475, 1954.
32. Flerkó, B. and G. Illei, *Endokrinologie* **35**, 123, 1957.
33. Flerkó, B. and J. Szentágothai, *Acta endocr., Copenhagen* **26**, 121, 1957.
34. Foà, C., *Arch. ital. biol.* **34**, 43, 1900. (Quoted from Parkes, A. S., *The Internal Secretions of the Ovary*, Longmans, Green & Co., London, 1929.)
35. Fortier, C., G. W. Harris and I. R. McDonald, *J. Physiol.* **136**, 344, 1957.
36. Friedman, M. H., *Amer. J. Physiol.* **89**, 438, 1929.
37. Ganong, W. F., in *Reproduction in Domestic Animals*, p. 185, Academic Press, New York and London, 1959.
38. Green, J. D., *Amer. J. Anat.* **88**, 225, 1951.
39. Greep, R. O., H. B. van Dyke and B. F. Chow, *Endocrinology* **30**, 635, 1942.
40. Greep, R. O. and I. C. Jones, *Recent Progr. Hormone Res.* **5**, 197, 1950.
41. Hair, G. W. and J. F. Mezen, *Endocrinology* **25**, 965, 1939.
42. Hammond, J. Jr., *Nature, Lond.* **167**, 150, 1951.
43. Harris, G. W., *Proc. Roy. Soc. B* **122**, 374, 1937.
44. Harris, G. W., *J. Physiol.* **107**, 418, 1948.
45. Harris, G. W., *J. Physiol.* **111**, 347, 1950.
46. Harris, G. W., *Neural Control of the Pituitary Gland*, Edward Arnold, London, 1955.
47. Harris, G. W., *Bull. Johns Hopk. Hosp.* **97**, 358, 1955.
48. Harris, G. W. and D. Jacobsohn, *Proc. Roy. Soc. B* **139**, 263, 1952.
49. Haterius, H. O., *Proc. Soc. exp. Biol., N.Y.* **31**, 1112, 1934.
50. Haterius, H. O. and A. J. Derbyshire, Jr., *Amer. J. Physiol.* **119**, 329, 1937.
51. Heape, W., *Proc. Roy. Soc. B* **76**, 260, 1905.
52. Hellbaum, A. A. and R. O. Greep, *Amer. J. Anat.* **67**, 287, 1940.
53. Herbert, J. and S. Zuckerman, *Nature, Lond.* **180**, 547, 1957.
54. Herbert, J. and S. Zuckerman, *J. Endocrinol.* **17**, 433, 1958.
55. Hill, M. and A. S. Parkes, *Proc. Roy. Soc. B* **113**, 537, 1933.
56. Hinsey, J. C. and J. E. Markee, *Proc. Soc. exp. Biol., N.Y.* **31**, 270, 1933.
57. Hohlweg, W. and M. Dohrn, *Wein. Arch. inn. Med.* **21**, 337, 1931.
58. Jefferson, J. M., *J. Anat., Lond.* **75**, 106, 1940.
59. Jöchle, W., *Endokrinologie* **33**, 129, 1956.
60. Jöchle, W., *Endokrinologie* **33**, 190, 1956.
61. Kallas, H., *C.R. Soc. Biol., Paris* **100**, 979, 1929.
62. Kallas, H., *Klin. Wschr.* **9**, 1345, 1930.
63. Luce-Clausen, E. M. and E. F. Brown, *J. Nutr.* **18**, 551, 1939.
64. Markee, J. E., J. W. Everett and C. H. Sawyer, *Recent Progr. Hormone Res.* **7**, 139, 1952.
65. Markee, J. E., C. H. Sawyer and W. H. Hollinshead, *Endocrinology* **38**, 345, 1946.
66. Marshall, F. H. A., *Quart. J. micr. Sci.* **48**, 323, 1904.
67. Marshall, F. H. A., *J. exp. Biol.* **17**, 139, 1940.
68. Marshall, F. H. A. and F. B. Bowden, *J. exp. Biol.* **11**, 409, 1934.
69. Marshall, F. H. A. and E. B. Verney, *J. Physiol.* **86**, 327, 1936.
70. Martini, L., L. Mira, A. Pecile and S. Saito, *J. Endocrinol.* **18**, 245, 1959.
71. Mazzi, V., *Z. Zellforsch.* **48**, 332, 1958.
72. McCann, S. M., R. Mack and C. Gale, *Endocrinology* **64**, 870, 1959.
73. Nikitovitch-Winer, M. and J. W. Everett, *Endocrinology* **63**, 916, 1958.
74. Pfeiffer, C. A., *Amer. J. Anat.* **58**, 195, 1936.
75. Popa, G. T. and U. Fielding, *J. Anat., Lond.* **65**, 88, 1930.
76. Popa, G. T. and U. Fielding, *J. Anat., Lond.* **67**, 227, 1933.
77. Rasmussen, A. T., *Endocrinology* **23**, 263, 1938.
78. Rowan, W., *Proc. Boston Soc. Nat. Hist.* **38**, 147, 1926.
79. Thomson, A. P. D., *Proc. Roy. Soc. B* **142**, 126, 1954.

80. THOMSON, A. P. D. and S. ZUCKERMAN, *Proc. Roy. Soc. B* **142**, 437, 1954.
81. VIVIEN, J. H. and J. SCHOTT, *C.R. Acad. Sci., Paris* **244**, 1263, 1957.
82. VOGT, M., *J. Physiol.* **100**, 410, 1942.
83. WALKER, D. G., C. W. ASLING, M. E. SIMPSON, C. H. LI and H. M. EVANS, *Anat. Rec.* **114**, 19, 1952.
84. WALKER, D. G., M. E. SIMPSON, C. W. ASLING and H. M. EVANS, *Anat. Rec.* **106**, 539, 1950.
85. WEINBERGER, L. M. and F. C. GRANT, *Arch. intern. Med.* **67**, 762, 1941.
86. WELLS, M. J. and J. WELLS, *J. exp. Biol.* **36**, 1, 1959.
87. WINGSTRAND, K. G., *The Structure and Development of the Avian Pituitary*, p. 316, C. W. K. Gleerup, Lund, Sweden.

DISCUSSION

Chairman: DR. WARREN O. NELSON

DR. VAUGHN CRITCHLOW: We have followed the work of Donovan and van der Werff ten Bosch, reviewed this morning by Professor Harris, with a great deal of interest. In collaboration with Miss Elwers, we have undertaken a series of experiments in the rat to examine the anatomic specificity of lesions that hasten puberty, and to determine

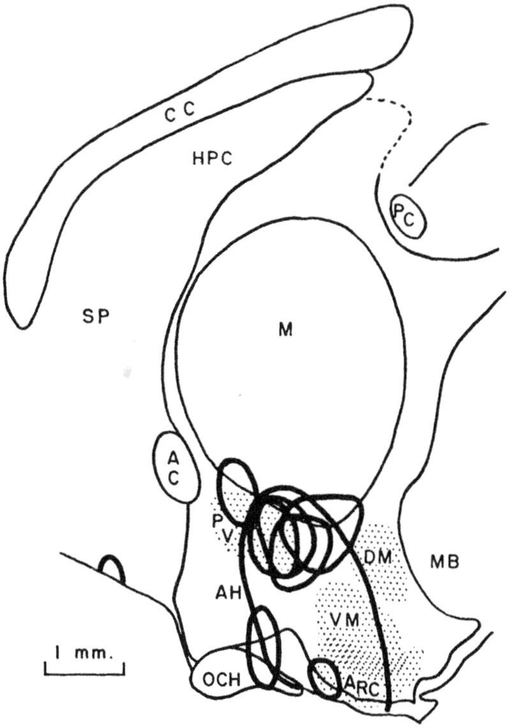

FIG. 1. Projections of effective hypothalamic lesions on a midsagittal diagram of the diencephalon. Abbreviations used: AH, anterior hypothalamic area; ARC, arcuate nucleus; CC, corpus callosum; DM, dorso-medial nucleus; M, massa intermedia; OCH, optic chiasm; MB, mammillary body; PV, paraventricular nucleus; VM, ventromedial nucleus.

whether the amygdaloid complex might be implicated in the neural mechanisms which are postulated to inhibit gonadotropin secretion. A more complete account of this work was published recently (1).

The methods used were similar to those outlined by Bogdanove and Schoen (2) who also observed the puberty-inducing effects of anterior hypothalamic lesions. All animals were lesioned at 18 to 20 days of age, examined daily for vaginal opening, weighed 2 to 3 times a week and killed at 33 days of age. Littermates were used as controls.

In brief, the results obtained with a series of 23 hypothalamic lesions and 7 blank operated rats were similar to those discussed this morning by Dr. Harris: lesions in the anterior hypothalamus were associated with precocious stimulation of the reproductive system.

TABLE 1. EFFECTS OF AMYGDALOID LESIONS ON BODY AND ORGAN WEIGHTS AND VAGINAL OPENING

	Body weights at autopsy	Organ weights—mg/100 gm body weight			Number of open vaginas
		Uterus	Ovaries	Adrenals	
Controls (24 rats)	105.1 ± 1.65* 93–118	86.8 ± 3.08 56–120	21.9 ± 0.81 16–29	23.1 ± 0.86 17–35	0
Ineffective lesions (27 rats)	100.0 ± 1.92 74–116	79.8 ± 3.12 55–117	22.7 ± 0.96 11–31	22.8 ± 1.40 16–31	0
Effective lesions (16 rats)	101.7 ± 2.95 77–124	169.9 ± 8.88 128–241	27.4 ± 2.09† 15–41	24.4 ± 0.63 18–29	6

* Mean $\pm$ standard error.
† Probably significantly different from controls ($P < 0.05$).

Figure 1 summarizes the antero-posterior locations of the nine lesions that were judged effective on the basis of uterine weights that were significantly heavier ($P < 0.01$) than those of 18 control rats. As illustrated, one lesion was large and involved most of the structures in the anterior hypothalamus. The remaining lesions were more discrete and, with the exception of one in the basal septum, involved parts of the medial anterior hypothalamus. It should be noted that several of these lesions were effective without sharing a common area of destruction.

Of the 14 ineffective lesions in this series, bilaterally symmetrical destruction was found in the thalamus, lateral hypothalamus, lateral preoptic region and olfactory bulb. Four ineffective lesions were grossly asymmetrical.

These data are in agreement with previously published work regarding the following points: (1) lesions placed in the rostral hypothalamus induced precocious sexual development, (2) no single hypothalamic structure could be implicated, (3) some degree of anatomic specificity was suggested by the number and location of ineffective lesions, and (4) the stress of cerebral trauma did not appear to be an adequate stimulus for early ovarian stimulation.

In contrast to the observations of Bogdanove and Schoen, the presence of corpora lutea in ovaries of rats bearing effective hypothalamic lesions was not indicative of damage to the arcuate nucleus: three of the four rats of this series that had corpora lutea in their ovaries had lesions that spared the arcuate nucleus. Also, a small effective lesion in this nucleus did not result in ovulation and luteinization. It appeared that effective lesions, regardless of location, triggered prematurely an orderly sequence of events which culminated in ovulation and corpora lutea formation, and autopsy at day 33 might interrupt this sequence at any one of several stages.

Having established some confidence in the specificity of this lesion response, we next directed our attention to the amygdaloid complex. Table 1 summarizes some of the results obtained. Twenty-four control rats had a mean uterine weight of 86.8 mg/100 gm body weight. Sixteen rats with lesions had uteri which were significantly

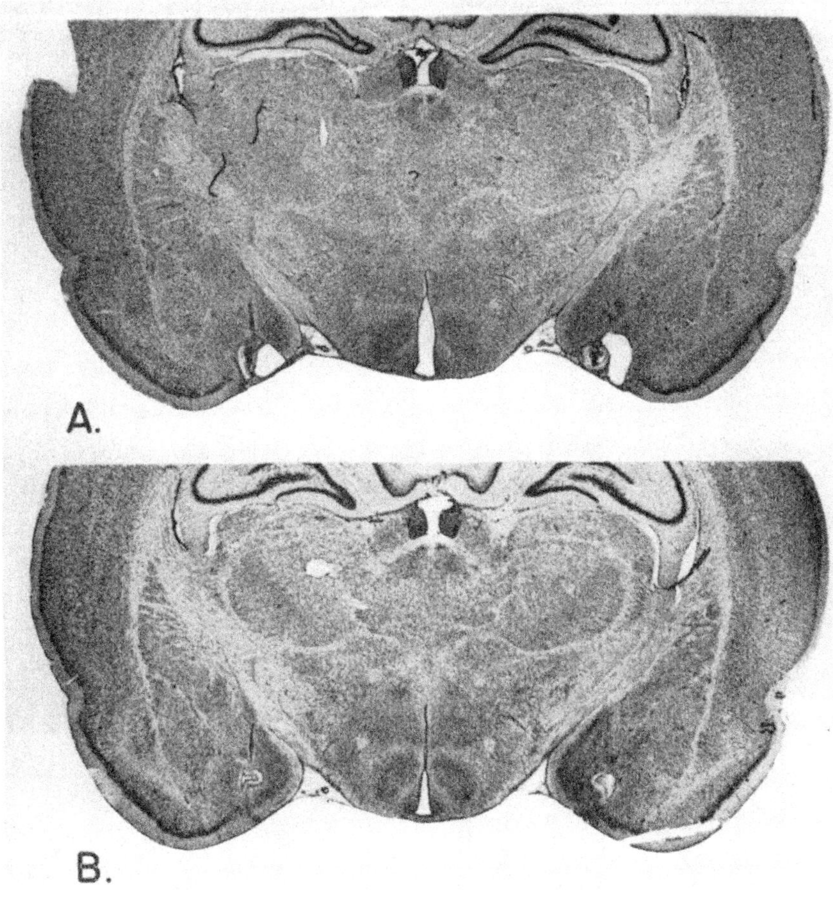

FIG. 3. Amygdaloid lesions effective in increasing ovarian and uterine weights.

heavier ($P < 0.01$) than the controls and were considered effectively lesioned. Twenty-seven lesioned rats had uteri which were comparable to those of the controls and were designated as ineffectively lesioned. The mean ovarian weight of the effectively lesioned animals was significantly greater ($P < 0.05$) than the mean of the controls; three pairs of these ovaries had corpora lutea. No differences were observed in body or adrenal weights.

Figure 2 shows on a composite diagram the bilateral destruction produced by all amygdaloid lesions associated with increased uterine weight. The area included portions of the cortical, medial and basal medial nuclei and had a longitudinal extent of about 1 mm. In contrast to the results obtained in the hypothalamus, these lesions

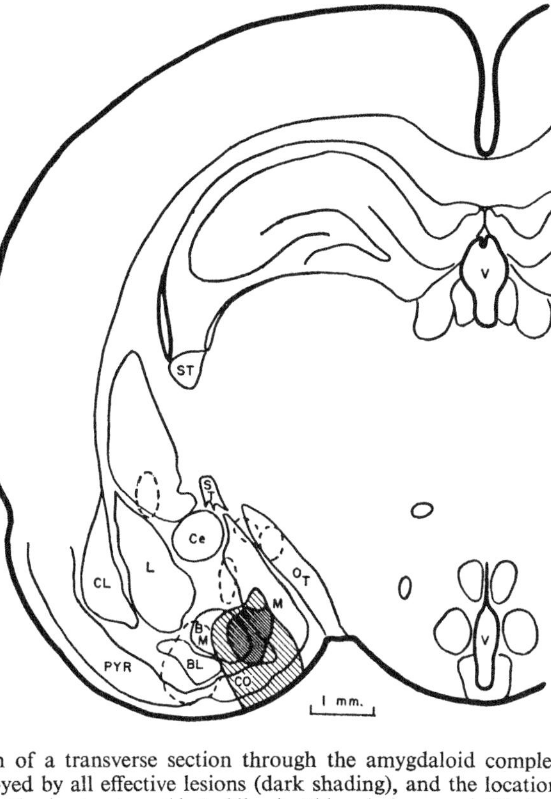

FIG. 2. Diagram of a transverse section through the amygdaloid complex showing the total area destroyed by all effective lesions (dark shading), and the location of ineffective lesions in adjacent brain structures (dotted lines). Abbreviations used: BL, basal amygdaloid nucleus, lateral part; BM, basal amygdaloid nucleus, medial part; C, claustrum; CE, central amygdaloid nucleus; CO, cortical amygdaloid nucleus; L, lateral amygdaloid nucleus; M, medial amygdaloid nucleus; OT, optic tract; PYR, pyriform cortex; ST, stria terminalis.

all shared a common area of destruction, indicated by the dark shading, that included parts of the medially located nuclei and the area between which contains the converging fibers of the stria terminalis. Bilateral involvement of this composite area was questionable in one effective lesion, and one was located in the anterior caudato-putamen complex. The dotted lines mark locations of all ineffective lesions placed bilaterally in the immediate vicinity of the effective amygdaloid area with the exception of one that was located in the composite area. In addition, bilaterally symmetrical ineffective lesions were located in the posterior extreme of the amygdala and in the thalamus. Eleven ineffective lesions were clearly asymmetrical. Two representative effective amygdaloid lesions are shown in FIG. 3.

These data suggest that a selected part of the amygdaloid complex may be included in neural mechanisms which are active in the inhibition of gonadotropin secretion in immature female rats. We have just begun to look for the anatomical connections that may relate this temporal lobe structure with the anterior hypothalamic area. In a few preliminary experiments, lesions in 24 rats that have failed to destroy the stria terminals bilaterally have been ineffective while two rats with lesions that conclusively destroyed this tract on both sides have shown precocious gonadal stimulation.

REFERENCES

1. ELWERS, M. and V. CRITCHLOW, *Am. J. Physiol.* **198**, 381, 1960.
2. BOGDANOVE, E. M. and H. C. SCHOEN, *Proc. Soc. Exp. Biol.* **100**, 664, 1959.

INTERACTIONS BETWEEN THE CENTRAL NERVOUS SYSTEM AND HORMONES INFLUENCING OVULATION*

CHARLES H. SAWYER and M. KAWAKAMI

Department of Anatomy, University of California, Los Angeles and Veterans Administration Hospital, Long Beach, California

INTRODUCTION

EVEN before the essential role of pituitary hormones in the process of ovulation was suspected, it was recognized that activation of ovulation in certain species required the nervous stimulation related to coitus. Haighton (1) suggested this as early as 1797, but Heape (2) is generally credited with the discovery of this reflex type of ovulation, which is the rule in rabbits, cats and several other species. After the convincing demonstration of hypophysial involvement in the ovulation process over 30 years ago by Smith and Engle (3) numerous attempts were made to analyze the mechanisms by which the nervous system activates the release of pituitary gonadotropin—not only in the reflex ovulators but also in the more numerous spontaneously ovulating forms. These experiments, involving central and peripheral nerve lesions, pituitary stalk sections, hypophysial transplants, electrical stimulation techniques, neurohumoral stimulants and pharmacological blocking agents, have been reviewed comprehensively by Benoit and Assenmacher (4).

During the 1920s and early 1930s, the physiology of the ovarian hormones, estrogens and progesterone, was also being elucidated (5). The secretion of these steroids was shown to be under the control of pituitary gonadotropins and the latter, in turn, were visualized by several workers, including Moore and Price (6) in 1932, to be influenced by a direct feed-back of target organ steroids to the hypophysis. However, because castration cells did not develop in transplanted pituitary glands, Hohlweg and Junkmann (7) proposed the existence of a hypothalamic "sex center" which controlled the release of pituitary gonadotropins and which was affected by the sex steroids in their feed-back circuit. Recently Flerkó and Szentágothai (8) have provided evidence in the rat of a direct antigonadotropic action of ovarian steroids at the hypothalamic level by observing the action of ovarian fragments transplanted into the region of the paraventricular nuclei.

* Supported in part by a grant (B-1162) from the National Institutes of Health.

That sex steroids do, directly or indirectly, influence the central nervous system is evidenced also by their obvious effects on reproductive behavior (9, 10). A direct action is implied by the results of experiments of Kent and Liberman (11), Fisher (12) and Harris, Michael and Scott (13) in which they injected steroids directly into the brain. Whether the hypothalamic area controlling gonadotropic function is identical to the area controlling reproductive behavior and whether either is a primary focus of steroid action are questions to be considered in the present paper.

In this report the authors attempt to summarize their recent experiments on the effects of pituitary and gonadal hormones on thresholds of central nervous activity as assessed by electroencephalographic (EEG) recording methods. These effects are correlated with changes in estrous behavior and thresholds of pituitary activation in the rabbit. Earlier results obtained with electrical stimulation and lesioning techniques are presented as an introduction to the anatomy of the hypothalamus, rhinencephalon and brainstem.

STIMULATION–LESION EXPERIMENTS; THE ANATOMICAL SUBSTRATE

Activation of the release of pituitary ovulating hormone in the rabbit by localized electrical stimulation of the hypothalamus and preoptic area, respectively, was achieved in 1937 independently by Harris (14) and Haterius

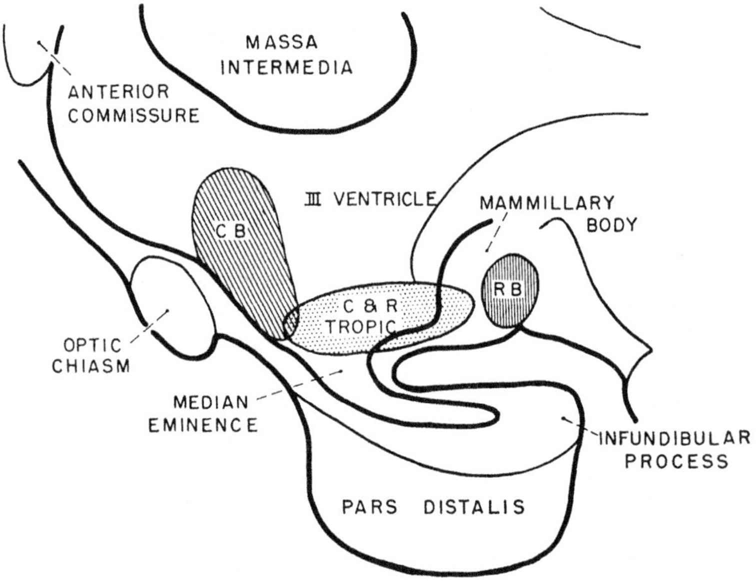

FIG. 1. Location of gonadotropic and sex behavioral areas in the hypothalamus of the female rabbit and the female cat. C&R TROPIC, common area controlling release of pituitary ovulating hormone in the cat and rabbit. CB and RB, areas in which lesions induce permanent anestrus in the cat and rabbit respectively.

and Derbyshire (15). Their findings have been confirmed repeatedly during the past 20 years, and a basal tuberal area especially sensitive to this type of stimulation has been outlined by Saul and Sawyer (16, 17) (FIG. 1). Localized electrolytic lesions in the middle of this area block copulation-induced ovulation in the rabbit with or without causing ovarian atrophy (18 ,19). An almost identical site, extending from ventromedial nuclei to mammillary bodies, has been delineated in the cat hypothalamus by Robison and Sawyer

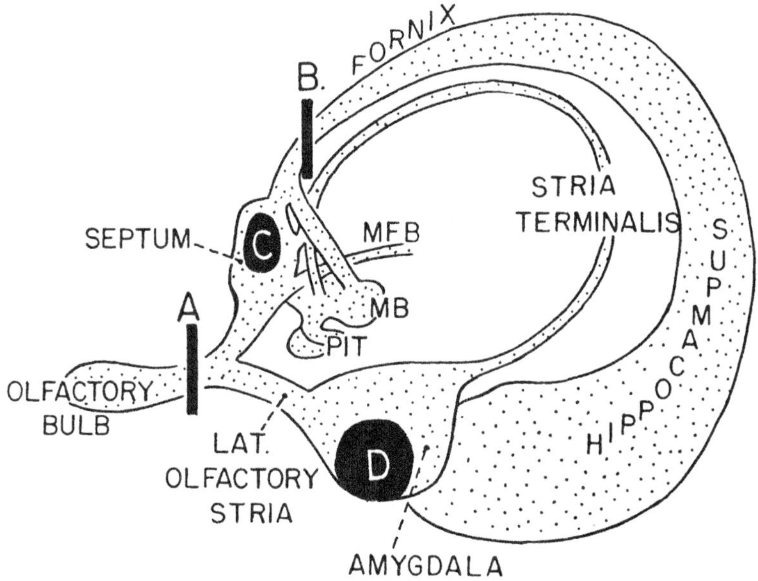

FIG. 2. Relationships of rhinencephalic structures and sites of lesions. A, transection of olfactory tracts or removal of bulbs; B, transection of fornix; C, septal lesion; D, amygdaloid lesion. MB, mammillary body; MFB, medial forebrain bundle; PIT, hypophysis. From Sawyer (19).

(20, 17) (FIG. 1) in which stimulation during estrus induces ovulation and lesions cause ovarian atrophy. Differential regions have been outlined which appear to control reproductive behavior in the two species (FIG. 1). Stimulation of these areas does not induce ovulation, and lesions do not lead to ovarian atrophy but do produce a condition of permanent anestrus which cannot be reversed by exogenous estrogen; ovulation can still be induced by direct stimulation of the gonadotropic area.

Projecting into the hypothalamus are numerous fiber tracts from the rhinencephalon or limbic lobe, the part of the brain which Papez (21) proposed as the anatomical substrate of emotion. These pathways include the medial forebrain bundle from olfactory and other rostral areas, the fornix from the hippocampus and the stria terminalis from the amygdala. The projections are now considered two-way circuits (22), but evidence of their involvement with reproductive behavior and neuroendocrine function persists. Koikegami *et al.* (23) were the first to report that stimulation of medial amygdaloid nuclei induces ovulation, and olfactory activity has been implicated in pharmacological induction of ovulation in the rabbit (24). Lesions in the amygdala and underlying pyriform cortex lead to hypersexualism in males of various species (25, 26). The lesions in the female rabbit rhinencephalon depicted in FIG. 2 did not inhibit reproductive behavior or block copulation-induced ovulation (19). However, there were some indications that removal of the olfactory bulbs and section of the fornix (combined lesions A and B) lead to a condition of behavioral hypersexualism in these females. The mammillary body, which receives projections from these areas and in which lesions lead to anestrus, will assume a position of considerable importance in the estrous behavior of the female rabbit if later experiments confirm these preliminary findings.

The brainstem reticular activating system (27) is also morphologically and functionally closely related to the hypothalamus and its activity. This system is especially sensitive to several of the drugs found to block ovulation in the rabbit and rat (28, 29). However, these drugs have been shown to be capable of blocking ovulation at the hypothalamic level (16), and Critchlow's (30) midbrain lesions which blocked ovulation in the rat did not necessarily destroy the reticular activating system.

AFTERREACTION TO COITUS; FEED-BACK HYPOTHESIS

In an effort to obtain neural correlates of pituitary activation by recording EEG activity simultaneously from several regions of the brain under conditions stimulatory to the adenohypophysis, chronic depth electrodes were implanted in the brains of many female rabbits. While continuous EEG records were being made these rabbits were free to move about, eat, drink and even to copulate with or fight other rabbits. Copulation in the estrous rabbit or vaginal stimulation in the estrous, estrogen-treated rabbit (31) was used to trigger the release of pituitary ovulating hormone. An example of the type of EEG change seen under these conditions (32) is contained in FIG. 3. During the stimulation period the changes were almost entirely artifacts attributable to movement. Within several minutes, however, the record characteristically assumed a "sleepy" appearance with spindle bursts in the frontal cortex and related areas (FIG. 3, B). The "sleepy" record continued from several minutes to half an hour or more and was replaced by a most unusual EEG pattern (FIG. 3, C–E). What appeared to be a hyperaroused record, with 8-sec sinusoidal waves predominant in several rhinencephalic areas related to the hippocampus, was associated with behavioral depression. The rabbit lay prone with her head on the floor (FIG. 4, c–e), her ears bent back, eyes partially closed, pupils constricted, bradycardia and depressed respiration. On recovery her EEG record reverted to a pattern of ordinary arousal (FIG. 3, E); she raised her head, stood up and usually went to the food bowl or extracted a pellet of feces from her anus and chewed it (FIG. 4, f).

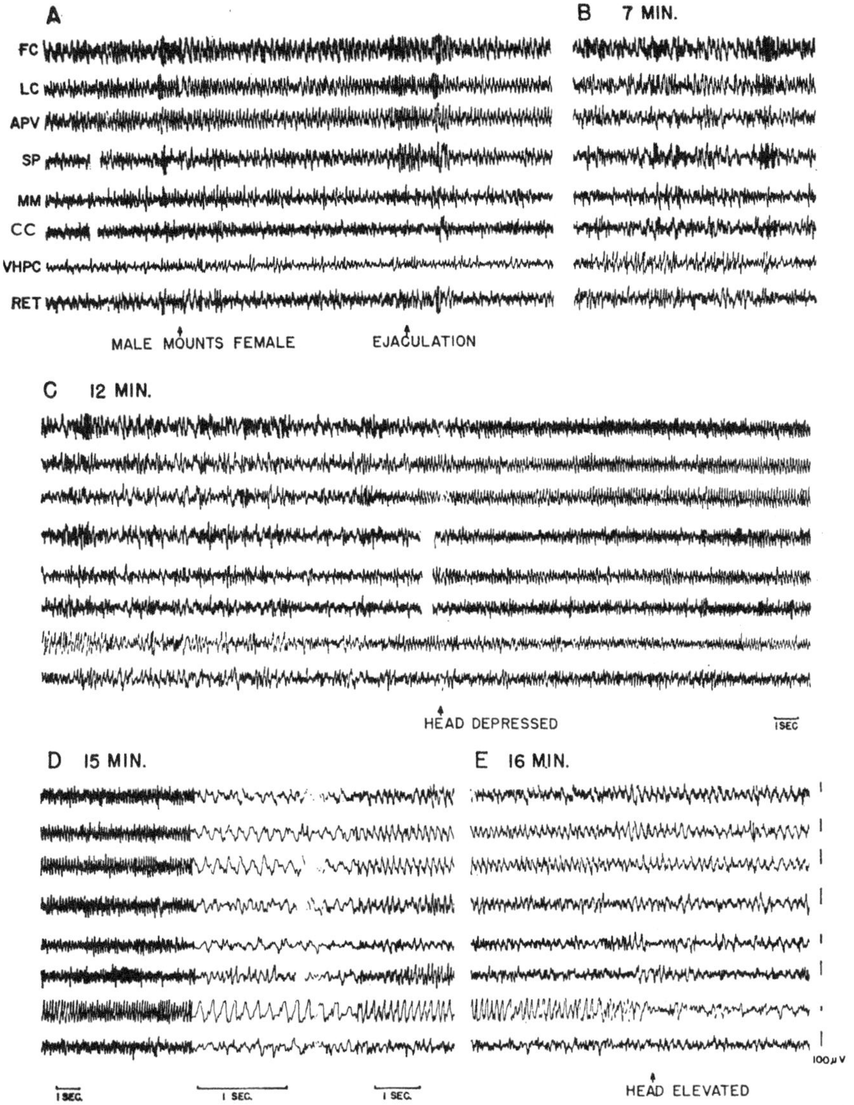

FIG. 3. Effects of coitus on the EEG of an unanesthetized unrestrained female rabbit with electrodes permanently implanted in her brain. EEG channels: FC, frontal cortex; LC, limbic cortex; APV, anterior paraventricular nucleus (thalamus); SP, septum; MM, medial mammillary nuclei; CC, corpus callosum; VHPC, ventral hippocampus; RET, midbrain reticular formation. From Sawyer and Kawakami (32).

This afterreaction to coitus, whose EEG characteristics were observed simultaneously with the behavioral changes, seems to occur ordinarily in the undisturbed female rabbit. It does not develop in a noisy room and it was missed in earlier observations probably because its behavioral characteristics, in the absence of a simultaneous recording of the unusual EEG pattern, are not dramatic. It cannot be induced in the anestrous rabbit by vaginal stimulation but it is readily evoked by this method in the estrous, estrogen-treated female. It does not occur in the male rabbit as a sequel to copulation.

At first it was thought that the EEG afterreaction did in fact represent correlates of nervous activation of the hypophysis. However, it soon became apparent that the time course was too late for such a relationship. An anti-nervous blocking agent must be injected within a minute post coitum to prevent ovulation (33) whereas the period of "EEG hyperarousal" or hippocampal hyperactivity may not appear for half an hour or more post coitum. By this time presumably considerable ovulating hormone has already been released, for enough has reached the circulation within an hour to make the further presence of the pituitary gland unnecessary for ovulation (34–36). So if the EEG afterreaction is more than coincidentally linked to the release of ovulating hormone it is more likely related to the discharge process itself or perhaps to the action of the released hormone on the brain as a direct feed-back mechanism. The reaction occurs in ovariectomized rabbits so the principal target organ of ovulating hormone is not involved in the feed-back mechanism (32).

This feed-back hypothesis led to attempts to induce a spontaneous EEG afterreaction, in the absence of coitus or vaginal stimulation, with the use of exogenous pituitary hormones and placental gonadotropins (37). The attempts were successful with purified preparations of pituitary luteinizing hormone (LH) (FIG. 5, A–D), human chorionic gonadotropin (HCG), equine gonadotropin (PMS) and also with lactogenic hormone (LTH) and the neurohypophysial principles, oxytocin and vasopressin. The other adenohypophysial tropins, follicle stimulating hormone (FSH) (FIG. 5, A^1–D^1), thyrotropin (TSH), adrenocorticotropin (ACTH) and growth hormone (somatotropin), all gave negative results. Interestingly all of the pituitary principles whose injection resulted in an EEG afterreaction are released in response to coitus. The results are consistent with the hypothesis that the post-coital EEG afterreaction is functionally related to the feed-back of these released pituitary hormones. Teleologically such a system would serve a useful purpose in shutting off the hypothalamo-hypophysial mechanism for activation of release of ovulating hormone.

The essential nature of the EEG afterreaction is incompletely understood. It has certain characteristics of a psychomotor seizure, and it appears to be related to the condition of adynamia described by Hess (38) and the "arrest reaction" of Hunter and Jasper (39). The latter is likened to a petit mal attack.

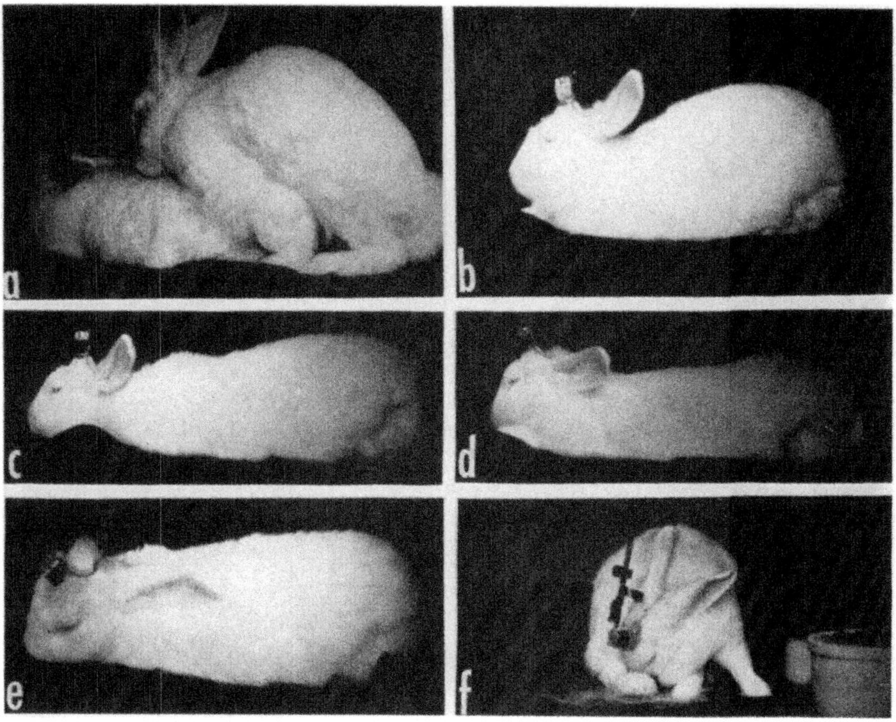

FIG. 4. Behavior of the female rabbit during and after coitus. From Sawyer and Kawakami (32).

Whether the latter conditions are influenced by hormones was not reported. Hormonally-induced changes in the rabbit EEG and behavior have been

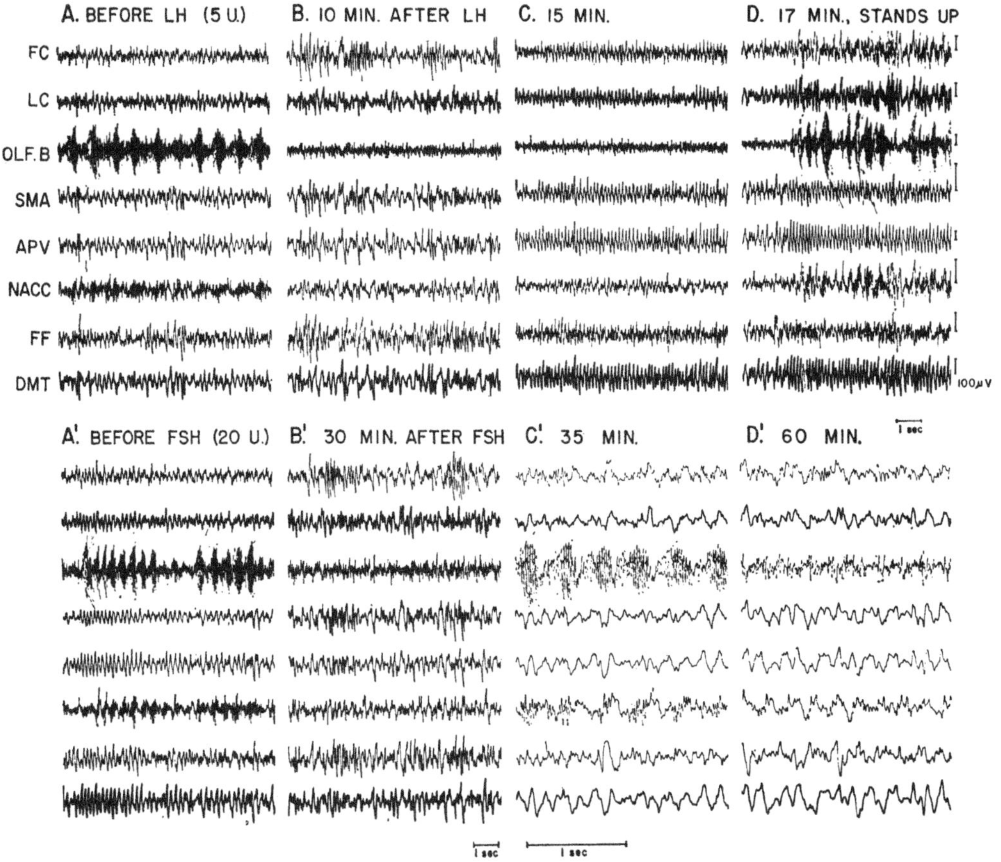

FIG. 5. Effects of intraperitoneal injections of LH and FSH on the EEG. Abbreviations (cf. FIG. 3): OLF.B, olfactory bulb; SMA, supramammillary area; NACC, nucleus accumbens; FF, fimbria of fornix; DTM, nucleus dorsomedialis thalami. From Kawakami and Sawyer (37).

reported extensively by Faure (40, 41). His olfacto-bucco-ano-genito-sexual syndrome has certain phases similar, if not identical, to stages in the EEG afterreaction sequence.

THRESHOLDS OF EEG AROUSAL AND EEG AFTERREACTION

It was soon discovered that the EEG afterreaction could readily be evoked in the estrous, but not in the anestrous, rabbit by low frequency (5/sec) electrical stimulation of the hypothalamus or rhinencephalon (37). The afterreaction often occurred too quickly to have been mediated by the release and feed-back of pituitary hormones and it must have been induced by more direct means. In FIG. 6, B the sleep spindles appeared within 30 sec of stimulating the septum for 30 sec at 5/sec, pulse duration 0.5 millisec; the phase of hippocampal hyperactivity started within one minute. The threshold

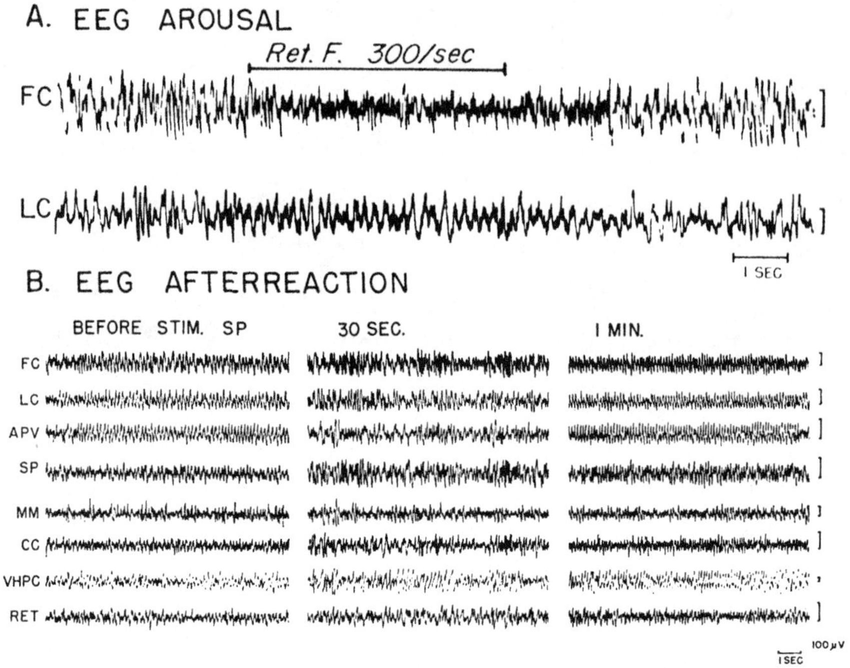

FIG. 6. EEG records of arousal (A) and afterreactions (B). Abbreviations: cf. FIG. 3. Explanation in text.

is defined as the lowest voltage which will induce a complete EEG afterreaction within 30 min of a single 30-sec period of 5/sec stimulation. If a positive response occurs in considerably less than 30 min it is considered appropriate to test a lower voltage without waiting for the full half-hour to elapse.

A completely different phenomenon is the EEG arousal response (FIG. 6, A). Here a short, five-second burst of high frequency (300/sec) stimulation applied to the midbrain reticular formation or related areas will, if above threshold, cause a desynchronization of the frontal cortex EEG pattern and a theta synchrony in the limbic cortex. If far above threshold, the response will outlast the stimulus, and behavioral arousal may occur: the rabbit may sit up or stand and look alert.

The "alert" theta rhythm of the limbic cortex, hippocampus and other areas is of lower frequency (4–6/sec) than the afterreaction phase of hippocampal hyperactivity (7–9/sec). During the latter phase the rabbit is so depressed behaviorally that the threshold of EEG and behavioral arousal is elevated even higher than during sleep.

With the techniques of measuring the two thresholds available for registering indices of the functional state of the brain, the effects of sex steroids on these thresholds were assessed and correlated with their known effects on behavior and on pituitary activation.

EFFECTS OF PROGESTERONE

Some years ago at Duke University, in work only recently published in detail (42), it was discovered that progesterone in the estrous or estrogen-treated rabbit exerts a diphasic effect on the threshold of pituitary activation. During the first few hours after injection of progesterone (2 mg s.c., in oil) the threshold is lowered, as evidenced by the finding that the ovulatory sequence can be initiated by vaginal stimulation, a method which is practically ineffective in the absence of progesterone. By 24 hr after progesterone treatment, however, the pituitary activation threshold is highly elevated: not only is vaginal stimulation ineffective but so is the coital stimulus itself, provided the rabbit will mate. Behaviorally during this latter period the rabbit is distinctly less estrous whereas during the first few hours after progesterone she seems to be "hotter" than when only estrogen is supplied. Thus there appears to be a diphasic effect of progesterone both on estrous behavior and on pituitary activation, the second or inhibitory phase of which is much better known than the earlier phase of facilitation.

The curve in FIG. 7 shows the diphasic effect of an injection of progesterone on the EEG arousal threshold and the continued elevation of the threshold following a second injection of the steroid 24 hr after the first (43). This curve is paralleled by the changes in EEG afterreaction threshold tabulated at the bottom. During the period of lowered thresholds, the rabbit attacked another female, mated with a male and revealed EEG afterreactions to coitus and to vaginal stimulation as well as to the electrical stimulation employed to assess the afterreaction threshold. As the threshold rose the rabbit became anestrous and EEG afterreaction became difficult or impossible to achieve even with electrical stimulation of the hypothalamus.

Figure 8 shows not only the two threshold curves during the first 10 hr after a single injection of progesterone to an ovariectomized estrogen-primed rabbit but also depicts the duration of the phases of the EEG afterreactions. Both thresholds remained depressed from one and one-half to four and one-half hours after the steroid injection. It is apparent that the rabbit, although estrogen-primed, was anestrous prior to, and later than six hours after progesterone treatment, but that during the period of lowered thresholds she mated and revealed the EEG afterreaction to coitus and to vaginal stimulation. During this stage the sleep spindles of the EEG afterreaction started immediately on electrical stimulation and once post-coitally.

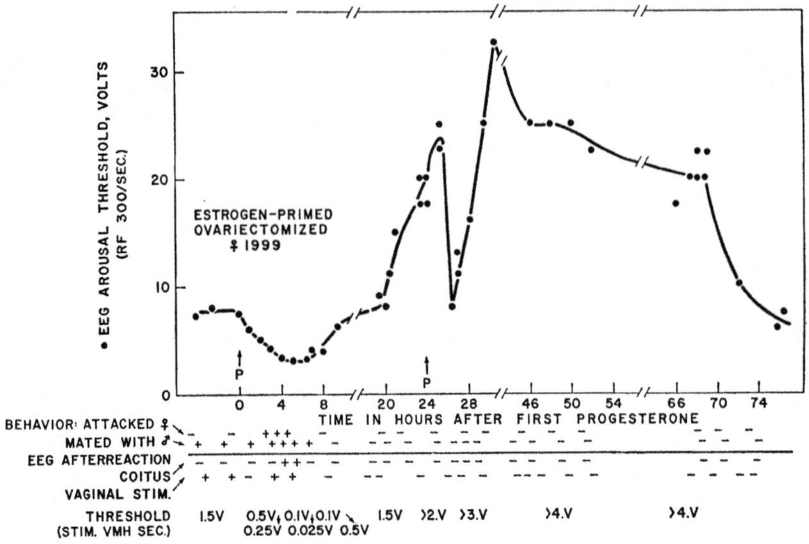

FIG. 7. Diphasic effect of progesterone on thresholds of EEG arousal (curve) and EEG afterreaction (tabulated below), and prolonged elevation of thresholds following second injection of progesterone. From Kawakami and Sawyer (43).

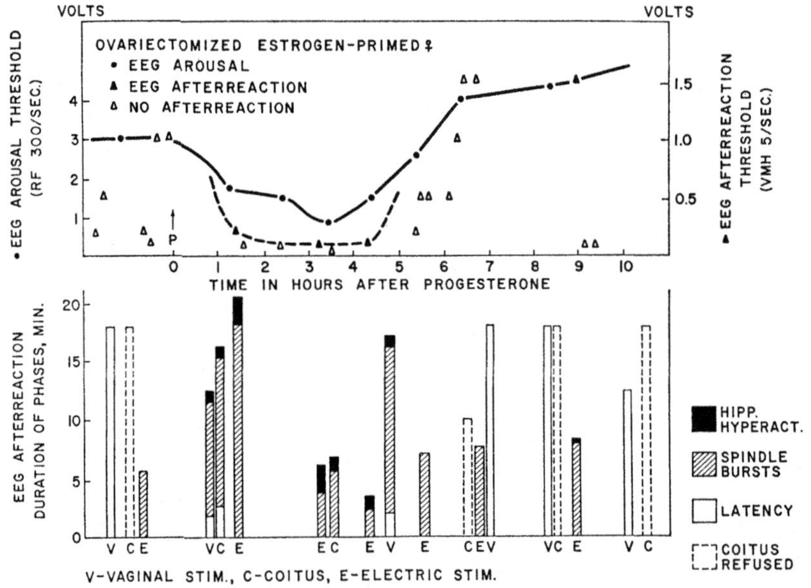

FIG. 8. Thresholds and EEG afterreaction data during the first 10 hr after progesterone treatment of an ovariectomized estrogen-primed rabbit. Open triangles represent unsuccessful attempts to elicit the EEG afterreaction. From Kawakami and Sawyer (43).

EFFECTS OF ESTROGEN, LOW DOSAGE

In the progesterone experiments described above the ovariectomized rabbits were primed for two days with estradiol benzoate (0.08–0.1 mg s.c., in oil) daily. This treatment usually neither lowered the thresholds appreciably nor brought the rabbits into heat. However, in the intact anestrous rabbit, possibly through synergism with endogenous progesterone, treatment with exogenous estrogen often lowered both thresholds. An example of this is

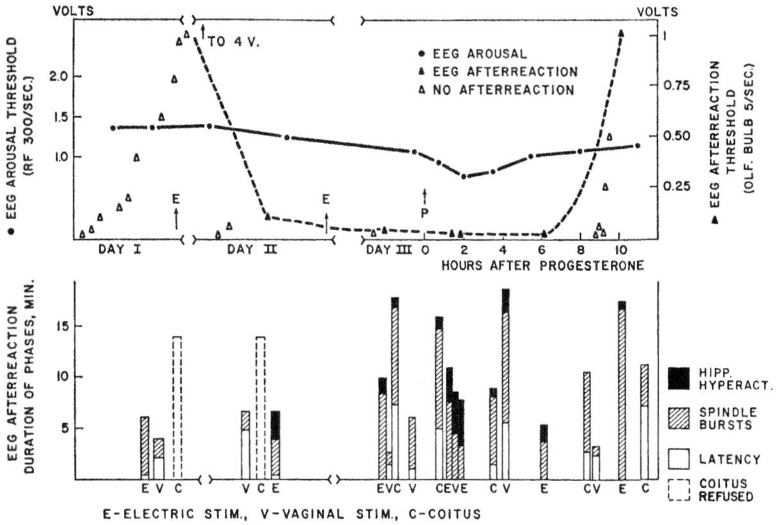

FIG. 9. Thresholds and EEG afterreaction data following estrogen and subsequently progesterone treatment of an intact (non-castrate) female rabbit. From Kawakami and Sawyer (43).

seen in FIG. 9. On the day after the first injection of estrogen, the still anestrous rabbit reveals a lowered EEG afterreaction threshold to electrical stimulation. On the day following the second estrogen injection the EEG afterreaction threshold is depressed still further and the arousal threshold somewhat lowered. At this time, prior to treatment with progesterone, the now estrous rabbit copulates and reveals an EEG afterreaction which is not, however, fully evocable by vaginal stimulation. Progesterone lowers the thresholds still further and during the next few hours even vaginal stimulation induces the EEG afterreaction. Between six and eight hours after progesterone administration the afterreaction threshold rises sharply while the arousal threshold slopes upward gradually.

Treatment of estrous rabbits with exogenous estrogen for two days or anestrous rabbits for four days lowered the threshold of pituitary activation to such an extent that ovulation could be induced in 40–50% of the cases by vaginal stimulation (31). When apparently estrous rabbits were treated for four days with estrogen, an appreciable number of them ovulated "spontaneously" during the winter and spring months but not during the summer (44) (FIG. 10). In a limited number of rabbits with chronically implanted electrodes, the EEG afterreaction and arousal thresholds, and the effects of

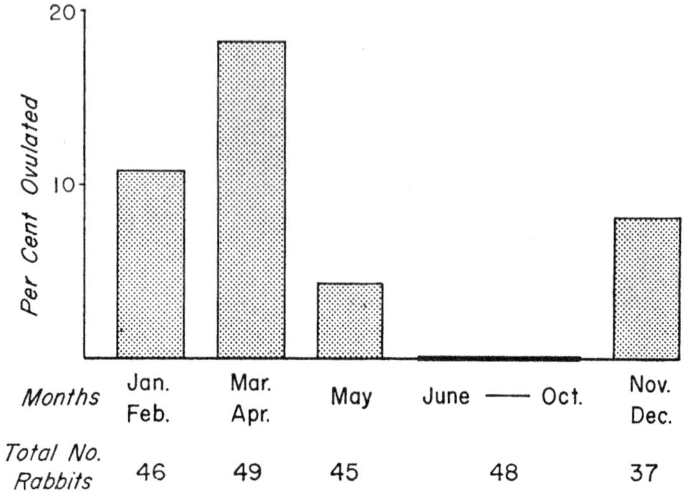

FIG. 10. Relative incidence of estrogen-facilitated spontaneous ovulation in the rabbit during various seasons of the year. From Sawyer (44).

steroids upon them, were assessed throughout the year (43). The most dramatic difference between February and June thresholds lay in the very low values of EEG afterreaction threshold in late February; even after progesterone the higher June threshold did not come down to the pre-progesterone value in February. In some of these experiments coitus in June was not followed by an afterreaction.

EFFECTS OF HIGH DOSAGES OF ESTROGEN OR TESTOSTERONE

In experiments such as those illustrated above in which progesterone and low dosages of estrogen were tested, the EEG arousal and afterreaction thresholds generally changed in a quite parallel manner. Under conditions in which both thresholds were minimal the pituitary activation threshold was also lowest and the rabbit was in heat; the elevation of both thresholds was correlated with anestrus and an elevated pituitary threshold.

It is possible with high dosages of estrogen or testosterone to separate the two thresholds in a given animal and to study the resultant changes in behavior and pituitary threshold. Five daily injections of 0.5 mg estradiol benzoate or 5 mg testosterone propionate (FIG. 11) result in lowered EEG arousal thresholds and elevated EEG afterreaction thresholds. At the end of treatment with either steroid, the rabbits are highly estrous but copulation is not followed by ovulation. The latter condition may be described as an elevated pituitary activation threshold; this may be correlated with the

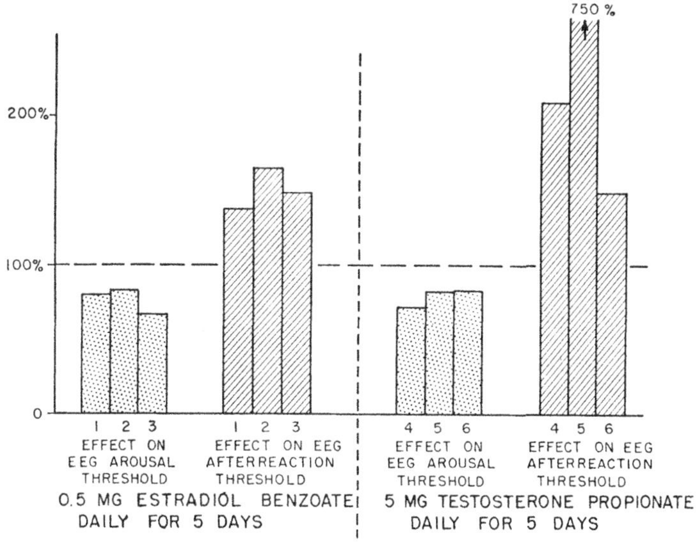

FIG. 11. Relative thresholds (expressed as percentages of pretreatment levels considered to be 100%) of EEG arousal and EEG afterreaction after prolonged treatment with high dosages of estrogen and treatment with androgen. The numbers (1–6) under the bars identify individual rabbits.

elevated afterreaction threshold while continued estrus may be correlated with the lowered EEG arousal threshold. Zondek and Sklow (45) noted the inhibitory effect of high dosages of estrogen and testosterone on electrically stimulated ovulation in the rabbit.

EFFECTS OF CERTAIN PITUITARY AND PLACENTAL HORMONES

As was mentioned earlier, treatment with certain pituitary or placental gonadotropins, lactogen and neurohypophysial hormones was often followed by the appearance of a "spontaneous" EEG afterreaction. It was proposed that the response might represent a natural feed-back mechanism to shut off further neural activation of the hypophysis. It was, therefore, of interest to study the effects of these agents on the two thresholds.

Figure 12 illustrates a representative response to these substances. Exerting little effect on the EEG arousal threshold, the gonadotropin caused a rapid lowering of the EEG afterreaction threshold to the point at which a "spontaneous" afterreaction occurred. For some hours thereafter the threshold remained at relatively low levels but ordinarily only one spontaneous afterreaction followed such an injection. In this particular case (FIG. 12) the rabbit had been pretreated with estrogen and a temporary condition of

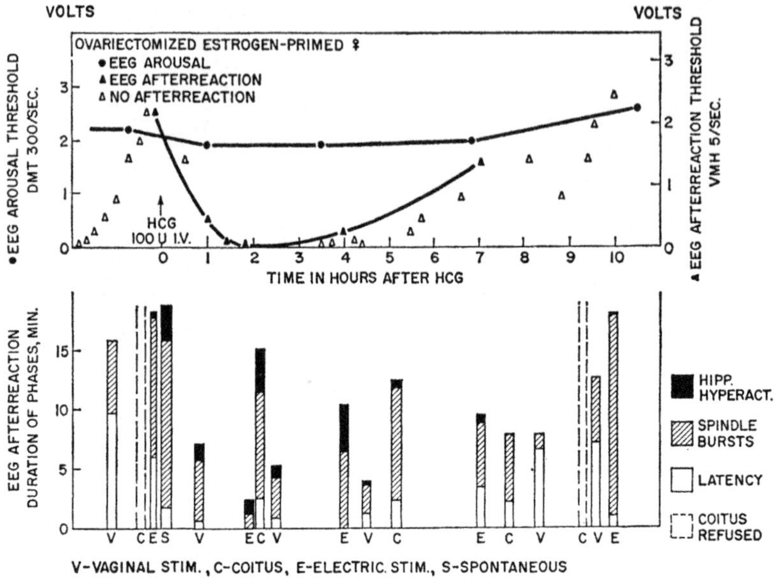

FIG. 12. Effect of human chorionic gonadotropin (HCG) on EEG thresholds in the estrogen-primed ovariectomized rabbit. In the unprimed castrate rabbit HCG still depresses the EEG afterreaction threshold but the occurrence of estrus and the slight depression in arousal threshold seen here do not occur in the absence of exogenous estrogen. From Kawakami and Sawyer (43).

estrus followed HCG treatment, although the arousal threshold was only slightly depressed. In the absence of estrogen neither estrus nor any effect on the arousal threshold was usually seen, although the EEG afterreaction threshold was reduced to the level at which a spontaneous response occurred. The results support the concept of a close relationship between the EEG afterreaction threshold and pituitary activation and indicate that the influence of these hormones on the nervous system, as well as that of the steroids, is one of altering thresholds rather than acting as stimulants *per se*.

EFFECTS OF THE NEW PROGESTOGENS

Some of the newer progestational compounds have been reported to have very prolonged actions (46) and to be strongly inhibitory to ovulation (47). Their effects on the two thresholds were naturally of considerable interest.

The progestational effects of 17α-hydroxyprogesterone caproate (Delalutin) are particularly long lasting (48). Interestingly enough (FIG. 13) this esterified steroid exerts a diphasic effect on both EEG afterreaction and arousal thresholds and both phases are very much prolonged. By way of contrast the effect on the EEG afterreaction threshold of a single injection of 25 mg

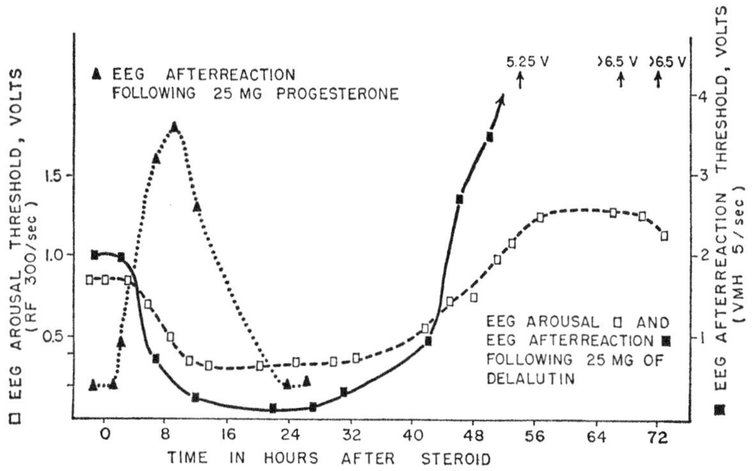

FIG. 13. Prolonged diphasic effect on EEG thresholds of treating an estrogen-primed ovariectomized rabbit with a single injection of 17α-hydroxyprogesterone caproate (Delalutin). The figures (5.25 V, >6.5 V) at the upper right refer to off-limits values of EEG afterreaction thresholds. The time course of changes in EEG afterreaction threshold following a similar dosage of progesterone is included for comparison.

progesterone is included in FIG. 13. Its phase of elevated threshold is terminated long before the completion of the first phase (lowered threshold) following Delalutin. In keeping with the functional concepts relative to these phases expressed above, during the Delalutin-prolonged first phase the rabbit will mate and ovulate; whereas she remains in an anestrous anovulatory condition during the phase of elevated thresholds.

Of the 19-nor steroid gestagens which have proven such potent inhibitors of ovulation as to receive extended clinical trial as contraceptives, the following have been tested for their effects on the two EEG thresholds: 17α-ethynyl-19-nortestosterone (Norlutin), 17α-ethyl-19-nortestosterone (Nilevar) and 17α-ethynyl, $\Delta^{5(10)}$-estrenolone (norethynodrel, which with added estrogen is known as Enovid). All of these agents affected the two thresholds in the differential manner illustrated in FIG. 14, prepared from norethynodrel data: they left the EEG arousal threshold essentially unchanged but rapidly raised the EEG afterreaction threshold. In confirmation of Pincus *et al.* (49) we found that the rabbits would readily mate 24 hr after the injection of 1 mg of any of these steroids but that such copulation was not followed by ovulation. Their differential elevation of the particular EEG threshold which we have come to associate with the threshold of pituitary activation, while leaving estrous behavior and its associated EEG threshold unaffected, makes these gestagens ideal antifertility agents, at least for the

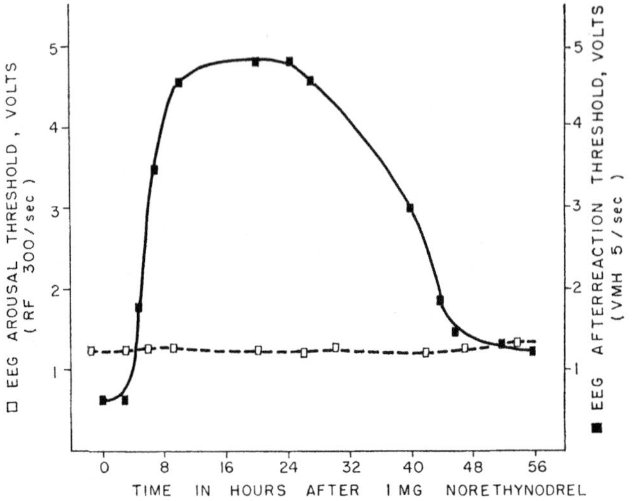

FIG. 14. Differential effect of norethynodrel on the EEG afterreaction and EEG arousal thresholds. Norlutin and Nilevar exerted similar effects.

rabbit. It is conceivable that the record of effects of new steroids on the two EEG thresholds in the rabbit might prove a useful index in screening antifertility agents.

DISCUSSION

The results of the present experiments, as well as those in which injections of hormones directly into the brain influenced behavior (11, 12, 13), leave little doubt that hormones can act directly on elements within the brain. Ralph and Fraps (50), for example, have reported that the intrahypothalamic injection of tiny amounts of progesterone will induce premature ovulation in the hen.

It may be that the hormone receptors within the brain, the areas most sensitive to the endocrine agents, are identical to the hypothalamic "centers" whose destruction eliminates behavioral or gonadotropic function. It should be possible, under this hypothesis, to activate the "centers" individually by localized hormone injections, and such appears to be the case (12, 13). With systemic treatment with effective dosages of estrogen and progesterone the two systems, behavioral and gonadotropic, are associated with EEG thresholds that change in a remarkably parallel manner. Such parallel changes coordinate coital behavior with a responsive pituitary–gonad axis. Gonadotropins, testosterone, the 19-nor gestagens and high dosages of estrogen affect the thresholds, and perhaps the receptors, differentially, thus permitting estrous behavior without ovulation and ovulation without estrous behavior.

It would appear that both the facilitory and the inhibitory influences of the sex steroids on the adenohypophysis are attributable to, or mediated by, their actions on the nervous system. There may be multiple receptors within the brain which are influenced in a coordinated manner by endogenous hormones or systemically administered exogenous hormones. Bodily needs, according to Dell (51), demand a nonspecific excitatory state for appetitive behavior; this condition is induced by the effects of elements in the internal environment on the brainstem reticular system. Consummatory behavior then produces changes which depress the generalized reticular activity and vigilance. The present results are consistent with this scheme, and they point to sex steroids as crucial elements of the internal environment responsible for the vigilant appetitive phase. Consummatory depression of the arousal system is effected by, or coordinated with, unusual activation of a rhinencephalic-hypothalamic circuit, probably involving actions of pituitary hormones on the nervous system.

SUMMARY

The hormonal feed-back circuit in the rabbit by which ovarian steroids alter pituitary susceptibility for ovulation and coordinate this condition with the estrous state has been shown to include the action of the steroids on two thresholds of activity in the brain. The EEG arousal threshold appears to be concerned with estrous behavior while the EEG afterreaction threshold parallels the threshold of pituitary activation. The natural EEG afterreaction, which is a common sequel to coitus in the rabbit, seems to represent an effect of the released pituitary hormones on the nervous system, perhaps in the nature of a negative feed-back to stop further release of gonadotropin. Certain steroids appear to be excellent antifertility agents by virtue of a differential elevation of the EEG afterreaction threshold and the absence of an effect on the EEG arousal threshold. The results are consistent with the concept that hypothalamic "centers" controlling sex behavior and gonadotropic secretion may represent important neuroendocrine receptors of hormonal influence on brain function.

Acknowledgments—The authors wish to thank the Schering Corporation for the estradiol benzoate (Progynon B), Dr. J. D. Fisher of Armour Pharmaceutical Corporation for the pituitary hormones, Dr. E. C. Reifenstein of E. R. Squibb and Sons for Delalutin, Dr. D. A. McGinty of Parke, Davis and Co. for Norlutin and Dr. F. J. Saunders of G. D. Searle and Co. for norethynodrel and Nilevar employed in the experiments. The figures were drawn by Charles Bridgman and photographed by Timothy Dodge.

REFERENCES

1. HAIGHTON, J., *Phil. Trans. Roy. Soc.* **87**, 159, 1797.
2. HEAPE, W., *Proc. Roy. Soc. B* **76**, 260, 1905.
3. SMITH, P. E. and E. T. ENGLE, *Amer. J. Anat.* **40**, 159, 1927.
4. BENOIT, J. and I. ASSENMACHER, *J. Physiol. (Paris)* **47**, 427, 1955.
5. ALLEN, E., *Sex and Internal Secretions*, Williams and Wilkins, Baltimore, Md., 1932.
6. MOORE, C. R. and D. PRICE, *Amer. J. Anat.* **50**, 13, 1932.
7. HOHLWEG, W. and K. JUNKMANN, *Klin. Wochschr.* **11**, 321, 1932.
8. FLERKÓ, B. and J. SZENTÁGOTHAI, *Acta Endocrinol.* **26**, 121, 1957.
9. BEACH, F. A., *Hormones and Behavior*, Hoeber, New York, 1948.
10. SAWYER, C. H., in *Handbook of Physiology: Neurophysiology* (Edited by H. W. Magoun, J. Field and V. E. Hall), p. 1235, American Physiological Society, Washington, D.C., 1960.
11. KENT, G. C. and M. J. LIBERMAN, *Endocrinology* **45**, 29, 1949.
12. FISHER, A. E., *Science* **124**, 228, 1956.
13. HARRIS, G. W., R. P. MICHAEL and P. P. SCOTT, in Ciba Foundation Symposium on *Neurological Basis of Behavior*, p. 236, J. and A. Churchill, Ltd., London, 1958.
14. HARRIS, G. W., *Proc. Roy. Soc. B* **122**, 374, 1937.
15. HATERIUS, H. O. and A. J. DERBYSHIRE, *Amer. J. Physiol.* **119**, 329, 1937.
16. SAUL, G. D. and C. H. SAWYER, *Federation Proc.* **16**, 112, 1957.
17. SAWYER, C. H., in conference on *Endocrinology of Reproduction* (Edited by C. W. Lloyd), p. 1, Academic Press, New York, 1959.
18. SAWYER, C. H., in *Physiological Triggers* (Edited by T. H. Bullock), p. 164, American Physiological Society, Washington, D.C., 1957.
19. SAWYER, C. H., *J. Exper. Zool.* **142**, 227, 1959.
20. ROBISON, B. L. and C. H. SAWYER, *Physiologist* **1**, 72, 1957.
21. PAPEZ, J. W., *A.M.A. Arch. Neurol. Psychiat.* **38**, 725, 1937.
22. ADEY, W. R., in *The Reticular Formation of the Brain* (Edited by H. H. Jasper, L. D. Proctor, R. S. Knighton, W. C. Noshay and R. T. Costello), p. 621, Little, Brown, Boston, Mass., 1958.
23. KOIKEGAMI, H., T. YAMADA and K. USUI, *Folia Psychiat. Neurol. Japan* **8**, 7, 1954.
24. SAWYER, C. H., *Amer. J. Physiol.* **180**, 37, 1955.
25. SCHREINER, L. and A. KLING, *J. Neurophysiol.* **16**, 643, 1953.
26. GREEN, J. D., C. D. CLEMENTE and J. DEGROOT, *J. Comp. Neurol.* **108**, 505, 1957.
27. MAGOUN, H. W., *A. Res. Nerv. & Ment. Dis. Proc.* **30**, 480, 1952.
28. SAWYER, C. H., B. V. CRITCHLOW and C. A. BARRACLOUGH, *Endocrinology* **57**, 345, 1955.
29. SAWYER, C. H., in *The Reticular Formation of the Brain* (Edited by H. H. Jasper, L. D. Proctor, R. S. Knighton, W. C. Noshay and R. T. Costello), p. 223, Little, Brown, Boston, Mass., 1958.
30. CRITCHLOW, B. V., *Endocrinology* **63**, 596, 1958.
31. SAWYER, C. H. and J. E. MARKEE, *Endocrinology* **65**, 614, 1959.
32. SAWYER, C. H. and M. KAWAKAMI, *Endocrinology* **65**, 622, 1959.
33. SAWYER, C. H., J. E. MARKEE and B. F. TOWNSEND, *Endocrinology* **44**, 18, 1949.
34. FEE, A. R. and A. S. PARKES, *J. Physiol., London* **67**, 383, 1929.
35. SMITH, P. E. and W. E. WHITE, *J. Amer. Med. Assn.* **97**, 1861, 1931.
36. WESTMAN, A. and D. JACOBSOHN, *Acta obst. gynec. Scandinav.* **16**, 483, 1936.
37. KAWAKAMI, M. and C. H. SAWYER, *Endocrinology* **65**, 631, 1959.
38. HESS, W. R., *Das Zwischenhirn*, Basel, 1949.
39. HUNTER, J. and H. H. JASPER, *EEG Clin. Neurophysiol.* **1**, 305, 1949.
40. FAURE, J., *Rev. Path. Gen. et Physiol. Clin.* **57**, 1029, 1263, 1445, 1957.
41. FAURE, J., *J. Physiol. Paris* **48**, 529, 1959.
42. SAWYER, C. H. and J. W. EVERETT, *Endocrinology* **65**, 644, 1959.
43. KAWAKAMI, M. and C. H. SAWYER, *Endocrinology* **65**, 652, 1959.
44. SAWYER, C. H., *Endocrinology* **65**, 523, 1959.
45. ZONDEK, B. and J. SKLOW, *Endocrinology* **28**, 923, 1941.
46. JUNKMANN, K., *Recent Prog. Hormone Research* **13**, 389, 1957.

47. PINCUS, G., J. ROCK, M. C. CHANG and C. R. GARCIA, *Federation Proc.* **18**, 1051, 1959.
48. KESSLER, W. B. and A. BORMAN, *Ann. New York Acad. Sci.* **71**, 486, 1958.
49. PINCUS, G., M. C. CHANG, M. X. ZARROW, E. S. E. HAFEZ and A. MERRILL, *Endocrinology* **59**, 695, 1956.
50. RALPH, C. L. and R. M. FRAPS, *Endocrinology* **66**, 269, 1960.
51. DELL, P. C., in Ciba Foundation Symposium on *Neurological Basis of Behavior*, p. 187, J. and A. Churchill, London, 1958.

DISCUSSION

Chairman: DR. WARREN O. NELSON

DR. WILLIAM HANSEL: Among the previous speakers, Harris in particular has pointed out the importance of the hypothalamus in regulating the secretion of the gonadotropins necessary for follicular growth and ovulation. Sawyer has described a typical electroencephalographic (EEG) arousal pattern, which occurs after stimulation of the mid-brain reticular formation and an EEG afterreaction which occurs following stimulation of hypothalamic and rhinencephalic loci in rabbits. A lowered arousal threshold was correlated with the induction of estrous behavior; a lowered afterreaction threshold appeared to be related to the release of pituitary ovulating hormone. Everett has shown that stimulation of the preoptic area consistently induces ovulation in rats given appropriately-timed injections of the ovulation-blocking drugs atropine and pentobarbital.

These results inevitably raise two major questions. The first of these concerns the nature of whatever humoral substances act between the hypothalamus and the adenohypophysis. The second concerns the afferent pathways, particularly those from the uterus, normally involved in activating those elements of the central nervous system which affect the neurohumoral regulation of the anterior pituitary.

The results of some of our recent studies on ovulation in the bovine are of particular interest in regard to both of these questions. Impressed with the possibility that oxytocin of hypothalamic origin might be involved in some way in the regulation of the secretion of anterior pituitary gonadotropins, Hansel *et al.* (*Proc. IIIrd Symposium on Reproduction and Infertility* (Ed. Gassner), Pergamon Press, 1958) tested the effects of injecting this hormone at the beginning of estrus on ovulation time in heifers. Ovulation in the bovine normally occurs about 12 hr after the end of an 18-hr estrous or "heat" period. In the oxytocin-treated heifers, the average time of ovulation was hastened by 5 hr, a result which might have been predicted on the basis of the recent finding by Sawyer and Kawakami that this hormone lowers the EEG afterreaction threshold, which appears to be related to the release of pituitary ovulating hormone.

Armstrong and Hansel (*J. Dairy Sc.* **42**, 533–542, 1959) later studied the effects of daily doses of oxytocin given at various times during the estrous cycle on ovarian function and cycle length in heifers. It soon became apparent that oxytocin administered on days 1 to 7 or 3 to 6 inclusive of the normal 22-day estrous cycle inhibited the development of the corpus luteum and produced a precocious estrus by the 8th–10th day of the cycle.

These results provided the first direct evidence for an effect of a neurohypophysial hormone on estrous cycle regulation and ovarian function in any species and, further, suggested that the administered oxytocin inhibited the production or release of luteotropin. However, in a subsequent experiment, oxytocin produced precocious estrus even when given concurrently with a prolactin preparation of bovine origin.

More recent results (*J. Dairy Sc.*, 1960 (In press) have served to emphasize the fundamental role played by the uterus in regulating cycle length and ovarian functions in the bovine. As in several other species, corpora lutea persist and estrous cycles do not occur in cattle after hysterectomy. Oxytocin injections proved incapable of inducing estrus in hysterectomized heifers.

This result led to studies of the effects of uterine dilatation and irritation on ovarian function and cycle length. Dilatation of the uterus by self-retaining rubber catheters, held in the uterus during the first 7 days of the cycle by small inflatable balloons, caused shortened estrous cycles, often 8 to 12 days in length, in a large proportion of the treated cows and heifers. In a similar experiment it was found that the infusion of 2 to 5 ml of raw semen, or the sediment obtained by centrifuging raw semen and preputial fluids containing large numbers of bacteria, into the uteri of heifers during estrus also induced precocious heat.

All of these treatments involving uterine insults also resulted in marked inhibition of the development of the corpus luteum. In some cases cystic corpora lutea resulted; in others the corpora lutea were simply quite small. Relatively few normal functional luteal cells were present in either case.

The physiological role which oxytocin plays in the regulation of the estrous cycle in cattle has not yet been established. It is conceivable that oxytocin injections, uterine dilatation, and the infusion of materials containing large numbers of bacteria into the uterus all cause luteal inhibition and precocious estrus by interfering with the normal production of some luteotropic substance by the bovine endometrium during the first half of the estrous cycle. Experiments now being carried out in which bovine endometrial extracts are injected into normal and pseudopregnant rats should provide an answer to this question.

Uterine stimulation in the bovine causes oxytocin release (Hays, R. L. and N. L. Van Demark, *Endocrinology* **52**, 634–637, 1953) and it is tempting to assume that the uterine dilatation and irritation in these experiments caused oxytocin release, which in turn inhibited luteotropin secretion either directly, or indirectly by influencing the hypothalamic release of some other neurohumor. The failure of oxytocin to induce estrus in hysterectomized heifers argues against such an interpretation, but this subject needs further study since the ovarian changes in these animals were not carefully followed and since it has also been found that multiple ovulations can occur in the ovaries of gonadotropin-treated, hysterectomized heifers in the absence of estrus.

Although these experiments indicate that oxytocin injections inhibit luteotropin secretion in the bovine, there are indications that exogenous oxytocin has the opposite effect in the rat (Benson, C. K. and S. J. Folley, *J. Endocrinol.* **16**, 189, 1957; and Desclin, L., *Ann. Endocrinol.* **17**, 586, 1956). In some preliminary experiments (unpublished) we have produced deciduomata in 4 of 8 oxytocin-treated rats by passing threads through their uteri 6 days after estrus and stimulation of the cervix, as compared to 0 of 6 rats treated in the same way but given no oxytocin injections. These results again suggest a luteotropic response to injected oxytocin in the rat.

Although it has not been possible to produce ovulation in the rabbit by oxytocin injections or by continuous infusion of oxytocin into the carotid artery over a period of 2 hours, there are some indications of increased gonadotropin secretion in the rabbit as a result of oxytocin injections. Armstrong and Hansel (*Internat. J. Fertil.* **3**, 296–306, 1958) have reported increased testis weights and seminiferous tubule diameters, and increased interstitial cell development in immature rabbits injected daily with oxytocin for 11 weeks. Martini *et al.* (*J. Endocrinol.* **18**, 245, 1959) have reported an increased urinary gonadotropin excretion in rabbits injected with oxytocin-containing preparations. Preliminary results indicate that oxytocin injections have no effect on estrous cycle length in normal ewes and guinea-pigs.

One of the most perplexing problems related to this subject has been the apparent lack of specific and repeatable effects of the various ovulation-blocking drugs. This has perhaps been more obvious in our work with cattle than it has been in experiments with other species. Atropine given at the beginning of estrus blocks ovulation in about 75% of the treated animals, but the blockage is temporary and ovulation usually does occur a few days later and in the absence of a second estrus. Concurrent injections of atropine or reserpine reduce the percentage of heifers that respond to daily oxytocin injections by a precocious estrus, but some heifers do have shortened cycles. Results such as these have been difficult to interpret, and may even suggest that the blocking drugs accomplish their effects in some non-specific manner such as by reducing blood flow through the portal vessels. Worthington (*Endocrinology* **66**, 19–31, 1960) has recently reported a reduced blood flow in the portal vessels in the mouse after injections of certain blocking drugs.

The reports of Sawyer and Kawakami are of particular importance in that they provide for the first time a common physiological effect of all the blocking drugs and steroids, i.e. they all elevate the EEG afterreaction threshold. These findings fit many of the known facts and can be used to explain many of our most puzzling experimental results. They are particularly impressive, for example, when applied to our results of experiments on the effects of progesterone on ovulation in the bovine. Small doses of progesterone injected within 2 hours after the beginning of estrus hasten ovulation, presumably by lowering the threshold for the release of pituitary ovulating hormone, so that this event occurs at an earlier than normal time. On the other hand, daily injections of larger amounts of progesterone from the 15th day of the cycle onward delay both estrus and ovulation until 4 to 5 days after cessation of the injections, presumably by maintaining elevated arousal and afterreaction thresholds.

Evidence has been accumulating to suggest that the neurohumors involved in anterior pituitary gonadotropin secretion are of hypothalamic origin, and that the blocking drugs exert their effects at more remote sites in the central nervous system. Perhaps the best of this evidence is Everett's demonstration of ovulation in the atropinized rat in response to electrical stimulation of the preoptic region. These results all suggest that the next major advance in our knowledge of the mechanism of ovulation is very likely to come about as a result of preparing hypothalamic extracts and injecting these into suitably prepared experimental animals, as Harris has already suggested.

THE PREOPTIC REGION OF THE BRAIN AND ITS RELATION TO OVULATION*

JOHN W. EVERETT

NEARLY thirty years ago Hohlweg and Junkmann (23) postulated the existence of a sex center in the hypothalamus. Today there is no doubt that many of the sexual, as well as non-sexual, functions of the adenohypophysis are under control of the central nervous system through the mediation of the hypothalamus and the special neurovascular linkage afforded by the hypophysial portal veins. Theory has moved on and now one postulates multiple mechanisms separately controlling diverse aspects of adenohypophysial function. One may question whether anatomically discrete "centers" exist; there is good reason to think that elements of several mechanisms may be anatomically interwoven and that each may involve an interplay among several parts of the brain.

We are concerned here with only one of these mechanisms and with only one basic method of experimental study, electrical stimulation of the brain. No attempt will be made to review in detail the historical background for the induction of ovulation by this means. It is only necessary to call to mind a series of studies by naming the investigators: Marshall and Verney (28); Haterius and Derbyshire (21); Harris (19, 20); Markee, Sawyer and Hollinshead (27); Kurotzu, Kurachi and Ban (26). Whereas these several investigations were carried out in the rabbit, a species that ovulates "reflexly", more recent studies have shown that ovulation can be induced by similar means in the rat, an animal that normally ovulates spontaneously. The first published record is the abstract of a paper by Critchlow (6), noting that proestrous cycling rats, in which the spontaneous ovulation was prevented by the administration of pentobarbital, could be induced to ovulate by electrical stimulation of the hypothalamus with electrodes resting close above the median eminence. This work was reported in full in 1958 (7). Meanwhile, Bunn and Everett (4) had been successful in inducing ovulation by stimulation of the amygdaloid complex in rats that had been made constant-estrous by continuous illumination.

The experiments that will be reported here are directly based on Critchlow's work, which in turn was based on the work of Everett and Sawyer (13). These

* These investigations were partially supported by grants from the National Science Foundation (G4431 and G9841).

workers had demonstrated that pentobarbital sedation of the cycling rat during a certain "critical period" on the day of proestrus will predictably block the expected ovulation for a 24-hr period. In rats that have been subjected to controlled illumination of 14 hr daily the critical period extends from 2.00 p.m. until after 4.00 p.m. It had first been defined by the use of atropine, a potent and predictable blocking agent for ovulation in both the rabbit and the rat (15, 32, 33).

In the summer of 1958 R. L. Riley and J. W. Everett set out to repeat Critchlow's experiment in a small series of rats, in preparation for attempts to induce ovulation during pseudopregnancy. We were gradually led into exploration of more and more rostral regions, eventually finding that the preoptic area could give more predictable results than had been possible in the tuberal region. We were briefly joined by Dr. C. D. Christian. During the summer of 1959 J. R. Harp joined us and undertook a study of thresholds in the preoptic region.

METHODS

The methods employed can best be described by giving an account of the standardized procedures that were used in the late phases. Departures from these standards will be noted whenever they are of significance.

As in previous investigations in this laboratory we employed rats of an inbred strain derived from Osborne–Mendel stock. The animals were regularly cycling adult females characteristically in the age range of 5 to 10 months and weighing 200 to 250 g. It is our practice to maintain at all times a group of 50 to 70 potential experimental subjects, from which vaginal smears are prepared daily 6 days a week. As animals are removed for experiments, others are added from time to time. Thus we have at all times a large control group. In the selection of an experimental subject it is demanded that she have a vaginal smear history of at least two 4-day cycles or two 5-day cycles in sequence immediately preceding the cycle in progress (9). Unless otherwise stated, it will be understood that subjects in proestrus were 4-day cyclic rats and had just experienced a diestrous interval of 2 days. Subjects said to be in diestrus day 3, on the other hand, were 5-day cyclic rats. Inasmuch as spontaneous "pseudopregnancy" occasionally occurs in this stock, inevitably a few "diestrous" rats turned out to have a leucocytic vaginal smear on the day after experimental treatment. Data from such animals are excluded for present purposes. Unless otherwise specified, all stimulations were confined to the interval between 2.00 and 4.00 p.m. Even on diestrus day 3 it has been shown that sensitivity to progesterone (as an ovulation incitor) is maximal during the afternoon hours (12). Predictability of the hours of the "critical period" is assured by a régime of 14 hr of daily illumination.

All animals were anesthetized with pentobarbital, 35 mg/kg body wt., injected intraperitoneally. In proestrous rats the injection was given at 1.50 to 2.00 p.m. In the diestrous rats, the time of injection was often advanced to 1.30. Sometimes as many as four rats were operated upon during the following two hours and, thus, stimulation of the brain was brought about at necessarily varying intervals after injection of the barbiturate. There were no indications of variable results because of this.

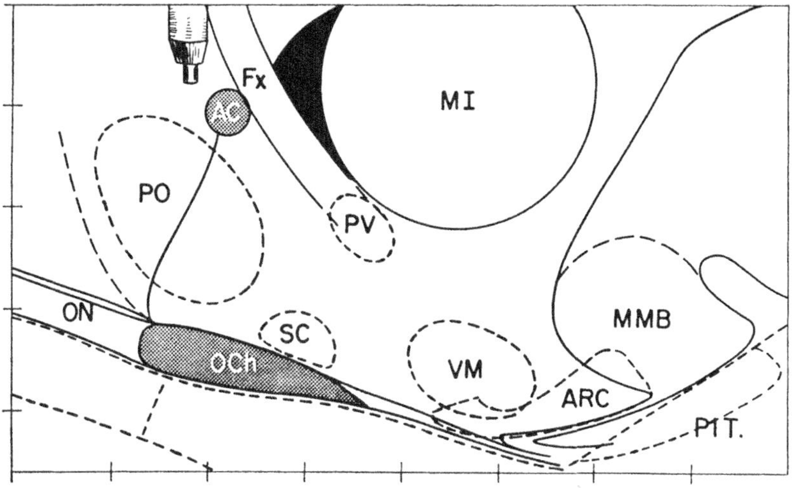

FIG. 1. Diagrammatic representation of the rat hypothalamus in sagittal section, from a camera lucida tracing of a hemisected head. A concentric electrode is drawn to scale at the upper left. Scale markings are in millimeters. The cranial floor and pituitary gland are shown in broken lines, as are the midline projections of several nuclei. Key: AC—anterior commissure, ARC—nucleus arcuatus, FX—fornix, MI—massa intermedia, MMB—mammillary body, OCh—optic chiasma, ON—optic nerve, PIT—pituitary, PO—preoptic nucleus, PV—paraventricular nucleus, SC—suprachiasmatic nucleus, VM—ventromedial nucleus.

While the animal was being placed in the stereotaxic apparatus, brief supplementary anesthesia with ether was administered. This was sufficient to inhibit reaction to exposure of the skull and drilling.

Electrodes were stainless steel 36 gauge wires, Teflon insulated, in 0.40 mm stainless steel tubing insulated with FormVar. Each element was bared at the tip (cf. FIG. 1), and the wire extended slightly beyond the shield (< 0.5 mm). Dual assemblies were prepared by soldering two of the concentric units in parallel to opposite sides of a shaft of steel tubing whose diameter was appropriate to give the desired spacing of 1.2 to 1.5 mm.

The stimulating current was taken from a Grass S-4C stimulator and isolation unit with a 200 kΩ resistor in each lead and with the electrode core anodic. For monitoring current an oscilloscope was connected across a low value resistor in series with one of the leads, and the system was calibrated with a precision microammeter and continuous d.c. current. Unless otherwise stated it will be understood that the stimulus consisted of monophasic, 1-msec pulses, at a frequency of 100/sec, in 30-sec trains at 30-sec intervals.

On the morning after stimulation the reproductive tracts were removed under ether anesthesia. The ampullas and adjacent turns of the oviducts were microscopically explored for ova (9). The ovaries were examined in physiological saline under the dissecting microscope. When fewer than 7 or 8 ova appeared in the ampullas, special attention was paid to the ovaries for signs of partial activation. No rigorous histological search was made, however. The brain was fixed by perfusion of the head with 10% formalin in saline. Paraffin sections were cut at 25 micra and these were subsequently stained by the Luxol fast blue–cresyl fast violet technique.

EXPERIMENTS AND OBSERVATIONS

Exploratory Studies

The early phases of the investigation were reported briefly to the Endocrine Society (11). These experiments are of interest at the present time largely because they eventually led us to explore the region between the rostral margin of the optic chiasma and the anterior commissure. The technique was at first relatively crude: the electrodes were comparatively coarse and stimulation parameters were quite different from those described above. The pulse duration was unnecessarily long (15 msec at 30/sec), as was the over-all period of stimulation, alternate 30 sec for 30 min. Voltages were not excessive, ranging from 3 to 5.

There were 29 proestrous rats in which electrode tips rested within 2 mm above the floor of the diencephalon or preoptic region (Series I). Sixteen rats ovulated during the following night. In 6 cases the electrodes lay in the preoptic region and 5 of the 6 ovulated, a fact that was especially interesting because of the implication from Critchlow's study that the electrodes must be close to the median eminence to be effective under pentobarbital anesthesia. Figure 1 shows the preoptic nucleus projected on the mid-sagittal plane of the rat brain.

Advanced Ovulation in Diestrous Rats

In rats that experience regular 5-day cycles the time of ovulation can be advanced 24 hr by injection of progesterone on the third day of diestrus (9). This effect, like spontaneous ovulation, is subject to blockade by atropine and is presumably mediated through the central nervous system (12). The latter study demonstrated that during the afternoon of diestrus day 3 there is a limited period of sensitivity to progesterone approximately 24 hr in advance of the "critical period" on the day of proestrus. There was thus excellent reason to expect that electrical stimulation of the hypothalamus in late diestrus would induce ovulation one day early, especially if the stimulus was administered during the late afternoon.

With techniques like those in Series I, 25 rats were stimulated on the third day of diestrus during 5-day cycles (Series II). In fact these two sets of experiments were carried out in parallel. Nine of the 25 rats ovulated during the night following stimulation and, significantly, among them were all 6 rats that had been stimulated in the preoptic region. When considered with the results in the proestrus series, these observations demonstrated that in this region one can work with a high degree of predictability.

To supplement the preliminary findings of Series II, 9 rats were stimulated on diestrus day 3 with dual concentric electrodes placed in the preoptic area (Series III). Parameters of stimulation were modified as follows: pulses of 1 msec, 100/sec, 30 sec on and off for 10 min. Voltage dial readings ranged from 1.5 to 4.0. Series resistors were not employed. Ovulation was induced in the 5 rats that were stimulated with voltages of 2.8 or more. Negative results were obtained with 2.5 volts or less.

A normal number of eggs was shed in 8 of the 9 ovulated rats of Series II and in all 5 of the ovulated rats of Series III. The exceptional animal produced only one tubal ovum. The ovaries closely resembled those normally found on the morning after spontaneous ovulation. The uteri were characteristically contracted in the animals that had shed the full complement of ova, whereas in the anovulatory specimens distended uteri were the rule. The vaginal smears of all animals, whether ovulation had occurred or not, were of the proestrous type. There was no evidence that the release of ovulating hormone modified the vaginal sequence in any degree.

Comparative Thresholds, Diestrus vs. Proestrus

The next step was to determine, if possible, whether any difference in threshold to electrical stimulation could be detected between late diestrus and proestrus. It seemed especially appropriate to compare proestrus in the 4-day cycle with the third day of diestrus in the 5-day cycle. Earlier work (12, 13) had suggested that in the latter type of animal a physiological block delays the spontaneous ovulating stimulus to the pituitary 24 hr longer than in the 4-day cyclic rat.

It was decided to monitor all stimuli for current by use of the oscilloscope. A further change in circuitry was the introduction of the 200 kΩ resistors in the electrode leads to give a rectangular pattern on the oscilloscope screen. In the absence of the resistors electrode capacitance creates a wave form that is difficult to evaluate, with a high initial spike that falls logarithmically to the end of the pulse and a negative spike after the break.

Two series of experiments were carried out, Series IV-A by James Harp and Series IV-B by J. W. Everett. The two series will be presented in parallel.

Stimulus parameters were identical in respect to pulse duration (1 msec) and frequency (100/sec). The differences were as follows: In IV-A, the dual electrode assembly was employed, the stimulus isolation unit was not used, and the over-all stimulation period was 10 min. In IV-B, the single concentric electrode and the isolation unit were employed, and stimulation lasted for only 5 min. In IV-A there were 50 rats, equally divided between diestrus and proestrus. In IV-B there were 21 rats in groups of 10 and 11, respectively.

TABLE 1. RESULTS OF PREOPTIC STIMULATION RELATIVE TO CURRENT AND TO STAGE OF THE ESTROUS CYCLE

Current, μA	Diestrus*	Proestrus*
A. 100	+	
70–75	+++	
60–65	+++++00	++
50	++++0000	+++++
40	+++000	++++0
30		++000
20		++0000
B. 70–75	++000	
50	00000	++++++
40		++000

* Each + and 0 indicates a rat with or without tubal ova.

Table 1 summarizes the results. The two sets of experiments point to a real difference between diestrus and proestrus. In IV-A alone there is a considerable overlap and comparisons of the 40–50 μA categories in the two columns (7/14 vs. 11/12) or of the 50–65 μA categories (9/15 vs. 10/10) show that in neither case is the difference between the ratios significant at the 5% level.* In IV-B, however, the difference between 6/6 and 0/5 in the 50 μA categories is significant at 1%*.

Statistics are perhaps less convincing, however, than the fact that the data from both IV-A and IV-B trend distinctly in the same direction. It seems especially noteworthy that in IV-B currents of 70–75 μA were less uniformly effective in diestrous rats than were currents of 50 μA in proestrous rats.

Effects of Various Parameters

At this point it is appropriate to discuss the effect of variation of the several parameters of stimulation (Series V): *frequency*, *pulse duration*, *current* and *total time*. The survey is still far from exhaustive and will be extended from time to time. It has two objectives: (1) to find an effective combination that produces minimum brain damage, for subsequent use with indwelling

* The estimates of significance were obtained by use of the tables of Mainland and Murray (*Science* **116**, 591, 1952).

electrodes, and (2) to determine the shortest over-all time of stimulation that will be predictably effective.

Table 2 lists some of the combinations that were tried. The animals represented were all 4-day cyclic rats in proestrus, with a single concentric electrode in the preoptic region. For purposes of later discussion attention is called to the first three lines of the table, which clearly show that a stimulus of no longer than 60 sec can be fully effective. The one positive case among

TABLE 2. RESULTS OF CERTAIN MODIFICATIONS OF THE PARAMETERS OF STIMULATION

Pulses per sec	Pulse duration	Current, μA	Time	Coulombs $\times 10^{-4}$	Result*
	msec		continuous		
100	1	100	90 sec	9.0	++
100	1	100	60 sec	6.0	+++
100	1	100	15–20 sec	1.5–2.0	+000
			on and off		
100	0.5	50	5 min	3.75	0
100	0.5	50	10 min	7.5	0
100	0.5	100	10 min	15.0	+
100	0.25	100	5 min	3.75	0
100	0.25	200	5 min	7.5	+
50	1	50	5 min	3.75	+0
300	0.3	50	5 min	6.75	+

* Each + or 0 indicates a rat with or without tubal ova.

the four in which the stimulus lasted only 15–20 sec was only a partial ovulation (5 tubal ova). The 60-sec examples constitute clear evidence of a triggering action.

In addition to the sets of parameters given in the remainder of Table 2 there are those used in Series I and II, a pulse frequency of 30/sec and pulse duration of 15 msec. Ovulation has thus been evoked, at least in some cases, by pulse frequencies of 30–300/sec, pulse durations of 0.25–15 msec, currents as low as 20 μA and stimulation periods as short as 15 sec. Any statement about the relative amounts of brain damage associated with the various combinations of parameters would be premature at this time, inasmuch as not all of the brains have been examined histologically.

Atropine Experiments

Experiments which pertain to the site of action of atropine as an agent blocking the release of ovulating hormone (Series VI) were carried out by J. R. Harp. The 11 subjects were 4-day cyclic rats in proestrus. Pentobarbital in the usual amount was given at 1.30 p.m. and was followed about 15 min later by a subcutaneous injection of atropine sulfate (350 mg/kg) in physiological saline. Everett and Sawyer (14) had shown that this dosage of atropine is uniformly effective in blocking spontaneous ovulation. We are indebted to Dr. C. D. Christian for determining that the combination of pentobarbital and atropine is non-lethal.

The dual electrode assembly was employed and, again, the site of stimulation was the preoptic region. Stimulus parameters were like those in Series IV-A. Current varied from 50 to 150 μA (Table 3).

TABLE 3. PREOPTIC STIMULATION UNDER THE COMBINED INFLUENCE OF PENTOBARBITAL AND ATROPINE

Current, μA	Results*
150	+++
65	++0
50	++++0
controls	0000000

* Each + and 0 indicates a rat with or without tubal ova.

The result was clear cut. All but two of the rats ovulated. Eight other animals served as controls to show that the ovulations could not have been the result of mutual counteraction of the drugs. All control animals were treated with pentobarbital and atropine in the same manner as were the experimental subjects; two of the group were subjected to stimulation (65 μA), but the electrodes lay outside the intended location.

DISCUSSION

Without question the preoptic region of the rat remains sensitive to electrical stimulation in spite of pentobarbital anesthesia, and as we have just seen, in spite of the blocking action of atropine as well. Examination of Critchlow's (7) diagram discloses three cases in which the electrode tips were near the anterior end of the optic chiasma in a basal location; two were positive. Although the electrode loci are represented in sagittal projection within the chiasma itself, they presumably rested in the diagonal band on either side of it. In many of our own cases the electrodes have also impinged on the diagonal band. Yet they were often just as effective when placed more dorsally.

Pentobarbital is thought to affect chiefly the multisynaptic pathways such as those within the reticular system (2, 17). Sawyer, Critchlow and Barraclough (31) reported that pentobarbital, atropine and morphine, in doses adequate for blocking ovulation in the rat, all have similar action in depressing the extralemniscal reticuloactivating system. Critchlow later observed that lesions which selectively destroy the mammillary peduncle tend to block ovulation in rats, supposedly by destroying the fibers of that system which ascend into the posterior hypothalamus. Sawyer, Critchlow and Barraclough proposed that the reticular formation may act permissively upon hypothalamic mechanisms that are more specifically in control of the release of ovulating hormone from the hypophysis. It would be interesting to test the effect of interrupting the mammillary peduncle on the results of preoptic stimulation. Very possibly such lesions would have no more effect than the addition of atropine to the pentobarbital-blocked rat. The present data from experiments with atropine indicate that the introduction of this second "blocking agent" does not elevate the preoptic threshold above that seen with pentobarbital alone.

Unavoidably the stimulation experiments supply no firm assurance that the preoptic region normally plays any role in ovulation. It is within the realm of possibility that stimulating that part of the brain simply transmits impulses back to the tuberal region by fibers that do not ordinarily function in this way. One is reminded of Sawyer's observation (30) in rabbits subjected to the combination of histamine and a low dose of pentobarbital, which set up a characteristic pattern of electrical activity in the rhinencephalon. This was followed by ovulation. Under these extraordinary circumstances the olfactory bulbs and their connections to the hypothalamus were essential participants, whereas in coitally-induced ovulation the olfactory bulbs can be spared (3). Although the fact is generally recognized that bilateral lesions in the anterior hypothalamus characteristically result in constant estrus in rats (1, 16, 18, 22, 25, 34) as well as in the guinea-pig (8), it is also recognized that ovulatory cycles can be restored in such animals by the administration of progesterone. Studies by Kawakami and Sawyer (24) demonstrate that in rabbits the effects of progesterone are widespread within the brain, influencing thresholds in the mid-brain reticular system, hypothalamus and rhinencephalon. Greer (18) reported that many of his lesioned, progesterone-treated rats not only regained cyclic function while they were receiving the steroid, but continued to cycle after treatment was withheld. Thus, it appears that if cells and/or fibers of transit within the preoptic region do take part in the normal process of pro-ovulatory stimulation of the adenohypophysis their roles are not obligatory.

In the face of this uncertainty, we can nevertheless make use of the preoptic region in several ways. The data at hand bring out several new points of interest. It is now adequately demonstrated that on diestrus day 3 of the 5-day cycle the hypophysis is already prepared to release the full quota of ovulating hormone and will do so whenever it receives the necessary signal from the nervous system. The physiological "block" that ordinarily delays ovulation in these rats for another 24 hr is some factor operating within the central nervous system. That factor manifests itself in the elevated preoptic threshold of the diestrous rat. With fair certainty the prediction can be made that when put to the test progesterone or estrogen supplements will bring the diestrus threshold to the proestrus level.

The 60-sec stimulations in Series V, even better than the 5-min stimulations of Series IV, display a triggering effect. Closely allied with this may be the all-or-none effect observed at threshold levels of stimulation in Series IV. Heretofore it had been thought that in the rat, quite unlike the rabbit, the neural mechanisms that provoke release of ovulating hormone operate continuously in an obligatory way during the half-hour or so occupied in the discharge of the hormone (10, 14). That view was based on results of atropine injection at various times during the "critical period". Numerous cases of only partial interference with ovulation were encountered, as well as the cases of complete blockade or complete ovulation. The proportion of partial effects was strikingly like that observed in a parallel series of partial hypophysectomies during the critical period. On the other hand, the administration of a threshold dose of atropine before the critical period in another group of rats resulted in an essentially all-or-none response. Thus, it seemed that the partial effects obtained during the critical period either by the full dose of atropine or by hypophysectomy must have been the result of interruption of the discharge of ovulating hormone already in progress. The frequency of the partial effects indicated that the atropine-sensitive component must act for at least 10 min, and more likely about half an hour. Although circumstantial evidence led to the conclusion that the site of action of atropine lies in the central nervous system, there was no direct proof that this applied to this species. It was necessary to fall back on the proof furnished by experiments in the rabbit (33). There remained a shade of doubt, therefore. Because of species differences and the pronounced differences in dosage and route of administration, it was still possible that in rats there might be a direct blocking action on the hypophysial cells. The doubt has now been dispelled.

At the same time, however, the new experiments present us with a paradox. It is now evident that a triggering stimulus of 60 sec or less can be effective although it operates upon a part of the system less remote from the median eminence than the blocking sites of pentobarbital and atropine. It thus becomes necessary to inquire what happens within the hypothalamus in response to the trigger. Does it set up some prolonged electrical activity? This should be readily subject to direct test.

Finally, attention must be called to observations by Christian (5) who noted ovulation in 5 estrous rabbits that ovulated after electrical stimulation of the preoptic region, in spite of the fact that they had been pretreated with atropine in amounts adequate to block the ovulation reflex. Saul and Sawyer (29) reported negative results from similar experiments, stating that stimulations in the preoptic area were "completely ineffective". Christian's observations are now amply confirmed.

SUMMARY

The preoptic region, in spite of pentobarbital anesthesia and relative distance from the median eminence, remains highly sensitive to electrical stimulation.

Stimulation of the preoptic region on diestrus day 3 will advance ovulation approximately 24 hr.

The preoptic threshold is lower on the day of proestrus than on diestrus day 3. Approximately similar results were obtained with (*a*) dual concentric electrodes, no isolation, a 10-min stimulation period, and (*b*) single concentric electrode, with isolation, and a 5-min stimulation period.

Preoptic stimulation under pentobarbital anesthesia will readily induce ovulation in proestrous rats that have been given atropine in an amount adequate by itself to block ovulation.

Exploratory study with varied parameters has given positive results in proestrous rats with pulse frequencies of 30 to 300/sec, pulse durations of 0.25 to 15 msec, currents as little as 20 μA and stimulation periods as short as 60 sec (100/sec, 1 msec, 100 μA, single electrode). In controls with no current, results were negative.

The data on the ineffectiveness of atropine show that the atropine-sensitive components of the LH-release mechanism are more remote from the median eminence than are the elements that can be activated by electrical stimulation of the preoptic region.

COMMENT ADDED IN PROOF

Since this paper was presented, a direct correlation has been found between positive results and the amount of electricity introduced, without evident relationship to other parameters. In histologic sections of the brains, areas of mild electrolytic damage were observed about the electrode tips in all animals that ovulated. In negative cases, on the other hand, there was often no apparent electrolysis; when it did exist the volume of affected tissue averaged much less than in positive cases. Subsequently, good results have consistently been obtained by use of a *direct current* of 100 μA for 30 sec or less, whereas control lesions of comparable dimensions produced by high-frequency electrocautery have been ineffective. Thus, it seems that the positive effect stems from chemical changes caused by the electrolysis. Doubtlessly the irritative effects of the electrolysis persist long after the current is turned off. This eliminates the paradox mentioned with respect to the atropine experiments, but complicates interpretation of the difference in "threshold" between diestrous and proestrous rats.

REFERENCES

1. ALLOITEAU, J. J., *Compt. rend. Soc. biol.* **148**, 875, 1954.
2. ARDUINI, A. and M. G. ARDUINI, *J. Pharmacol. & Exper. Therap.* **110**, 76, 1954.
3. BROOKS, C. McC., *Amer. J. Physiol.* **120**, 544, 1937.
4. BUNN, J. P. and J. W. EVERETT, *Proc. Soc. Exper. Biol. & Med.* **96**, 369, 1957.
5. CHRISTIAN, C. D. and J. E. MARKEE, *Anat. Rec.* **127**, 403, 1957 (Abstract).
6. CRITCHLOW, B. V., *Anat. Rec.* **127**, 283, 1957 (Abstract).
7. CRITCHLOW, V., *Amer. J. Physiol.* **195**, 171, 1958.
8. DEY, F. L., *Amer. J. Anat.* **69**, 61, 1941.
9. EVERETT, J. W., *Endocrinology* **43**, 389, 1948.
10. EVERETT, J. W., *Endocrinology* **59**, 580, 1956.
11. EVERETT, J. W., R. L. RILEY and C. D. CHRISTIAN, *Proc. of the Endocrine Society*, Atlantic City, N.J., June 1959.
12. EVERETT, J. W. and C. H. SAWYER, *Endocrinology* **45**, 581, 1949.
13. EVERETT, J. W. and C. H. SAWYER, *Endocrinology* **47**, 198, 1950.
14. EVERETT, J. W. and C. H. SAWYER, *Endocrinology* **52**, 83, 1953.
15. EVERETT, J. W., C. H. SAWYER and J. E. MARKEE, *Endocrinology* **44**, 234, 1949.
16. FLERKÓ, B. and V. BARDOS, *Acta neurovegetativa* **20**, 248, 1959.
17. FRENCH, J. D., M. VERZEANO and H. W. MAGOUN, *A.M.A. Arch. Neurol. & Psychiatr.* **69**, 519, 1953.
18. GREER, M. A., *Endocrinology* **53**, 380, 1953.
19. HARRIS, G. W., *Proc. Roy. Soc., London*, Series B, **122**, 374, 1937.
20. HARRIS, G. W., *J. Physiol.* **107**, 418, 1948.
21. HATERIUS, H. O. and A. J. DERBYSHIRE, JR., *Amer. J. Physiol.* **119**, 329, 1937.
22. HILLARP, N.-Å., *Acta endocrinol.* **2**, 11, 1949.
23. HOHLWEG, W. and K. JUNKMANN, *Klin. Wchnschr.* **11**, 321, 1932.
24. KAWAKAMI, M. and C. H. SAWYER, *Endocrinology* **65**, 652, 1959.
25. KOBAYASHI, T., S. HIROSHI, M. MARUYAMA, K. ARAI and S. TAKEZAWA, *Endocrinol. Japonica* **6**, 107, 1959.
26. KUROTZU, T., K. KURACHI and T. BAN, *Med. J. Osaka Univ.* **2**, 1, 1950.
27. MARKEE, J. E., C. H. SAWYER and W. H. HOLLINSHEAD, *Endocrinology* **38**, 345, 1946.
28. MARSHALL, F. H. A. and E. B. VERNEY, *J. Physiol.* **86**, 327, 1936.
29. SAUL, G. D. and C. H. SAWYER, *Federation Proc.* **16**, 112, 1957.
30. SAWYER, C. H., *Amer. J. Physiol.* **180**, 37, 1955.
31. SAWYER, C. H., B. V. CRITCHLOW and C. A. BARRACLOUGH, *Endocrinology* **57**, 345, 1955.
32. SAWYER, C. H., J. W. EVERETT and J. E. MARKEE, *Endocrinology* **44**, 218, 1949.
33. SAWYER, C. H., J. E. MARKEE and B. F. TOWNSEND, *Endocrinology* **44**, 18, 1949.
34. VAN DYKE, D. C., M. E. SIMPSON, S. LEPKOVSKY, A. A. KONEFF and J. R. BROBECK, *Proc. Soc. Exper. Biol. & Med.* **95**, 1, 1957.

DISCUSSIONS

Charles A. Barraclough: One of the principal difficulties encountered in an investigation of the neural factors concerned with the control of ovulation in the rat is the fact that this species ovulates spontaneously. Thus, the general approach used in investigations of this phenomenon has been to study factors which will inhibit ovulation and to correlate such inhibition with the destruction or depression of specific regions in the central nervous system. Another method of study has been described by Dr. Everett this morning in which the natural stimulus for ovulation is blocked by pentobarbital anesthesia and ovulation is then induced by electrical stimulation of various hypothalamic areas. Although this latter procedure permits a more accurate localization of the regions of the hypothalamus concerned with the ovulatory discharge of gonadotropin from the adenohypophysis, under these conditions the factor of central nervous depression with a drug is still present.

In our investigations we have used a preparation which does not require prior inhibition of ovulation to study central nervous control of ovulation, the androgen-sterilized rat. In previous studies we observed that administration of a single subcutaneous injection of 1.0 mg of testosterone propionate to the 5-day-old rat resulted in permanent sterility (Barraclough, C. A., *Anat. Rec.* **130**, 267, 1958). When autopsied at 100 days of age, the ovaries of these animals contained numerous large vesicular follicles as well as follicles in various other stages of development, but ovulation had not occurred and corpora lutea were absent (Figs. 1 and 2). Furthermore, these ovaries secrete estrogen as evidenced by the persistence of a cornified vaginal mucosa. Seemingly the particular malfunction in adenohypophysial gonadotropin secretion of the sterile rat does not reside in the inability of this gland to secrete FSH or LH (ICSH) but rather in the failure of this gland to release gonadotropin in sufficient quantity to cause ovulation, a function controlled by the hypothalamus. Thus, it may be that androgen administration during infancy alters hypothalamic-hypophysial interrelationships by rendering the hypothalamic areas responsible for the ovulatory discharge of gonadotropin refractory to intrinsic activation. As such, the proper impetus for the ovulatory release of gonadotropin is not supplied to the adenohypophysis and sterility ensues. To test this hypothesis, experiments were designed to determine whether the pituitary of the sterile rat would respond to hypothalamic activation by discharging sufficient gonadotropin to cause ovulation. Six adult sterile rats (235–250 gm body wt.) were given an intraperitoneal injection of 25 mg/kg of pentobarbital sodium. This dosage was selected as it does not block ovulation in the normal cyclic rat nor the stress-induced discharge of ACTH, but will keep the animals sufficiently subdued to be placed in a stereotaxis apparatus. In these rats, bipolar concentric electrodes were stereotaxically oriented in the median eminence region of the hypothalamus and stimulation was performed in this and subsequent experiments using the following parameters: 100 μA current delivered at a frequency of 100/sec with a duration of 1 msec, for 15-sec on/off periods over a 15-min total period. These parameters were selected as they had been shown previously by Critchlow (*Amer. J. Physiol.* **195**, 171, 1958) to be effective in inducing ovulation in the Nembutal-blocked rat, and they are quite similar to the parameters reported by Dr. Everett in his studies. At autopsy, 24 hr after stimulation, the Fallopian tubes were examined for the presence of ova and the ovaries for corpora lutea. All autopsy results and electrode placements were confirmed histologically. Under these circumstances, electrical stimulation of the median eminence failed to induce ovulation. However, considering the ovarian–pituitary axis of the persistent-estrous rat, in which pituitary gonadotropin is being released in response to the constant blood levels of estrogen, the possibility

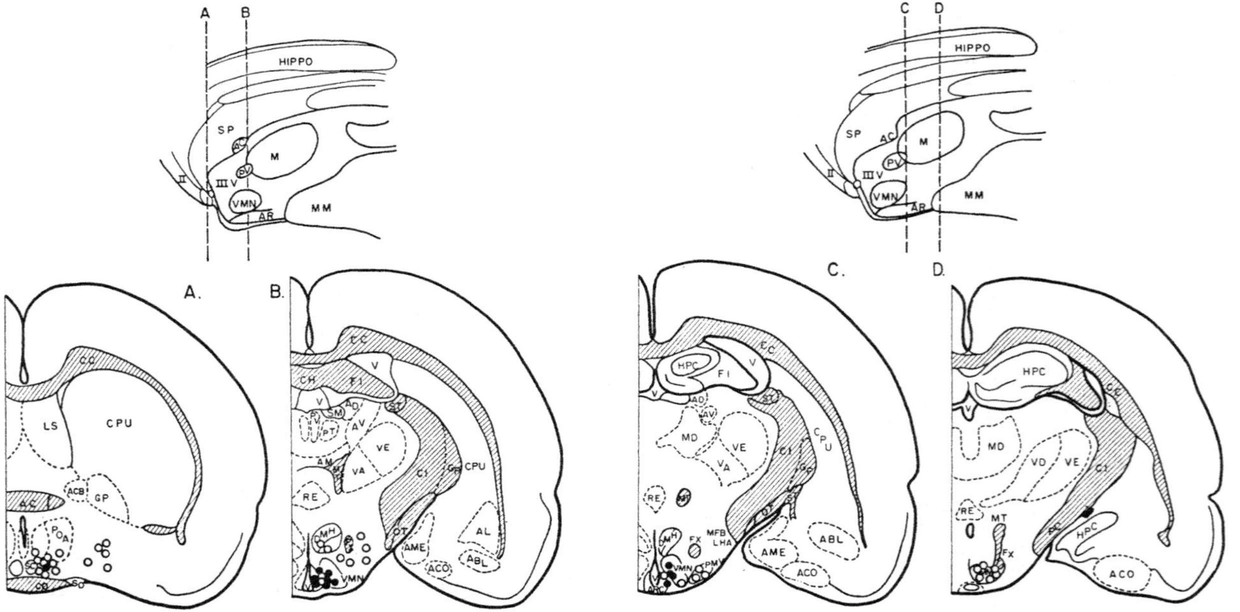

FIGS. 4, 5. Midsagittal and coronal sections of rat hypothalamus indicating points of stimulation. *Closed circles* indicate points where stimulation caused ovulation. *Open circles* represent areas where ovulation failed to occur on stimulation. Abbreviations used in this and subsequent figures: AC, Anterior commissure; ACB, Area parolfactoria lateralis; AR, Arcuate nucleus; CC, Corpus callosum; CPU, Nucleus caudatus/Putamen; CO, Optic chiasm; DMH, Dorsal medial nucleus; FX, Fornix; GP, Globus pallidus; LS, Lateral septal nucleus; MM, Medial mammillary nucleus; MT, Mammillothalamic tract; POA, Preoptic area; SC, Suprachiasmatic nucleus; SO, Supraoptic nucleus; V, Ventricle; VMN, Ventral medial nucleus.

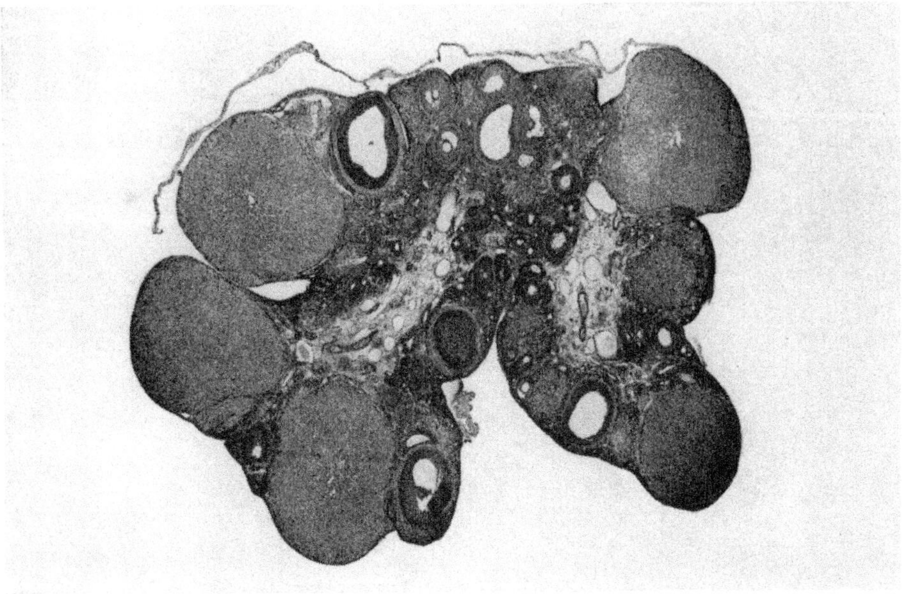

FIG. 1. Normal rat ovary at 100 days of age.

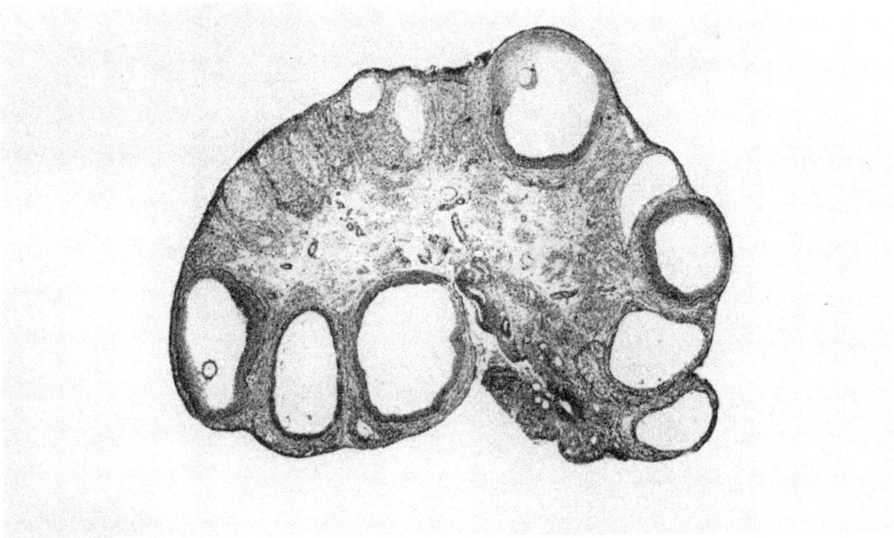

FIG. 2. Ovary of rat injected with 1.0 mg of testosterone propionate at 5 days of age and autopsied at 100 days of age.

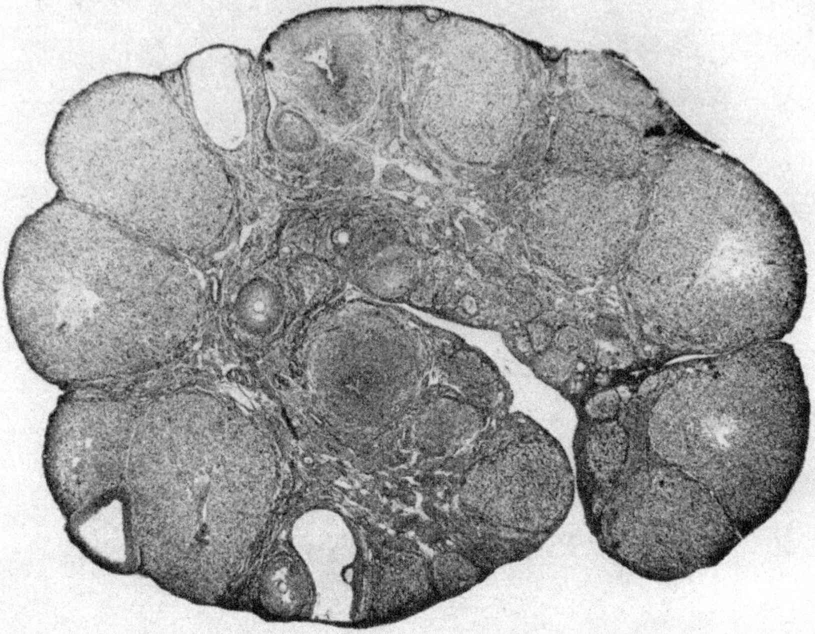

FIG. 3. Ovary of progesterone-primed, androgen-sterilized rat following median eminence stimulation on the day of proestrus.

existed that insufficient concentrations of gonadotropin were stored in the pituitary to cause ovulation when released on hypothalamic stimulation. In order to assure sufficient gonadotropin storage, six sterile rats were pretreated with progesterone in a dosage calculated to block the secretion of gonadotropin (2 mg s.c. in oil). This dosage of progesterone interrupted the persistent vaginal cornification and generally induced 3 days of diestrus followed by a single day of proestrus. When no further treatment was given, all rats returned to the persistent-estrous condition. If, however, the median eminence was stimulated on the day of proestrus, ovulation occurred in all animals (FIG. 3). Progesterone alone did not cause ovulation. It is apparent, therefore, that the sterile rat pituitary can function normally provided (*a*) proper gonadotropin storage is permitted and (*b*) an impetus for its release is *supplied* by the hypothalamus.

Once assured that the progesterone-primed sterile rat could be induced to ovulate on hypothalamic activation, we made a more specific study of the hypothalamic

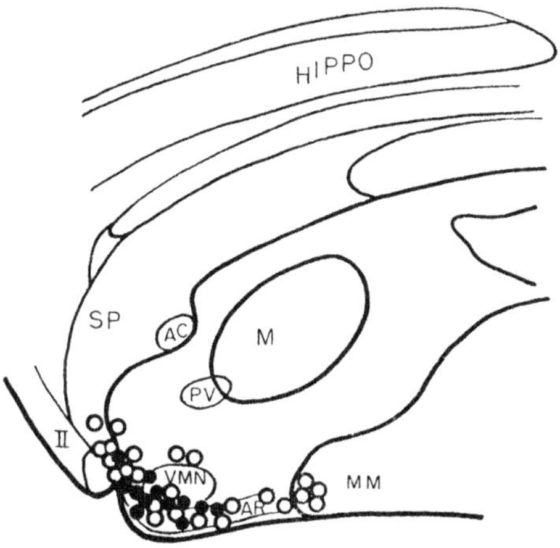

FIG. 6. Midsagittal reconstruction of rat hypothalamus indicating extent of area which when stimulated resulted in ovulation. Abbreviations: Hippo, Hippocampus; M, Massa intermedia; PV, Paraventricular nucleus; SP, Septum; II, Optic nerve.

regions which would cause ovulation when stimulated. In this preparation, the positive areas were found to occupy an area just rostral and caudal to the ventral medial and arcuate nuclei (FIGS. 4, 5, 6). Stimulation of the medial or lateral preoptic areas or the mammillary body regions did not induce ovulation nor did stimulation of the lateral hypothalamic or median forebrain bundle regions. These results are contrasted to those of Everett in which ovulation could readily be induced by stimulation of the preoptic area. This discrepancy raises several questions: (*a*) It has been demonstrated that the malfunction in the ovulatory mechanism of the androgen-sterilized rat is not resident in the adenohypophysis as such, but more likely at the hypothalamic level. Does the failure of the preoptic region of this animal to induce ovulation in response to stimulation indicate the site of "masculinization"? (*b*) What specific structures are being stimulated in the preoptic area to cause adenohypophysial activation in the normal rat? The amygdala is known to contribute efferent fibers via the stria terminalis to the hypothalamus and it has also been implicated in the control of ovulation. Is it this tract which is being stimulated, and if so can ovulation be induced by preoptic stimulation in animals with amygdaloid lesions in which fiber tract degeneration (stria terminalis) has occurred? With regard to the first question we have obtained some recent data which would further tend to support the hypothesis that the anterior hypothalamic area is the site of the deleterious androgen action.

The biphasic action of progesterone in first facilitating and then inhibiting the discharge of gonadotropin in the rat is well recognized. Everett (*Endocrinology* **43**, 389, 1948) has demonstrated that administration of progesterone to a normal cyclic

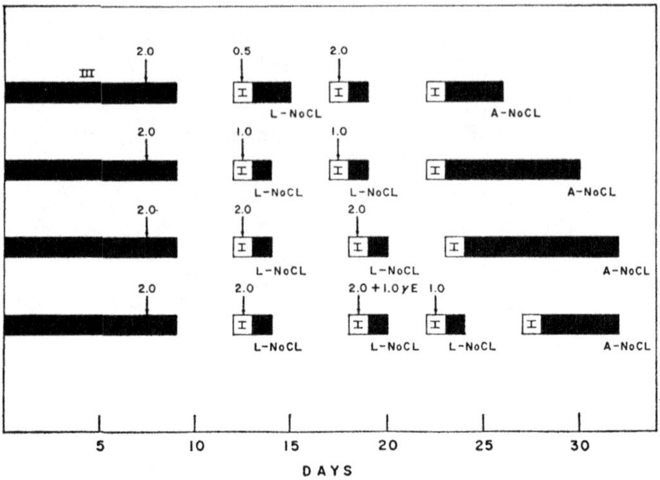

FIG. 7. Effects of spaced injections of progesterone on vaginal cycle of androgen-sterilized, persistent-estrous rat. Abbreviations used in this and FIG. 8: I, Proestrus; III, Estrus; L, Laparotomy; CL, Corpora lutea; A, Autopsy. Solid bars indicate persistent vaginal cornification; blank spaces represent days of diestrus.

rat on the last day of diestrus will advance ovulation one day. Spaced injections of progesterone when administered to the spontaneous persistent-estrous rat (DBN strain) will likewise induce ovulation (Everett, J. W., *Endocrinology* **32**, 285, 1943). We have attempted also to ovulate the androgen-sterilized rat by either spaced or daily injections of progesterone. Following the procedure described by Everett (1943) for the induction of ovulation in the spontaneous persistent-estrous rat, single "interrupting" dosages of 2.0 mg of progesterone were administered to each of 4 groups of 8 adult sterile rats. This injection generally resulted in a 3-day period of diestrus followed by one day of proestrus at which time a second "ovulatory" dose of progesterone was administered. Laparotomy was ordinarily performed 48 hr after the second injection, at which time the ovaries were examined for the presence of corpora lutea. Regardless of the dosage used, ovulation did not occur (FIG. 7). These results were confirmed at autopsy by histological examination of all ovaries. In a second series of experiments a single "interrupting" dose of 2.0 mg of progesterone was administered to each of 4 groups of 8 animals. Following this single injection, daily subcutaneous injections of either 0.25, 0.5, 1.0, or 2.0 mg were given to one or the other of the four groups for a 3-to 4-week period. Twenty-four to 48 hr after the last injection, the animals were sacrificed and the ovaries examined for the presence of corpora lutea. The effects of such treatment on the vaginal cycles are summarized in FIG. 8. Although the vaginal cycles could be restored with the lower dosages, ovulation did not occur in any of the groups studied.

These results suggest that progesterone does not facilitate ovulation by a direct action on the adenohypophysis. As demonstrated previously, the pituitary of the sterile rat, following the "interrupting" dose of progesterone, stores sufficient gonadotropin to be released on hypothalamic stimulation and cause ovulation. However, ovulation did not occur in any of the progesterone experiments regardless of the dosage employed. This would tend to support the hypothesis that progesterone facilitates ovulation in the rat by its action on the hypothalamus, perhaps in a fashion described by Kawakami and Sawyer (*Endocrinology* **65**, 631, 1959) for the rabbit.

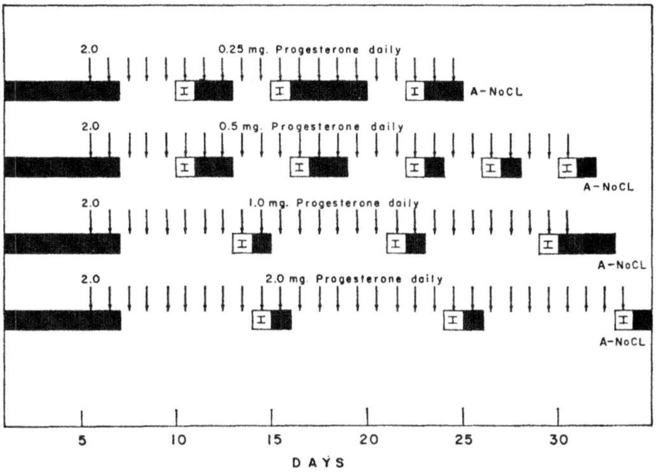

FIG. 8. Effect of daily injections of progesterone on the vaginal cycle of the androgen-sterilized, persistent-estrous rat.

The data further implicate the anterior regions of the hypothalamus as the specific sites of progesterone action. Thus, prepubertal treatment of rats with androgen may not only render the preoptic areas of the hypothalamus refractory to electrical stimulation but to progesterone as well. Further evidence suggesting that progesterone may exert its action at the preoptic area has been presented by Greer (*Endocrinology* **53**, 380, 1953) and Van Dyke *et al.* (*Proc. Soc. Exp. Biol. Med.* **95**, 1, 1956) who reported that rats in which ovulation had been interrupted by anterior hypothalamic lesions would not ovulate in response to progesterone.

These data, although in contrast to the observation reported by Everett for the normal rat, do support the hypothesis that the preoptic region of the rat may be the critical site for control of ovulation.

This work was supported by Grant Number RG-5496 from the United States Public Health Service.

CHAIRMAN NELSON: We shall now have a period of general discussion. I think perhaps I would like to call on Dr. Folley to contribute such remarks as he wishes to the discussion this morning.

DR. S. JOHN FOLLEY: First, may I say what I should have said yesterday afternoon, when Dr. Greep called on me. I want to express my sincere thanks to the appropriate people who made it possible for me to come all the way from England to be present at this wonderful meeting. It is particularly fortunate that arrangements could be made to hold it in such magnificent surroundings which provide a wellnigh perfect environment for the discussion of a specialized subject by a small group such as this. I regard it as a great privilege to be here.

I feel that I should do something to justify my presence by making a few remarks now regarding what we have heard this morning. We have had some most fascinating papers which fully maintained the high standards set by the papers yesterday afternoon.

I was most interested in Dr. Sawyer's paper, and in this connection I would like to refer to some observations on the ewe, which were reported in *Nature* last August by Raeside and McDonald (*Nature* **184**, 388, 1959), which seem to fit in very well with his conclusions. As you know, the ewe is a seasonal breeder and these workers investigated the threshold doses of estrogen required to induce estrus in spayed ewes primed with progesterone. They found that less estrogen was required for this response during the breeding season than during anestrum. This would seem to point to the existence of a built-in rhythmic variation in the sensitivity of the so-called hypothalamic "sexual center" which controls estrous behavior. On the other hand, the threshold doses of estrogen necessary to induce characteristic changes in the chemical properties of the cervical mucus were the same regardless of whether the treatment was given during the breeding or non-breeding season. Thus peripheral responses to estrogen appear to be constant irrespective of season.

Coming to Dr. Hansel's contribution, which interested me a great deal, I find it very difficult to reconcile his results with those of other workers and of ourselves on small animals. I think it is true to say that in laboratory animals, certainly rats and rabbits, the experiments with oxytocin almost exclusively point to the release of prolactin rather than gonadotropin. The best known exception is provided by the results reported in Japan by Shibusawa and his collaborators who claim that oxytocin releases gonadotropins as judged by an increased excretion of 17-ketosteroids in the urine. Dr. Hansel himself, in a recent review, has ably discussed the Japanese results and I thought he dealt with them admirably without appearing to be unduly critical. Obviously, as Dr. Hansel pointed out, we cannot accept these results without further confirmation. This being so, I think the balance of evidence from experiments on small animals would appear, at least to me, to indicate that oxytocin, rather than releasing gonadotropins, evokes the release of LTH, by which I mean prolactin. How then can Dr. Hansel's interesting results be reconciled with this conclusion? We know, as he made clear, that in the cow uterine interferences of various kinds almost invariably cause the release of oxytocin. In passing, it might be interesting in this connection to recall a curious custom practised by the women of certain primitive tribes in Africa when they milk their cows. The custom is to blow into the vagina of the cow just before milking, thus inflating it with air. This seems to favor the occurrence of the milk-ejection reflex which, as you know, involves the release of oxytocin. To return to our main theme, I cannot help wondering whether Dr. Hansel's results might not be due to the presence of some polypeptide, different from oxytocin but chemically related to it, which might have been present in the preparations he used. In any event, I was interested in his suggestion that administered oxytocin might feed back on the central nervous system. Especially is this so because we have thought along these lines ourselves, in relation to our own experiments on rats, in which we have evidence of prolactin release evoked by administration of oxytocin. It seems quite possible that the doses of oxytocin used in Dr. Hansel's experiments might inhibit the release of the animal's own oxytocin. Evidence indicating the possibility of such a feed-back mechanism was provided some years ago by Petersen and his colleagues (Donker, Koshi and Petersen, *Science* **119**, 67, 1954) who were studying the effects of regular injections of oxytocin in a cow just before milking in order to cause more complete evacuation of the udder. When the treatment was discontinued after 156 repetitions at hourly intervals the natural milk-ejection reflex was significantly inhibited and it took some days before it returned.

Professor Harris showed some beautiful slides and I would like to refer to one in particular, the one which illustrated various types of humoral mechanisms. There is one other type of mechanism which he did not include, that I have often thought might apply to the anterior pituitary. This is the direct chemical action of one type of cell upon another by means of a cellular secretion. Looking in a general way at the picture of anterior-pituitary function, as understood at present, the secretion of gonadotropins on the one hand and of LTH (or prolactin) on the other, at any rate in the rat, seemed to be alternative functions. There are various circumstances in which one can inhibit the secretion of gonadotropins, for instance by administering reserpine or by high doses of estrogen, or especially by transplanting the pituitary into the anterior chamber of the eye or under the capsule of the kidney. Here one gets inhibition of gonadotropin release or virtual disappearance of gonadotropic function while at the same time the release of prolactin is unhindered or even enhanced. On the other hand, if the transplanted pituitary is replaced in its natural position LTH secretion ceases and regular estrous cycles are re-established. Can it be that the gonadotropes, nourished as they seem to be by their natural proximity to the median eminence, exert by local humoral action an inhibitory influence on the acidophils, including those which secrete prolactin? This idea should be susceptible of experimental test.

I should like to end these remarks by asking Professor Harris, referring to his very interesting experiments with median eminence extracts, whether he has tried the administration of extracts of whole posterior pituitary lobe by his very fascinating and elegant pituitary plumbing technique? In addition I would like to know whether he has made any pituitary infusions with adrenalin, noradrenalin, histamine or serotonin?

DR. GEOFFREY HARRIS: We have started preliminary experiments infusing posterior pituitary preparations. We started with "Pitressin", but since this may be contaminated with anterior pituitary hormones we have recently obtained a highly purified preparation of lysine vasopressin from Dr. A. V. Schally in Houston, and also some synthetic arginine vasopressin from Dr. V. du Vigneaud. The results at the moment are too few to warrant any comment.

With regard to the other point raised, concerning intra-pituitary infusions of adrenalin and noradrenalin, Dr. B. T. Donevan and myself worked a few years back on this point (*J. Physiol.* **132**, 577–585, 1956). The technique differed a little in the previous experiments from that presently used. Infusions were made under anesthesia and through glass needles. However, we found that such infusions into the pituitary glands of rabbits did not result in ovulation.

DR. WILLIAM HANSEL: Dr. Folley has raised two interesting questions which deserve comment. The first of these concerns the role of prolactin in the cow. There are at least two experiments suggesting that prolactin is not luteotrophic in the bovine. Wisconsin workers have attempted and failed to prolong the length of the estrous cycle by daily injections of prolactin beginning at about the 15th day of the cycle and continuing through the 22nd day. In some of our own experiments we have attempted and failed to overcome the ability of oxytocin to produce precocious estrus by giving concurrent prolactin injections. The prolactin used was of ovine origin. It is possible that the dosages used in both of these experiments were too low.

Dr. Folley has also raised a question concerning the purity of the oxytocin preparations used in our work. In most of the experiments Armour's purified preparation was used. In addition, the estrous cycle was shortened in several cases by injections of a synthetic oxytocin preparation (Syntocinon, Sandoz Corp.). This preparation was free of vasopressin, but probably contained some peptides other than oxytocin. None of the preparations used possessed any measurable gonadotropic potency.

CHAIRMAN NELSON: I know that Dr. Segal wants to say something at this time, but I am going to ask him to be brief.

DR. SHELDON SEGAL: I think it is worthwhile spending more time on the subject of androgen-sterilized rats for several reasons. This experimental condition bears on our understanding of the normally occurring differences in pattern of gonadotropin release between males and females of a given species. As Dr. Barraclough has indicated, it also suggests important considerations with respect to localization of neural areas controlling gonadotropin release. In addition, a complete analysis of this experimental situation provides good evidence for the action of steroids on neural tissue, directly. The Japanese workers, Takewaki and Tagasuki, have shown that the steroid-induced sterility follows the post-natal administration of corticoids and estrogens, as well as androgens. Pfeiffer (*Amer. J. Anat.* **58,** 195–225, 1936) described the same result with the implantation of new-born testes in litter-mate females.

The need for pre-treatment with progesterone to cause electro-stimulated ovulation in these anovulatory animals has been interpreted by Dr. Barraclough to indicate that without progesterone the anovulatory female pituitary is deficient in stored LH. We have assayed these gonadotropins with respect to both total gonadotropins, based

TABLE 1. GONADOTROPIN CONTENT OF PITUITARY GLANDS

Group	Number of glands	Average pituitary weight* (mg)	Average ovarian weight† (mg)	Weaver-Finch test. Positive reactions total number
Normal ♂	4		212	20/20
60-day-old	2		184	18/20
	1	8.7±4	112	12/20
	1/2		65	2/20
Anovulatory ♀	4		226	10/10
60-day-old	2		194	8/10
	1	10.8±8	103	6/10
	1/2		68	0/10
Normal ♀	4		194	8/20
60-day-old	2		126	2/20
	1	11.6±5	66	0/20
	1/2		40	—

* Averages ± standard deviation calculated from the weights of 20 pituitary glands of each type.

† Assay animals were immature female rats; control ovaries average 32 mg. All weights represent average of 3 pairs of ovaries following a three-day injection period.

TABLE 2. THREE MONTHS MATING RECORD OF ANOVULATORY RATS

Reaction to male	No. of females	Post-coitus vaginal smears	Indicated ovarian events
Non-receptive	42		
Receptive:			
2 or 3 matings	2	Prolonged anestrus*	Ovulation functioning C.L.§
3 or 6 matings	4	Short diestrus†	Ovulation
4 or 9 matings	12	CVC‡	No ovulation

* Pregnancy-type of vaginal smear, 13–22 days' duration.

† Diestrus smear, 3–5 days' duration, followed by continuous vaginal cornification.

‡ Constant vaginal cornification.

§ Corpora lutea.

on ovarian weight increase in immature female rats, and specific LH content using the Weaver-Finch test (Segal, S. J. and D. C. Johnson, *Arch. d'Anat. Micros. et Morphol. Exper.* **48 bis,** 261–274. 1959).

The assays show that, like the normal male, the anovulatory female pituitary is richer in gonadotropins, both total and specific LH content, than the normal female. (Table 1.)

In the same article (*ibid.*) we have reported on the mating reactions of anovulatory females (Table 2). About 30% accept males. Some (about 10% of the total group tested) will respond to the mating by spontaneous ovulation. The total results of these studies indicate that the androgens administered post-natally have a direct inductive effect on the neural centers controlling gonadotropin release and the extent of this effect can vary among the treated animals. In some cases a partial induction of the total gonadotropin-releasing neural mechanism(s) results from the androgen treatment. Varying degrees of effect could be distinguished.

MECHANISMS CONTROLLING OVULATION OF AVIAN AND MAMMALIAN FOLLICLES*

A. V. NALBANDOV
University of Illinois, Urbana

IT IS generally conceded that mature follicles rupture in response to the action of an ovulation-inducing hormone (commonly considered to be the luteinizing hormone, LH), but the mechanism of ovulation remains unknown (7). In many mammals the interval between LH release (or injection) and ovulation is about 10 hr, but the changes which take place in the follicle wall between the time when LH first bathes the follicular cells and the time when these cells part along the stigma and allow the ovum to escape are practically unknown.

It should be kept in mind that LH release from the pituitary is a relatively sudden event which lasts 30 min in the rat (4), 60 min in the rabbit (5) and 26 to 150 min in the chicken (12), and that all protein hormones, and LH is no exception, are destroyed very rapidly after they enter the circulation. Thus, whatever influence LH has on mature follicles causing them to rupture about 10 hr later is of transient nature and is certainly not sustained over the whole interval between LH-release and ovulation. It seems that LH *initiates* a change which then runs its course and terminates in ovulation. The purpose of this paper is to present data on the ovulability of follicles and to propose a theory of the mechanism of ovulation based on these data.

Several older theories on the mechanism of ovulation have been summarized and reviewed by Hartman (6). Follicles do not rupture because their "ultimate" size has been reached or because the interior pressure of the liquor folliculi bursts the follicular wall. It is known that follicles can continue to grow long past the time when they should normally rupture. Cysts are often many times larger than follicles of ovulatory size and the internal pressure in cysts is much greater than it is in follicles; yet, cysts may persist for weeks or months without rupturing. In pigs, cattle and sheep, follicles become flabby a few hours before ovulation even though there is no visible break in the follicle wall and no detectable oozing of its contents. These facts certainly do not argue in favor of intra-follicular pressure as being the cause

* Data presented were taken from the Ph.D. Thesis submitted by Howard Opel (University of Illinois), 1960.

of ovulation. Similarly, one can discount the massaging effects of the fimbria as aiding in ovulation since follicles rupture normally in animals in which the fimbriae have been amputated or in which the whole reproductive tract has been removed. Neither can intestinal pressure on the ovaries be called upon as an aid in follicular ruptures since in sheep and rabbits ovulation proceeds normally in exteriorized ovaries not in contact with the gut.

Rugh (11) and Wright (14) have found that in hypophysectomized frogs follicles can be made to ovulate more readily than in intact frog females (sample responses: 100% ovulation in hypophysectomized females vs. 30–40% ovulation in intact control frogs). To Wright this observation suggested the possibility that the pituitary gland, due to unavoidable trauma at the time of hypophysectomy, may release a substance which sensitizes follicles and makes them more susceptible to the effects of ovulation-inducing hormones. Although this sensitizing substance was not identified, it was assumed to be the follicle-stimulating hormone (FSH). In another study Wright (13) confirmed earlier observations that frog ovaries taken from intact females can be made to ovulate *in vitro*. His data are of interest in view of the discussion to follow. Wright found that, as the amount of frog pituitary tissue added to the vessels containing frog ovaries *decreased* from two to one and on down to 1/16th of one gland, efficiency of ovulation *increased* from about 20 to 80%. Wright proposed that this decrease in the efficiency of ovulation could be due to an excess of LH in the vessels containing the higher concentration of pituitary gland tissue. When the concentration of pituitary tissue in the fluid bathing the ovaries was kept constant, efficiency of ovulation gradually increased with time, being 0% at 5 to 10 hr after the start of the *in vitro* trials and approaching 100% at 24 hr.

Most recently Bergers and Li (1) showed that ovaries of frogs pretreated with extracts of frog anterior pituitary tissue ovulated *in vitro* in response to ovine LH (ICSH) or growth hormone with about equal efficiency. However, this is not as great as that obtained with frog pituitary gland extracts. No *in vitro* ovulations were obtained with either prolactin or FSH. Progesterone was also able to induce *in vitro* ovulations but the number of eggs shed was below that obtained from the hypophysial hormones.

Chicken follicles too may ovulate *in vitro* provided they are exposed to the endogenous hormones for an as yet undetermined minimum time prior to being excised. According to Neher *et al.* (10), follicles removed one hour prior to normally expected ovulation can ovulate *in vitro*, while preliminary data (unpublished) suggest that removal 3 to 5 hr prior to expected rupture is not followed by dehiscence.

In women, follicles are surrounded by a network of reticular fibers and reticular cells which resemble smooth muscle cells without fibrils. In rabbit, pig and sheep follicles, true smooth muscle cells are present either in both the theca interna and the theca externa, or only in one of them but not in the other. In the follicle walls of chicken and frog ovaries true smooth muscle cells are present. The occurrence of smooth muscle cells in these and probably other species made it reasonable to think that their presumed ability to contract may play a role in bursting ripe follicles. Many abortive attempts have been made to induce ovulation by substances known to cause contraction of such fibers or by the electrical stimulation of the follicle wall (3). Oxytocin, injected systemically into rabbits, not only does not hasten ovulation but prevents it completely (2).

The injection of LH-containing gonadotropins may hasten ovulation by several days in mares, or by several hours in chickens, pigs and cows. Similarly, ovulation may be delayed by the use of such blocking agents as atropine in rabbits and cows or dibenamine in chickens. Thus, the follicle seems to become capable of ovulating long before it is normally called upon to do so by endogenous LH. It also retains its ability to ovulate past the normal time of rupture, if the release of LH is blocked or delayed by experimental means. The follicle of the mare remains ovulable for three to seven days and in the hen, under certain experimental conditions, it retains its ability to ovulate for as long as three weeks after it has reached ovulatory size (8).

Considering the data briefly summarized thus far, it appears justifiable to conclude that follicles reach ovulability before their "destined" time to rupture and retain their ability to ovulate for a considerable time after this event should have normally occurred. The follicle, not unlike a sound sleeper who will be awakened by an alarm clock, is unaware of its fate but, like the well-rested sleeper, it is physiologically ready and waiting passively for the signal to begin the final transformations leading to its ultimate fate—ovulation. For the follicle the signal is the arrival of LH. This signal is comparable to the ringing of an alarm clock which, having run down, leaves no memory of its sound other than the effect it produces on the suddenly altered metabolism of the awakened sleeper.

The data to be presented are concerned with the possible nature of the transformations which take place in the follicle between the time it receives the order to ovulate and ovulation itself.

Before discussing further the theoretical aspects of the problem of the ovulability of the follicles, data will be presented bearing on this problem in laying hens. Similar work is in progress in mammals but it is not sufficiently conclusive to permit discussion at this time. The experimental work to be presented involves laying hens which were hypophysectomized after they had laid the first two eggs (C_1 and C_2) of their clutch which in these birds normally consists of four or more eggs. Since, in the hen the interval between LH release and ovulation is variously estimated to be 8 to 12 hr in length, all hypophysectomies were performed about 18 hr before the expected ovulation of the C_3 follicle. Thus, there was a good margin of safety to make certain

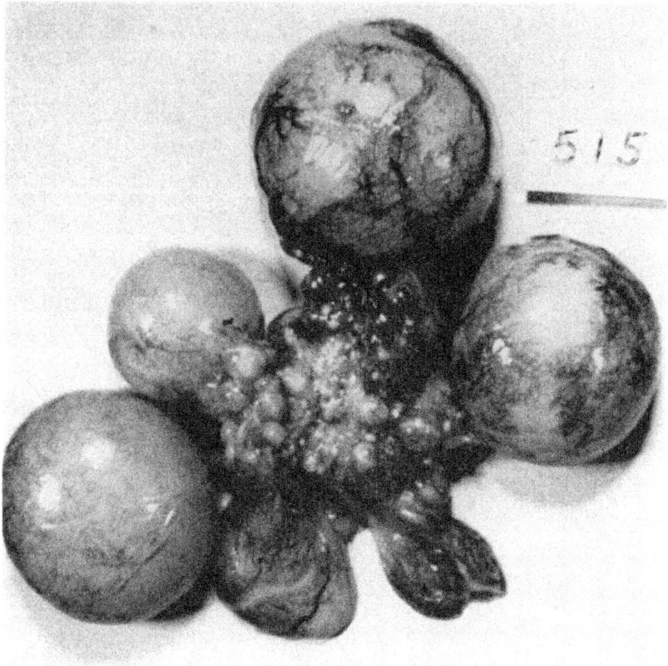

FIG. 1. Ovary of normal intact laying hen.

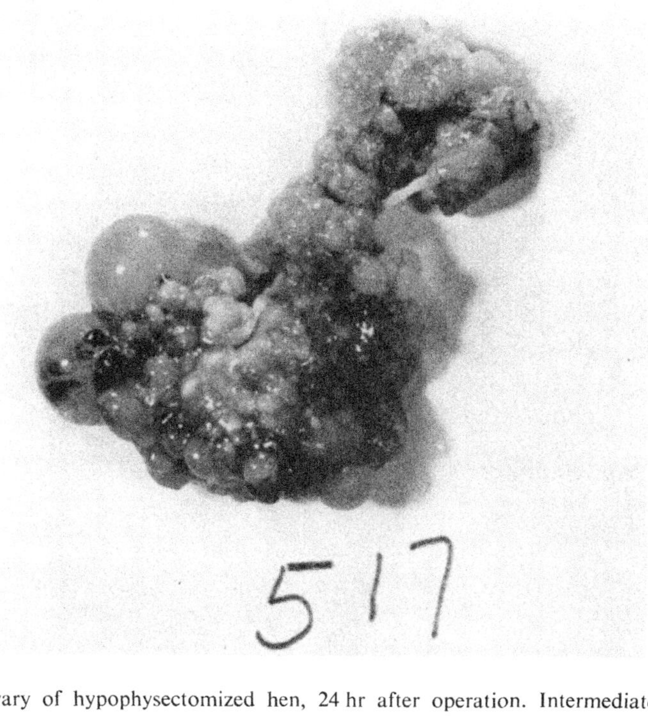

FIG. 2. Ovary of hypophysectomized hen, 24 hr after operation. Intermediate atresia.

that ovulations induced after hypophysectomy were caused by exogenous hormones rather than by the release of the hen's own LH. Success of treatment was judged either by laid eggs or by the presence of ovulated ova at autopsy which was performed at appropriate times following treatments.

In the absence of hormonal support the ovary of hypophysectomized hens undergoes extremely rapid atrophy (Table 1; compare FIGS. 1 and 2).

TABLE 1. EFFECT OF HYPOPHYSECTOMY ON RATE OF FOLLICULAR ATRESIA OF LAYING HENS

Hours after operation	No. of hens	% Follicles atretic in weight class (g)					
		15+	10–14.9	5–9.9	1–4.9	0.4–0.99	0.09–0.39
6	6	0	0	0	0	0	19.7
12	6	50.0	10.0	20.0	1.2	0	47.5
18	6	100.0	57.0	20.0	0	0	60.7
24	6	100.0	100.0	67.0	100.0	100.0	100.0
48	2	All follicles of measurable size					
72	3	All follicles of measurable size					

Attention is called to the fact that atresia begins not with the largest but with the smallest follicles (Table 1, 6 hr). By 12 hr after operation it includes the large follicles, but even by 18 hr the medium-sized follicles are not as hard hit as are the two extreme size classes. By 24 hr after hypophysectomy virtually all follicles of measurable size have become atretic.

On the basis of these data we know that, in the absence of exogenous hormone support, we can count on an interval of about 12 hr after hypophysectomy during which most follicles of ovulable size can be caused to ovulate with appropriate exogenous hormonal stimulus.

We shall first consider experiments in which an ovulating dose of LH was injected into laying hens which were hypophysectomized after lay of the C_2 follicle and 18 hr prior to the next anticipated release of their own LH. A single intravenous injection of LH was given to some hens as early as 2 hr, to others as late as 24 hr after hypophysectomy. The results of this experiment proved to be as interesting as they were unexpected. It will be seen (Table 2) that while at 2 hr all hens ovulated only one ovum, at 6 and 12 hr after the operation the majority of hens ovulated two, and in one case even three ova. The changes in the efficiency of ovulation, with increasing time after hypophysectomy, are further shown in the following comparison:

Hours after hypophysectomy:	2	3	4	6	12	15	18	24
Average No. of ovulations/hen:	1.00	1.25	1.25	1.88	1.63	1.38	0.63	0.13

In the intact laying hen it is not possible to induce more than one ovulation which is always the largest follicle in the ovary. But, in hypophysectomized hens even immature follicles ovulate and all follicles appear to become progressively more ovulable the longer they remain without gonadotropic hormone support other than the ovulatory dose of LH. This holds true only up to 12 hr after the operation, since after that time most follicles of even remotely ovulable size become physically atretic and thus are incapable of ovulating (Table 1). Of further interest is the fact that while most ova

TABLE 2. EFFECT OF TIME ON OVULABILITY OF FOLLICLES OF HYPOPHYSECTOMIZED LAYING HENS INJECTED I.V. WITH 4.0 mg OF LH AT TIME SHOWN

Hours after operation	No. of hens	No. single ovulations	No. double ovulations	Average weight of ova (g)			
				C_1	C_2	I_1	I_2
2	8	8	0	18.4	17.7	16.3	—
3	8	6	2	17.0	16.3	14.9	7.7
4	8	6	2	18.4	17.4	15.0	11.1
6	8	1	7	17.6	17.0	15.4	13.7
12	8	2	5*	17.5	17.2	14.9	10.2
15	8	5	3	14.9	14.6	12.1	9.8
18	8	5	0	17.1	16.8	10.2	—
24	8	1	0	17.0	16.8	11.3	—

LH preparation (Armour Lot No. R377201) contains FSH. C_1, C_2—last ova shed prior to hypophysectomy. I_1, I_2—ova induced by LH injection.
* One hen ovulated 3 follicles, one weighing 2.1 g.

induced to ovulate after hypophysectomy (I_1) weighed less than their normally ovulated predecessors, their weights are still within the normal range. All I_2 ovulations, however, are very significantly below normal ovulatory size. In spite of frequent and systematic attempts to induce ovulation of immature follicles in intact laying hens with a gamut of doses of LH, this has never been achieved in this laboratory or reported in the literature. It is interesting that intact laying hens treated with progesterone will ovulate very immature follicles with relative frequency. The reasons for this and the conditions under which it occurs remain unknown.

In a second experiment the question was asked whether the sensitivity of follicles to LH increases with time elapsing since hypophysectomy. Accordingly hens were injected with graded doses of LH at 6 or 12 hr after operation. This trial showed (Table 3) that at 6 hr no ovulations were induced with doses below 0.50 mg of LH, while at 12 hr 0.20 mg of LH was sufficient to cause single ovulations. Furthermore, double ovulations at 12 hr were produced with much lower doses of LH than the doses required to cause double ovulations at 6 hr. Attention is also called to the fact that even mammoth doses of LH (up to 20.0 mg) did not inhibit ovulation or reduce efficiency.

The observations presented in these experiments (Tables 2 and 3) led to the postulate that ovulation may be normally a hormone withdrawal phenomenon. To test this possibility further, a comparison was made between ovulability of follicles which were exposed to LH alone, with those which were given LH together with support by a gonadotropic hormone. Since the LH preparation used was known to be heavily contaminated with

TABLE 3. EFFECT OF TIME ON DOSE OF LH REQUIRED TO INDUCE SINGLE OR DOUBLE OVULATIONS IN HYPOPHYSECTOMIZED HENS

Dose of LH (g)	6 hr after operation			12 hr after operation		
	No. of hens	No. of ovulations		No. of hens	No. of ovulations	
		Single	Double		Single	Double
0.15	–	–	–	6	0	0
0.20	–	–	–	6	2	0
0.25	6	0	0	6	2	1
0.50	6	4	0	6	3	3
1.00	6	4	2	6	2	4
1.50	4	2	2	–	–	–
2.00	6	0	6	–	–	–
4.00	4	0	4	–	–	–
6.00	4	0	4	–	–	–
8.00	4	0	4	–	–	–
20.00	4	1	3	–	–	–

TABLE 4. EFFECT OF HORMONAL SUPPORT ON THE OVULABILITY OF FOLLICLES OF HYPOPHYSECTOMIZED HENS

No. of hens	First injection					Second injection			
	Hours after operation	LH (mg)	PMS (CNU)	No. ovulations		Hours after operation	LH (mg)	No. ovulations	
				Single	Double			Single	Double
10	6	0.5	0	8	1	30	4.0	1	7
6	6	0.5	6	6	0	30	4.0	0	1*
4	6	2.0	–	1	3	18	4.0	0	0
4	6	4.0	–	0	4	12	4.0	0	0
4	6	4.0	–	0	4	30	4.0	0	0

* Weight 0.81 g.

FSH, and since even small doses of FSH may be sufficient to provide support, it was decided to use the minimum effective dose of LH in order to minimize the FSH effect. Two groups of hens were each injected with 0.5 mg of LH

6 hr after operation. One of these groups received, simultaneously with LH, an intramuscular injection of six Cartland-Nelson units of pregnant mare's serum (PMS). Both groups responded to the LH injection by ovulations (upper part of Table 4). Thirty hours after operation, a dose of LH was injected which in previous experiments had been found maximally effective in inducing double ovulations (Table 3). It will be noted that, while 8 of the 10 hens injected with LH alone ovulated (7 of them twice), only one double and no single ovulations were obtained from the 6 hens supported with PMS.

If the initial ovulating dose of LH is high, no subsequent ovulations can be obtained when the second dose of LH is given 12, 18 or 30 hr after operation (bottom part of Table 4). While these results should be considered tentative they may mean that enough FSH was contained in the initial dose of LH to provide support and to prevent the ovulation of otherwise ovulable follicles which should have ruptured after the second LH injection.

DISCUSSION

The data presented lead to the conclusions that ovulability of follicles is greater in hypophysectomized hens than it is in intact control animals; that ovulability increases progressively with time after hypophysectomy until follicles become physically unable to ovulate; and that less LH is required to ovulate follicles which have not had gonadotropic hormone support for a longer time than those follicles which had been under the influence of gonadotropin more recently.

In view of these findings the theory is proposed that ovulation is normally a two-stage phenomenon. During the first stage follicles reach ultimate ovulatory size, which is determined by the total available circulating tropic hormones, distributed in the follicular circulatory system in accordance with the vascular capacity of individual follicles. One indication that the amount of circulating hormone limits follicular size is the fact that, in both mammals and birds, follicles can be caused to grow beyond their normal ovulatory size if exogenous gonadotropic hormone is injected. In the chicken the normal follicular size hierarchy can be easily obliterated by the injection of exogenous gonadotropins (Nalbandov, 1959). The individual vascular system of avian follicles is thus seen as playing a vital role in determining the rate of follicular growth. As the largest follicle approaches its ovulatory size, the amount of blood flowing through its vascular system is thought to be proportionally less than the amount available to smaller follicles. If this assumption is correct (preliminary observations support it) then the amount of hormone available per unit of follicular cells is also lower in the largest follicles than in the smaller ones. Because of this reduction in the concentration of gonadotropic hormones, the largest follicle is viewed as having reached a stage of "physiological atresia", during which hormone concentration is inadequate to maintain active proliferation of the cellular components

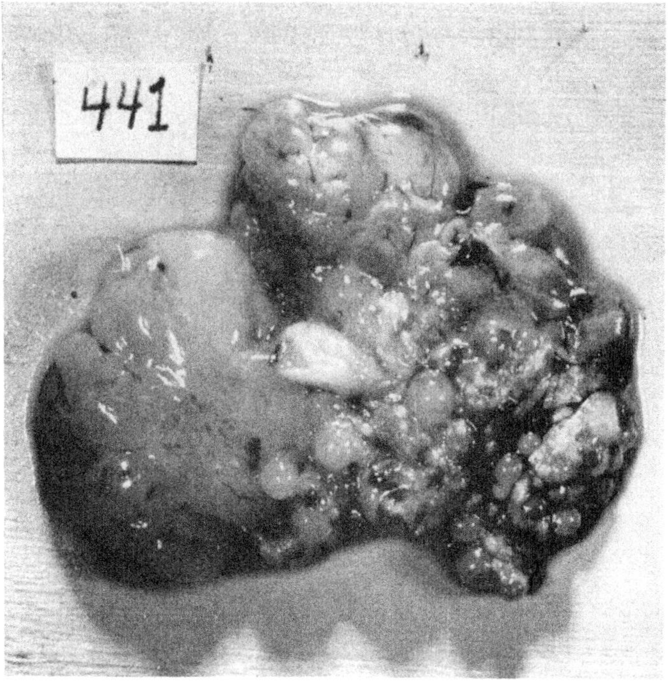

FIG. 3. Ovary of hypophysectomized hen remains atretic with inadequate gonadotropic hormone support (0.25 mg of chicken pituitary/day for 3 days).

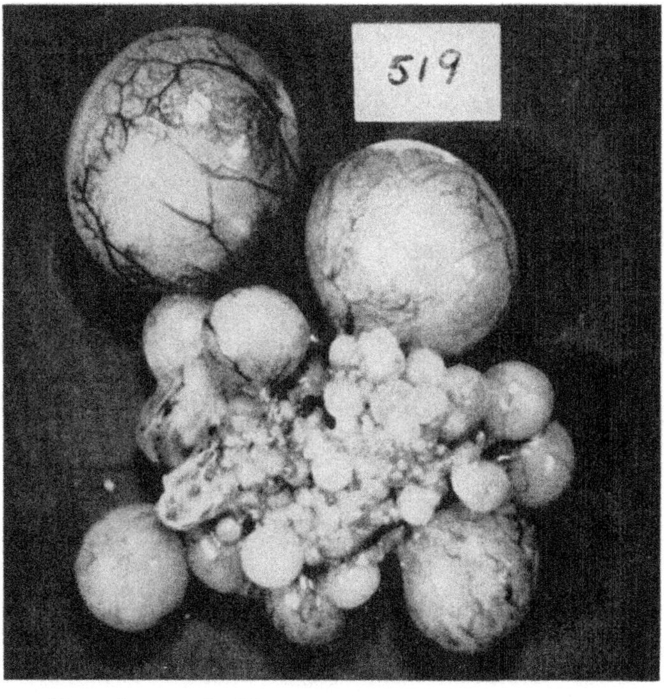

FIG. 4. Ovary of hypophysectomized hen restored to normal appearance with 4.0 mg of crude chicken pituitary/day for 3 days.

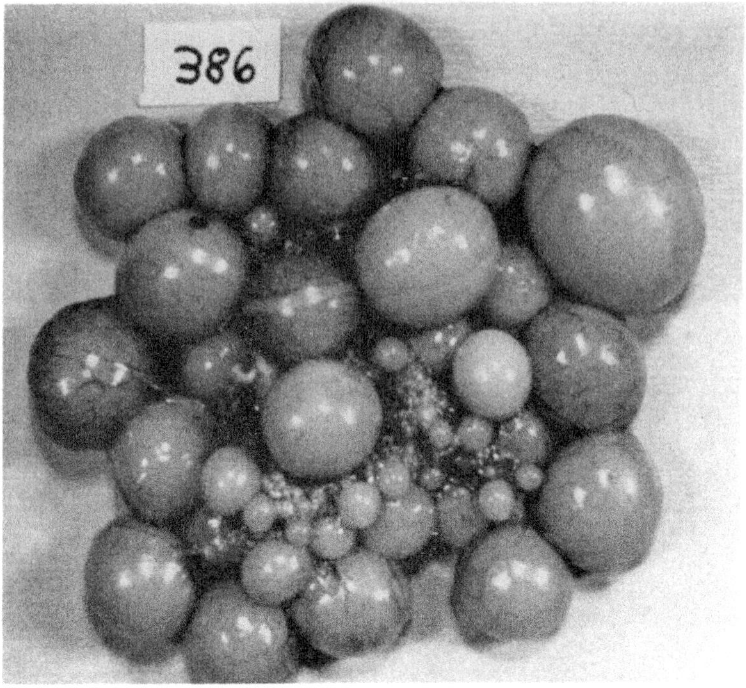

FIG. 5. Ovary of hypophysectomized hen overstimulated by injection of 2 I.U. FSH/day for 6 days.

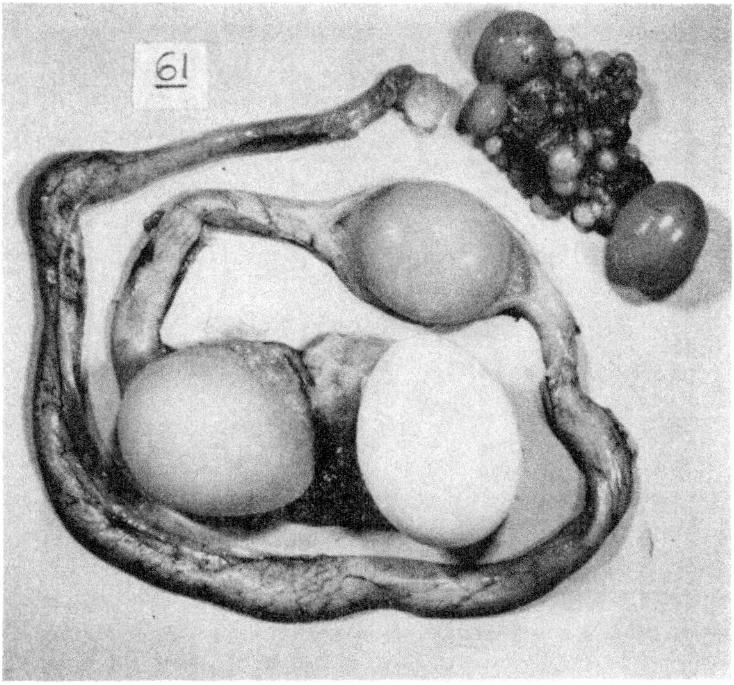

FIG. 6. Multiple ovulations induced in a hypophysectomized hen injected with mammalian LH 6 to 12 hr after operation.

of follicles. The distinction then is that during the hormone-adequate phase follicles are capable of rapid growth but are incapable of ovulating, while during the hormone-inadequate phase they are in a stage of physiological atresia when they can be made to ovulate because they are physiologically essentially "inactive". If follicles remain without adequate gonadotropic support too long, physical atresia sets in and they become incapable of ovulating for obvious reasons.

The stage of "physiological atresia" which, according to the theory proposed, is viewed as being due to a deficiency of gonadotropic hormone is relatively prolonged, lasting days in mares and rabbits, and hours in other mammals and in chickens. It is also distinguished by the fact that during this phase follicles can ovulate at any time after they receive the LH-born signal to do so. This view is supported by the experimental evidence presented which shows that follicles, which have become ovulable as a result of hormone withdrawal following hypophysectomy, can be made non-ovulable if they receive support in the form of small or moderate doses of FSH-containing hormones which presumably prevent them from becoming "physiologically atretic" and hence ovulable.

The question now arises what physiological changes take place in the follicle wall and especially in the stigma of follicles which are in the phase of physiological atresia and which have received the signal that ovulation shall occur about ten hours later.

The tentative theory is proposed that the effect of LH may be that of causing either general follicular ischemia, or local ischemia which is restricted to the stigma of follicles. In normal hens ovulation is demonstrably preceded by a blanching of the wall of the follicle destined to ovulate, the stigma widens measurably and the capillaries extending across it constrict. Eventually a small rip appears in one corner of the stigma and the ovum bulges through it. The rip widens and the ovum slips out of the follicular sac which collapses. These conclusions are based on subjective but numerous observations which do not lend themselves easily to quantitative measurements. Experiments now in progress are designed to test the theory that ovulation is the result of ischemia, although it is recognized that if ischemia is restricted to the stigma area of the follicle, it will be difficult to measure minor differences in the amount of blood present, especially in the smaller mammalian follicles.

In laying hens the mature follicle may be maintained in the ovulatory state over prolonged periods of time. In hypophysectomized hens this can be done by supporting the mature follicle with FSH-containing hormones. If the dose of supporting hormone injected is chosen correctly, the follicle will not ovulate nor will it become atretic. However, if an ovulatory dose of LH has been administered to hens containing follicles which have reached the "physiological atresia" stage, their ovulation cannot be prevented if supporting FSH treatment is begun at the time of hypophysectomy. These as yet incomplete observations are interpreted to mean that the process of "physiological atresia" is irreversible and that follicles which have reached that stage have three possible fates—they can be maintained in that phase with small doses of FSH-containing hormones, they can ovulate in the presence of LH, or they can become physically atretic in its absence.

If gonadotropic hormones are injected into laying hens, ovulations are stopped and, depending on the dose of hormone injected, the ovary will be slightly stimulated or overstimulated. Ovulations will be held in abeyance until LH injection which will cause the ovulation of one or more follicles, all of which will invariably be near normal ovulatory size. These observations are cited as additional evidence for the contention that immature follicles receiving adequate gonadotropic hormone support are incapable of ovulating. Only those follicles which have reached ovulatory size and are too large (or too numerous in cases of superovulations) to be adequately supplied by gonadotropic hormone are capable of ovulating in response to ovulatory doses of LH.

While additional work will have to be done, much of the evidence presented for birds appears applicable to mammals. Meanwhile it is impossible to discuss the subject in detail until additional evidence is obtained.

SUMMARY AND CONCLUSIONS

Data are presented to show that ovulability of follicles is significantly greater in hypophysectomized hens than it is in normal controls, and that the rate of ovulation increases as the interval from hypophysectomy to LH injection increases. The sensitivity of follicles to LH is increased in hypophysectomized hens and is significantly greater 12 hr after operation than at 6 hr.

While it is never possible to induce multiple ovulations or to cause ovulations of immature follicles in intact hens not treated with hormones, this can be done consistently in hypophysectomized laying hens.

On the basis of these data the theory is proposed that ovulation is normally due to non-support of the mature follicle by gonadotropic (FSH-containing) hormones. This hormone withdrawal makes them capable of ovulating if they receive the signal (LH) to do so.

The theory further proposes that LH acts on the ovulable follicle by causing general or localized ischemia which results in necrosis of the stigma and leads to its eventual rupture.

Comparative studies on the rate of blood flow through mammalian and avian follicles in relation to time of ovulation are being continued.

REFERENCES

1. BERGERS, A. C. J. and C. H. LI, Amphibian ovulation *in vitro* induced by mammalian pituitary hormones and progesterone, *Endocrinology* **66**, 225, 1960.
2. BRINKLEY, H., Unpublished data, 1960.

3. Dushkind, S., Observations on the mechanism of ovulation in the frog, hen and rabbit, *Western J. of Surgery Obst. and Gynec.* **55**, 424, 1947.
4. Everett, J. W., The time of release of ovulating hormone from the rat hypophysis, *Endocrinology* **59**, 580, 1956.
5. Fee, A. R. and A. S. Parkes, Studies on ovulation. I. The relation of the anterior pituitary body to ovulation in the rabbit, *J. Physiol.* **67**, 383, 1929.
6. Hartman, C. G., Ovulation, fertilization and the transport and viability of eggs and spermatozoa, *Sex and Internal Secretions*, 2nd Ed., Williams and Wilkins, N.Y., 1939.
7. Hisaw, F. L., Development of the Graafian follicle and ovulation, *Physiol. Rev.* **27**, 95, 1947.
8. Huston, T. M. and A. V. Nalbandov, Neurohumoral control of the pituitary in the fowl, *Endocrinology* **52**, 149, 1953.
9. Nalbandov, A. V., Neuroendocrine reflex mechanisms, Bird ovulation, *Comparative Endocrinology*, John Wiley & Sons, N.Y., 1958.
10. Neher, B. N., M. W. Olsen and R. M. Fraps, Ovulation of the excised ovum of the hen, *Poultry Sci.* **29**, 554, 1950.
11. Rugh, R., Relation of the intact pituitary gland to artificially induced ovulation, *Proc. Soc. Exptl. Biol. Med.* **40**, 132, 1939.
12. Van Tienhoven, A., The duration of stimulation of the fowl's anterior pituitary for progesterone-induced LH release, *Endocrinology* **56**, 667, 1955.
13. Wright, P. A., Factors affecting *in vitro* ovulation in the frog, *J. Exptl. Zool.* **100**, 565, 1945.
14. Wright, P. A., Sensitization of the frog ovary following hypophysectomy, *Physiol. Zool.* **19**, 359, 1946.

DISCUSSIONS

Dr. Roland K. Meyer: I shall begin with an analysis of the tissues that compose the wall of the follicle in the bird; the stratum granulosum is involved in the secretion of yolk and perhaps progesterone, the theca interna in the production of estrogen; the smooth muscle elements are contractile. Dr. Nalbandov has used menstruation as a model in describing his concept of the mechanisms involved in ovulation in the bird. I would like to use as a model the myometrium during pregnancy as it develops in preparation for the expulsion of the fetus.

The development of the myometrium is influenced by both estrogen and progesterone, as produced in early pregnancy by the ovary, later by the placenta. I suggest that the smooth muscle cells in the wall of the follicle are likewise stimulated by estrogen and/or progesterone produced in the adjacent theca interna and/or granulosum. The smooth muscle elements are thus developed in preparation for the expulsion of the ovum which is progressively increasing in size as the yolk is secreted. As in the pregnant uterus, the wall of the follicle is subjected to increasing tension as the ovum increases in size. Just prior to ovulation in the bird, under the influence of FSH and small amounts of LH, progesterone is increased causing the release of larger amounts of LH, which causes a further increase in distension of the follicle wall and tension of the smooth muscle. It is postulated, as in the uterus at parturition, that under the influence of estrogen and progesterone the muscle coat has become fully developed and begins to contract as the optimum degree of stretching is reached.

As a consequence the vessels in the wall of the follicle are compressed and ischemia occurs, especially in the stigma. The stigma disintegrates, and the contracting follicle wall expels the ovum through the opening.

This concept is based on the assumption that ovulation is the result of an integrated interaction of physical factors which are developed in the tissues of the follicle under the positive influence of hormones. Unlike Dr. Nalbandov's explanation it does not involve any elements of hormonal deprivation, or follicular atresia.

I have presented these thoughts as elements of a working hypothesis, even though Dr. Nalbandov has stated that intrafollicular pressure and the smooth muscle of the follicle are not considered to be very important factors in ovulation in birds.

Dr. Andrew V. Nalbandov: Well, in general, I am in sympathy with what Dr. Meyer has said. It is hard for me to conceive of an ischemia, which would not lead to some mild atresia, if you want to call it that.

I am grateful for your remarks, and the only thing I can say is that we will continue to work on it and see what come out of it.

OVULATION IN THE DOMESTIC FOWL

RICHARD M. FRAPS

Agricultural Research Service, U.S. Department of Agriculture
Beltsville, Maryland

OBSERVATIONS and experiments on many species have contributed much to our knowledge of various aspects of ovarian development and ovulation in birds. The common domestic fowl is, however, the only avian species for which we have today any fairly substantial and coherent perspective—incomplete though this may be in many respects—of processes directly and indirectly involved in ovulation.

A number of arguments might be advanced for the seemingly disproportionate concern with ovulation in the fowl, including such things as this bird's ready availability, adaptability to experimental conditions and procedures, and possession of convenient external indices of gonadal function (65). But in addition to these obviously desirable attributes, the domesticated hen continues to ovulate over much of the year, she does so in definite patterns so arrayed as to constitute recurring cycles of considerable experimental significance and, not least in importance, the time of most ovulations may be predicted with a high degree of accuracy.

With good cause the hen thus deserves its favored position in the study of ovulation in birds. Nevertheless, a sound knowledge of the physiology of ovulation in birds can scarcely be based on any single species, and it is regrettable that so little is known regarding these complex and undoubtedly diversified phenomena among other species, and more particularly in wild birds exhibiting restricted breeding seasons. This broader comparative knowledge seems all the more desirable in view of the suspicion that the domestic hen has been so highly selected for egg production that her reproductive processes can no longer be regarded as representative of birds generally and of wild birds more specifically.

It is true that broody and incubation behavior have been greatly reduced in many contemporary breeds of fowl, but the same can be said of those wild species, such as the American cowbird and the European cuckoo, in which brood parasitism has become established. It is also true that processes responsible for follicular growth, maturation and ovulation proceed more intensively in the contemporary domestic fowl than in her wild forebears, but this can hardly be held to signify any qualitative change in underlying mechanisms embodied, for example, in nervous, neuroendocrine and endocrine controls over ovarian function. These mechanisms may indeed be basically much alike in all avian (and mammalian) species, despite the great and obvious diversity of reproductive patterns exhibited by differing species. For the time being, therefore, it seems reasonable to suppose that ovulation and related processes in the domestic fowl proceed from and are mediated through mechanisms fundamentally similar in all avian species, however peculiar or unique or even artificial some final expressions of reproductive processes may appear to be.

FOLLICULAR–PITUITARY RELATIONSHIPS

Ovarian function in the fowl and in most birds differs in at least two obvious respects from that of mammals, as Nalbandov (44) has recently emphasized. The ovarian complement of developing follicles consists typically of an array which exhibits well-defined differences in size, not of a group comparable in size through successive developmental stages as is commonly seen in mammals. Of the bird's complement, only a single follicle, the largest of the series, matures and is ovulated at a time. In contrast, the simultaneous maturation and ovulation of a number of follicles is typical of mammals. Nalbandov has called attention particularly to the point that birds must be assured of "an endocrine mechanism permissive of the existence of a hierarchy of follicles of graded sizes, only one of which is capable of ovulating at any one time". Experiments directed toward the imposition and maintenance of the typical follicular hierarchy in the hypophysectomized hen by simulation of the naturally occurring "endocrine mechanism" are discussed by Nalbanov elsewhere in this volume. Of more immediate concern here are relationships between follicular development, maturation and ovulation in the intact hen, relationships which require, to begin with, some understanding of timing of these processes. Various aspects of the subject have been discussed earlier (15–17, 37).

The Ovulation Cycle

Under optimal (12–14 hr) photoperiods, the hen typically lays an egg on each of two or more consecutive days, does not lay on one day and then lays again on two or more consecutive days. The eggs thus laid on consecutive days constitute a sequence (often but wrongly called a clutch). In sequences of low to moderate length (2 to about 8 eggs), the first egg is laid during early morning (or lighted) hours, subsequent eggs at later hours on successive days until the sequence is completed with lay of a terminal egg during afternoon hours. The interval between successive eggs of a sequence is thus somewhat greater than 24 hr; the term lag has been proposed (15) to describe the difference between the interval separating lay of consecutive eggs and

24 hr. Stated differently, lag is simply the difference in times of day at which successive eggs are laid.

Time of oviposition, particularly in battery-caged hens, may be recorded within almost any desired limits of accuracy. From such records of lay, the time of ovulation of individual follicles constituting the corresponding ovulation sequence may be estimated with fair accuracy. Briefly, each ovulation except the first of a sequence occurs at a definite interval, of the order of 15–45 min and varying inversely with sequence length, following the preceding oviposition. The first ovulation of a sequence takes place on the day before the second, and earlier than the second by not less than the extent of lag between next to terminal and terminal ovipositions. These relationships have been described in detail elsewhere (17).

Times of ovulation so calculated for White Leghorn hens, maintained under lights from 6.00 a.m. through 8.00 p.m., and ovulating in sequences of two to six members, are recorded in Table 1. Ovulation of the first member of

TABLE 1. TIMES OF OVULATIONS IN SEQUENCES OF 2 TO 6 MEMBERS, WHITE LEGHORN HENS UNDER 14-HR PHOTOPERIOD (LIGHTS 6.00 A.M.–8.00 P.M.)

n	Ovulating follicles*					
	C_1	C_2	C_3	C_4	C_5	C_6
2	6.38*	11.10	—	—	—	—
3	5.58	9.56	**12.39**†	—	—	—
4	5.49	9.17	11.16	**1.12**	—	—
5	5.48	8.56	10.34	**12.02**	**1.33**	—
6	6.05	8.57	10.55	**12.02**	**12.49**	**2.14**

* From Fraps (17).

† Light faced figures, morning hours; bold faced figures, afternoon hours.

sequences at about 6.00 a.m., the hour of onset of lights, is of no significance. Under relatively lengthy photoperiods (e.g. 18 hr light), the first ovulation takes place well after onset of lights. Under relatively short photoperiods (e.g. 10 hr), it occurs sometime before onset of lights.

The extent of lag between successive members of the sequences for which actual times of ovulation were given in Table 1 are recorded in Table 2, together with total lag within the sequences—the difference, that is, in times of day between first and terminal ovulations. Total lag obviously increases with sequence length, but to a lesser extent in the longer sequences. In even the lengthiest of sequences, total lag rarely exceeds some nine hours.

Heywang (33) published extensive data on intervals between lay of successive eggs by White Leghorn hens maintained under natural photoperiods for a year at Glendale, Arizona. Lag in ovulation sequences of 2 to 13 members has been calculated from these intervals and is presented graphically in Fig. 1.

TABLE 2. LAG (IN HOURS) IN OVULATION SEQUENCES OF 2 TO 6 MEMBERS, BASED ON TIMES RECORDED IN TABLE 1*

n	Lag at successive places					Total lag
	h_2	h_3	h_4	h_5	h_6	
2	4.53	—	—	—	—	4.53
3	3.97	2.72	—	—	—	6.68
4	3.47	1.98	1.93	—	—	7.38
5	3.13	1.63	1.47	1.52	—	7.75
6	2.87	1.97	1.12	0.78	1.42	8.15

* From Fraps (17).

The solid columns of each vertical bar measure lag, in hours (ordinates), between successive ovulations; the solid plus superimposed open columns measure the cumulative lag at third and subsequent places in the several sequences; total lag is so indicated at the last place in each sequence.

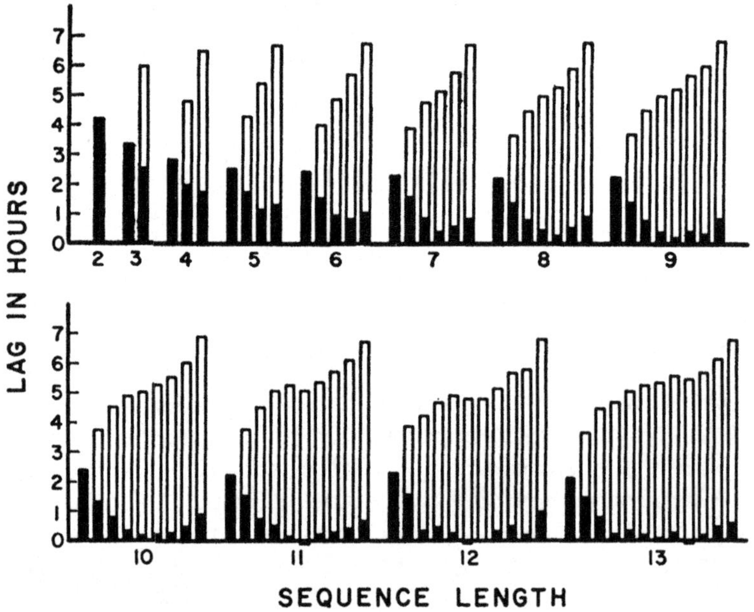

FIG. 1. Lag in ovulation sequences of 2 to 13 members. Solid bars, lag at successive places in each sequence; solid with lined bars, cumulative lag. (From Fraps (17).)

Several characteristics of ovulation sequences are illustrated by these histograms. The greatest value of lag appears in the two member sequences, where there is, of course, only one place of lag, that between first and second ovulations. In all other sequences the greatest value of lag is between first and second ovulations, though this decreases as the number of members in sequences increases from three to around seven or eight. But with this decrease in lag between first and second ovulations with increasing sequence length, there occur decreases in lag at subsequent positions, all of which become fairly constant in sequences of seven or eight or more members. At sequence lengths greater than seven or eight members, an increasing number of lag

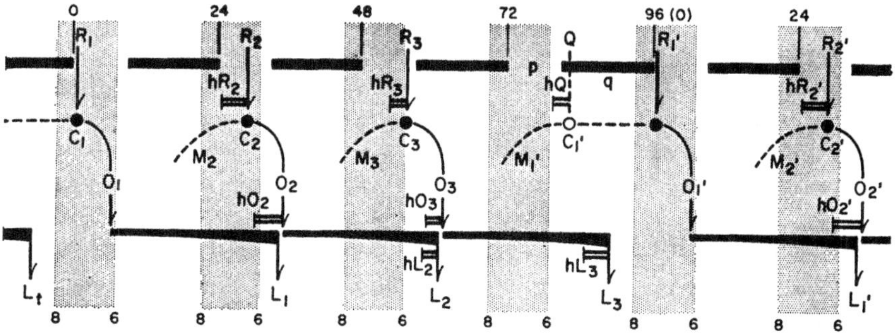

FIG. 2. Time relationships in a 4-day cycle ($n=3$). Hours of darkness (8.00 p.m.–6.00 a.m.) are set off by the vertical stippled bands. The days of the cycle, top of the figure, are each divided in an "open" period and a period of lapse, *p* and *q* respectively on the last day of the cycle (hours 72–96). Subscripts denote successive events or members: R, *onset* of OIH releases; C, follicles; O, ovulations; L, ovipositions; M, "maturation curves" of the follicles. Q indicates the approximate hour of excitation and onset of OIH release if the sequence were continued. Primed designations apply to the succeeding cycle. Other details in text. (Based on Fraps (16, 17).)

values approach or equal zero following decreasing order of lag in the first several places. The interval between successive ovulations is then 24 hr. Theoretically, at least, the number of members in a sequence may be increased indefinitely with little or no increase in total lag beyond that seen in sequences of some seven or eight members. It may be noted that lag always increases in the terminal place or two before these lengthy sequences are terminated.

In regularly ovulating hens, the termination of one ovulation sequence on a given day is followed almost invariably by the initiation of another sequence on the second day thereafter; ovulation fails to occur, that is, on only a single day. This single day on which ovulation fails to occur may be denoted conveniently as the day of lapse. Unless otherwise stated, we shall be concerned with the interim between the terminal ovulation of one sequence and the initial ovulation of a succeeding sequence only in this limited sense.

In Fig. 2, successive ovulations in a 3-member sequence are represented by O_1, O_2 and O_3, the first and second ovulations of a succeeding sequence by O_1' and O_2'. Lag of the second ovulation with respect to the first is indicated by hO_2, and of the third ovulation with respect to the second by hO_3. Ovipositions consequent upon successive ovulations are designated L_1, L_2 and L_3 and lag by hL_2 and hL_3. The time required for the egg to traverse the oviduct is practically, if not quite, equal to the interval between a given ovulation and the corresponding oviposition.

Ovulation Frequency

In hens exhibiting the typical "one day" lapse between sequences of n members, ovulation frequency (f) is defined as $f=n/(n+1)$, where $n+1$ is equal to cycle length in days. The limit approached by $n/(n+1)$ is unity. The equation $f=n/(n+1)$ therefore expresses, for differing values of n, the frequency of ovulation relative to the limit 1. In the 3-day cycle which has proved so useful in much experimental work, $n=2$ and $f=2/3$ or 0.67. The value of f becomes 0.75 in the 4-day cycle, 0.80 in the 5-day cycle and so continues to increase by constantly decreasing increments as cycle length increases. Since $n/(n+1)$ can only approach 1 as a limit, ovulation frequency in the lengthiest of cycles can never quite attain 1.5 times the value of f in the 3-day cycle. In the 2-day cycle, $n=1$ and $n/n+1=0.50$; birds so ovulating on alternate days are not considered here because of the difficulty in predicting continuation of the cycle. It is of interest to note, however, that hens ovulating at this minimal rate or frequency (for the 1-day lapse) are in fact ovulating at 0.5 the maximal attainable frequency. Ovulation frequency thus measures a fundamental aspect of the cycle which is obscured by sequence or cycle length as such. The significance of ovulation frequency in other connections will become apparent later.

Follicular Maturation and OIH Release

It has been assumed rather generally that the pituitary gonadotropin directly responsible for ovulation in the intact hen is the luteinizing hormone (LH), and further, the pituitary has been supposed by this author, at least, to release LH episodically, and specifically for ovulation, in greater than the "basal" quantities which, together with the follicle-stimulating hormone (FSH), are required for follicular growth and maintenance. Recently, however, Nalbandov (44) has postulated for birds the existence of a single gonadotropic complex with FSH- and LH-like properties. A similar view has been advanced by van Tienhoven (65) on somewhat different grounds.

Evidence for the view that LH is the pituitary gonadotropin immediately responsible for the induction of ovulation in the intact hen has been reviewed elsewhere (17). Briefly, LH preparations from sheep pituitaries were found to be much more effective than were FSH preparations from the same source, and the latter were effective only when administered at levels high enough to carry appreciable quantities of LH (23). Fractionation of male chicken pituitaries yielded an LH preparation roughly 500 times more effective than was the FSH fraction (26), and again, the ovulation-inducing effect of the

FSH preparation could well be attributed to contamination with LH. On the basis of these results, Fraps *et al.* (26) concluded that the luteinizing fraction was "identical with the avian ovulation-inducing gonadotropin".

It is of some interest in connection with the proposed unitary concept that similar ratios of gonadotropic activity were found in the pituitaries of cocks, non-laying hens and laying hens when the glands were assayed for FSH content mainly (55) or for ovulation-inducing effect (13).

Insofar as relationships between follicular maturation and release of ovulation-inducing hormone (OIH) are in question, it is perhaps of little importance whether we think in terms of LH or of the postulated gonadotropic complex. What is important is the timing of OIH release with reference to follicular maturation and, to anticipate the final issue, whether or not the timed release of OIH is under control of the central nervous system.

Returning to Fig. 2, the relationships believed to exist between follicular maturation, OIH release, and ovulation are represented schematically for the 4-day ovulation cycle described earlier. Onset of OIH release during the first "day" of the cycle is indicated by R_1; OIH acts on the mature follicle, C_1, to effect the first ovulation, O_1, of the cycle. In similar fashion, OIH releases associated with R_2 and R_3 induce ovulation of the C_2 and C_3 follicles. No release of OIH occurs on the following day, but does so on the day thereafter, R_1' initiating a succeeding cycle.

As thus formulated, the onset of OIH release is assumed to take place at an approximately constant interval before each corresponding ovulation of the cycle. It follows that lag at R_2 and R_3, indicated by hR_2 and hR_3, are the same as lag at O_2 and O_3. And since all ovulations, whatever the length of sequence, occur within restricted hours of the 24, the onset of corresponding OIH releases must occur within similarly restricted, but earlier, hours of the 24. Days of the cycle given in the topmost lines of Fig. 2 refer to this aspect of the OIH release cycle, not to ovulation as such. Onset of OIH release may occur within hours 0–8 or so of the cycle day, not during remaining hours of the 24, set off by the horizontal bars near the top of Fig. 2. The hours of the 24 during which onset of OIH release may occur have been denoted the release or open period, the remaining hours the period of lapse (17); these are indicated by *p* and *q* respectively between hours 72 and 96 (day 4) of the cycle.

To result in ovulation, the presence of a mature or ovulable follicle obviously must be posited at the time of each OIH release; it does not follow that the presence of an ovulable follicle is closely associated with OIH release. Once a cycle is initiated with OIH release for ovulation of the C_1 follicle, successive follicles of the sequence must mature within the interval (24 hr + lag) separating successive releases of OIH. The fact that this is so seems obvious in the observation that, at the time of a given OIH release (e.g. R_1 of Fig. 2), the follicle next due to ovulate remains completely indifferent to the ovulatory stimulus, yet the same follicle responds by ovulation to the succeeding OIH release, R_2 of the sequence.

In our early experiments on the induction of ovulation, injections were timed for effect on follicles subsequent to the first of a sequence (C_S follicles), since in these the hour of normally expected ovulation could be predicted accurately. When subsequently the response of the C_1 follicle was investigated, it was found—somewhat surprisingly at the time—that its ovulation could be induced at considerably greater intervals before normally expected ovulation than was possible with other follicles of the sequence (14, 21, 22). Or, following injection of appropriate gonadotropins at equal but considerable intervals before the hour of normally expected ovulation of C_1 and C_S follicles, the C_1 follicle was found to be much the more sensitive, as was confirmed by Bastian and Zarrow (3). A similar differential in ovulatory response of C_1 and C_S follicles to progesterone was described by Fraps and Dury (23, 24).

TABLE 3. APPROXIMATE QUANTITIES (MG/HEN) OF MALE CHICKEN ANTERIOR PITUITARY POWDER INDUCING OVULATION OF C_1 AND C_2 FOLLICLES IN ABOUT 50% OF INTRAVENOUSLY INJECTED HENS AT INDICATED HOURS FOLLOWING PRECEDING OVULATION ($n=2$ FOR ALL HENS)

Hours from preceding ovulation	"Best estimate" of 50% ovulation level	
	C_1 follicle	C_2 follicle
7	0.50	0.20
10	0.15	0.15
13	0.05	0.10–0.15
16	0.02	0.02
19	0.02	0.02

When the earliest hour at which notable sensitivity of the C_1 follicle could be demonstrated experimentally was considered with reference to time of preceding ovulation rather than to time of next expected ovulation, its high ovulability was seen to be attained at about the same interval following the preceding ovulation as did subsequent follicles of the sequence. This supposition was tested by ascertaining the quantity of dried male chicken anterior pituitary powder required to force ovulation of C_1 and C_2 follicles of 2-member cycles in about 50% of hens injected at increasing intervals following the preceding ovulation. [Unpublished experiments of Fraps, Rothchild and Neher; summarized by Fraps (17).] The "best estimate" of responses following closely upon preceding ovulation leaves much to be desired, but ovulability of C_1 and C_2 follicles clearly increases with increasing time from preceding ovulation (Table 3). The similar and high sensitivities at 19 hr seem of particular significance, for following injections at this interval after the preceding ovulation the C_2 follicle is forced to ovulate prematurely by no more than about 3 hr in contrast with a prematurity of some 17 hr for the C_1 follicle.

In an extensive series of experiments, Bastian and Zarrow (3) determined the quantities of luteinizing hormone required to induce ovulation of first and subsequent follicles of the sequence at stated intervals before the hour of expected normal ovulation. Their results were in important respects very similar to those described above, although they appear not to have recognized the possibility of similar courses in maturation of C_1 and C_S follicles with reference to hour of preceding ovulation. The possibility that failure of the highly ovulable C_1 follicle to ovulate earlier than it actually does because of "lack of release of ovulating hormone" (14) is noted, but Bastian and Zarrow consider also, and with greater favor, the possibility that the observed high degree of sensitivity could be the result of "a release of the ovulating hormone on the night prior to ovulation", but at levels inadequate to induce ovulation. If, however, the course by which the C_1 follicle attains ovulability is in fact substantially the same as that of C_S follicles, no special condition need be postulated for this fact, nor for its continuing and perhaps even slightly increasing sensitivity to OIH preparations as it approaches the hour of actual ovulation.

The foregoing observations are believed, in any event, to afford strong evidence for the conclusion that the C_1 follicle does in fact attain to ovulability by substantially the same course, with reference to time of preceding ovulation, as do other follicles of the sequence. In Fig. 2 the curves M_2, M_3 and M_1' are seen thus to stand in an approximately constant relationship with ovulations O_1, O_2 and O_3 respectively. But since the onset of OIH release is believed to take place at a constant interval before each ovulation of the cycle, the courses of increasing ovulability represented by M_2, M_3 and M_1' bear also an approximate constancy with respect to the postulated OIH releases, R_1, R_2 and R_3. The question might then be raised as to whether OIH, or endocrine factors associated with processes of follicular rupture, initiate maturation of the succeeding follicle of the cycle. This author has more or less tacitly assumed that OIH is the effective agent, but little evidence bears directly on the issue. If the pituitary gonadotropin secreted into the blood stream is in fact a single entity, as Nalbandov (44) and van Tienhoven (65) suggest, an episodic release of OIH would imply relatively high levels of FSH as well as of LH activity. The initiation of follicular maturation might then be attributed to such episodically recurrent periods of high FSH activity, but this must remain a matter of conjecture at the moment.

Pituitary Competence during the Period of Lapse

In Fig. 2, the C_1' follicle is seen to have become fully ovulable at about the time Q, the interval between R_3 and Q being made the same as between

R_2 and R_3. If the OIH release sequence were continued in correspondence with the follicular maturation sequence, OIH release should therefore be expected at or about the time of Q. Failure of OIH release to take place at this time, or at any time during the period of lapse, might signify lack of OIH reserves in the pituitary, or failure of the pituitary to respond to usual stimuli. The possibility of OIH secretion at subovulatory levels, one aspect of pituitary inadequacy, may reasonably be dismissed at the outset, since subovulatory levels of ovulation-inducing gonadotropin have been shown to result in follicular atresia (3, 21, 22), a condition rarely seen in the regularly ovulating hen.

TABLE 4. OVULATIONS ADDED TO ANTICIPATED 2-MEMBER SEQUENCES FOLLOWING SUCCESSIVE INJECTIONS OF MALE CHICKEN ANTERIOR PITUITARY TISSUE (AP) OR PROGESTERONE (Pg)

Group	Hens	Injection			Ovulations added	
	No.	Hormone	Quantity mg	Interval hr	Per hen No.	Range No.
A	10	AP	1.0	24	2.4	0–5
B	6	AP	1.0	26	3.0	1–5
C	10	Pg	0.3	24	2.0	0–5
D	10	Pg	0.6	24	2.5	1–5
E	10	Pg	0.9	24	2.5	1–4

From Neher and Fraps (45).

Evidence to be assessed later supports the view that progesterone effects ovulation in the hen by way of the central nervous system, stimuli from which cause the release of OIH from the pituitary. The induction of ovulation following the systemic administration of progesterone at or about the time of C_1 follicle maturation (Q of Fig. 2) should therefore signify pituitary competence. In an attempt to ascertain the extent to which the two-member ovulation sequence might be prolonged, Neher and Fraps (45) injected progesterone or male chicken anterior pituitary tissue some 24–28 hr following the presumed hour of terminal OIH release and repeated such injections at 24-, 26- or 28-hr intervals until the ovary failed to respond by ovulation. As is evident from results recorded in Table 4, progesterone was about as effective as was the pituitary preparation in extending the ovulation sequence, both in mean number of induced ovulations per hen and in the upper limit attained in some hens. Failure to induce more than about 5 successive ovulations following progesterone injection was most probably caused by failure to maintain the sequence of maturing follicles, not by failure of the pituitary to release OIH, since the same upper limit also was encountered following injection of the pituitary preparation. This view is borne out by the decreasing order of yolk weights in the lengthier successions of induced ovulations. Mean weights of the second normally ovulated and the succeeding four yolks for the 13 hens in which ovulation was induced 4 times or more were 17.4, 16.8, 16.2, 15.5 and 14.3 g. The mean difference between first and last members of the series, 3.1 g, suggests that the secretion of FSH (or of the gonadotropic complex) did not keep pace with the enforced demand for follicles capable of maturation and subsequent ovulation.

In any event, the level of pituitary response elicited repeatedly by progesterone at or near onset of the period of lapse lends no support to the view that the normal ovulation sequence is terminated by pituitary inadequacy, the period of lapse representing, as it were, a period of recovery (44). On the contrary, onset of the period of lapse seems to indicate the abrupt intervention of conditions which prevent response of an entirely competent anterior pituitary to stimuli which otherwise are closely associated with the presence of a mature follicle. And perhaps the resumption of ovulation, at a definite hour of the 24 under a given photoperiod, constitutes equally cogent evidence for a similarly abrupt termination of the conditions which impose the period of lapse. If the relationship between mature follicle and pituitary response seen during the course of the ovulation sequence depends upon a nervous relay, so to speak, this relay appears not to respond, during the period of lapse, to the usual stimuli associated with follicular maturation. OIH release therefore fails to occur for lack of nervous activation of the pituitary, not because of any defect in pituitary function. Evidence for this view will now be considered.

NERVOUS CONTROL OF OIH RELEASE

Basically, the anatomical and functional relationships between the hypothalamus and the pituitary appear to be much the same in birds and in mammals. The absence of direct nervous connections between hypothalamus and pars distalis and the existence of a well-developed portal system (30) is firmly established in birds (29, 67). In birds, the neurohypophysis is separated from the adenohypophysis by a connective tissue septum, thus eliminating, as Harris (31, 32) has emphasized, any possibility of vascular control of the anterior pituitary by the neurohypophysis. In his comprehensive monograph on the avian pituitary, Wingstrand (67) described the tracts from the hypothalamus to the neurohypophysis and along their course, a special region of the median eminence in the ventral wall of the infundibulum, notable for its content of neurosecretory material. From this region the pituitary portal vessels pass to the anterior pituitary. Wingstrand, as did Green and Harris earlier (30), concluded that hypothalamic control of the anterior pituitary was effected by transport of some neurohumor from this region of the median eminence to the secretory cells of the pituitary.

Experimental evidence, based largely on mediation of the effects of light to the gonads, strongly supports the conclusions of Wingstrand (67) and Green (29). From a series of experiments on the drake, the results of which were considered in two general papers, Benoit and Assenmacher (5, 6) conclude that lengthened photoperiod is no longer capable of inducing the usual gonadotropic response of the anterior pituitary deprived of blood from the specialized region of the median eminence. In two recent papers Assenmacher (1) and Benoit and Assenmacher (7) have emphasized again the dependence of gonadotropic function on the integrity of neurosecretory regions in the hypothalamus, of the hypothalamico-hypophysial tract to the special zone of the median eminence, and of the anterior portal vessels forming the final link with the anterior lobe.

Hypothalamic-pituitary relationships have been investigated recently in the male white-crowned sparrow, with special reference to neuroendocrine functions in relation to photoperiod and gonadal response (46). The observations described by Oksche *et al.* are in accord with those of earlier workers.

In the regularly ovulating hen, Shirley and Nalbandov (61) reported complete interruption of the portal vessels to result permanently in "a condition indistinguishable from hypophysectomy as far as the ovary and the sex hormone-dependent structures are concerned". Neurohypophysectomy, on the other hand, had no such effect and, following an adequate recovery period, ovulation proceeded at the same rate as in unoperated controls (62).

As was noted earlier, these and other investigations have been concerned mainly with seasonal or long-term gonadal responses, mostly to light, and therefore with control of continuing secretion of pituitary gonadotropins. The problem posed by OIH release may, at first sight, appear to be different in some respects. The release of OIH is believed to be episodic, and to occur in response to a specific stimulus of follicular or ovarian origin. It is at least conceivable that such a stimulus, of "internal origin", might act directly on the pituitary to cause the release of OIH. However, there is now good evidence that this is not the case: whatever the stimulus for OIH release, it appears to act initially at a neural level, thence over neuroendocrine pathways to the anterior pituitary gland. This is not to say that the ovarian hormones may not influence the anterior pituitary gland directly, but only that this appears not to be true of OIH release.

Photoperiod and the Period of Lapse

We have called attention earlier to the highly significant circumstance that, during most or all of the period of lapse, the ovary carries an ovulable follicle and the pituitary is responsive to progesterone. What seems to be lacking is some definitive connection between follicle and pituitary, a connection dependent upon some element which is responsive to the follicular (or ovarian) stimulus and which also can activate the anterior pituitary. Moreover, the period of lapse appears in a relatively constant relationship with certain phases of photoperiod; it is in fact one aspect of the diurnal rhythmicity so evident, under a wide range of photoperiods, in the restriction of ovulation or OIH release to certain hours of the 24. Considering these relationships together, one would almost inevitably have to conclude that the suspected non-functional link seen during the period of lapse between follicle and pituitary was nervous in nature. No other structure or entity could be expected to possess the characteristics apparently required to prevent OIH release during an interim so closely associated with photoperiod. One might therefore conclude that OIH release, when it occurs naturally, does so over nervous and neuroendocrine pathways, the nervous component becoming operative in association with specific phases of photoperiod. However simple and attractive such an argument may seem in retrospect, it does not afford rigorous experimental evidence that OIH release is in fact dependent upon neural activation of the pituitary, nor could it tell us what nervous structures are essential.

Effects of Pharmacological Agents

Presumptive evidence pointing to neural participation in the mechanism of OIH release is based on effects of pharmacological agents believed to act at a nervous level. Much of this work, it should be noted, was inspired by results described by the Duke University investigators in the rabbit and the rat.

Progesterone has been used extensively in these investigations, and effects on normally incident and progesterone-induced ovulation will be considered together.

Nembutal (pentobarbital sodium), amongst other barbiturates, was shown by Everett and Sawyer (11) to block LH release in the rat. Everett subsequently (10) demonstrated Nembutal blockade of the LH release induced by progesterone in 5-day cycling rats. In the hen, however, Bastian and Zarrow (2) were unable to prevent either normally incident or progesterone-induced ovulation by the administration of Nembutal. It was later observed by Fraps and Case (19) that Nembutal, Dial (diallylbarbituric acid) and Ipral calcium (probarbital calcium), following administration at 4.00 p.m. for effect on the C_1 follicle, caused premature ovulation in low to moderate (13 to 28) percentages of injected hens. Dial and Nembutal were found also to act synergistically with low levels of progesterone in the induction of premature ovulation, not to block its action.

Fraps and Case (19) suggested that the ovulation-inducing effects of these several barbiturates might result from neural excitation, secondary to depression, and consequent activation of the pituitary. But perhaps an alternative explanation may be based on the supposition that these barbiturates suppress activity in a region or "center" which inhibits, during the period of lapse, another hypothalamic "center" directly responsible for neurohumoral activation of the pituitary. Such a view is in accord with the observation that release of OIH for C_1 ovulation is most closely associated with onset of darkness (according to our calculations), and that light plus activity act to suppress OIH release (3). The discovery of the "stimulatory" effects of lesions by Donovan and van der Werff ten Bosch (8, 9), discussed elsewhere in these proceedings (p. 56), may afford grounds for speculation on the operation of such mechanisms on a diurnal scale.

Phenobarbital sodium, injected under the same conditions as were Nembutal, Dial and Ipral calcium, failed either to induce ovulation prematurely or to block ovulation of the C_1 follicle (19). The drug was found however to prevent some 40–50% of expected ovulations of C_8 follicles (Fraps and Conner, cited in (17)). Phenobarbital sodium also effectively blocks the ovulation-inducing action of progesterone and other steroids on the C_1 follicle when administered 30–40 min before injection of the steroids (17).

The action of other pharmacological agents has also been investigated in the hen. Zarrow and Bastian (70) reported blockade of both normally expected and progesterone-induced ovulation of the C_1 follicle by the parasympatholytic drug, atropine and the adrenolytic agent, SKF-501. Dibenamine (*N*,*N*-dibenzyl-B-chloroethylamine), presumably an adrenergic blocking agent, was shown by van Tienhoven, Nalbandov and Norton (66) likewise to block both normal and progesterone-induced ovulation. The drug was increasingly effective in preventing normal ovulation as the interval between injection and expected ovulation was increased from 6 to 14 hr, with the notable exception of an unaccountably low incidence of blocked ovulations at 12 hr. Their observations led van Tienhoven *et al.* to suggest that "the stimulus for LH release and hence ovulation takes place about 14 hours prior to follicle rupture", an interval considerably greater than that favored by this author—some 8 hr—on other grounds.

The increasing effectiveness of presumptive blocking agents with increasing interval from injection of submaximal levels to expected ovulation has been observed often in our laboratory. When administered 38 hr before expected ovulation of the C_1 follicle, Dial, Nembutal, phenobarbital sodium, Dibenamine, SKF-501 and atropine sulfate all effectively suppress ovulation (20), a result which may possibly stem from interruption of mechanisms other than those responsible for OIH release.

In a subsequent study, van Tienhoven (64) attempted to determine the duration of stimulation of the hen's anterior pituitary for progesterone-induced OIH release, using atropine and Dibenamine to block the release. He noted a longer duration of stimulation from the adrenergic than from the cholinergic component; for the adrenergic component the duration of stimulation was estimated to vary from about 26 min to 2.5 hr. van Tienhoven believed his results to indicate a concurrent stimulation and release of LH from the hen's pituitary.

Oviducal Suppression of OIH Release

Huston and Nalbandov (35) reported that interposition of various obstructions, or even of a surgical thread, in the lower magnum of the hen's oviduct interrupted ovulation without signs of other hormonal disruption. The combs of all hens remained throughout the period of observation like those of normally laying hens, betokening the continued secretion of estrogen and thus of some LH secretion. Upon sacrifice of hens carrying such irritants for as long as 20 days the ovary was found to bear a practically normal complement of follicles, with little or no evidence either of follicular overgrowth or of atresia. No recently ruptured follicles were seen, thus disposing of possible failure of the oviduct to engulf yolks from otherwise undetected ovulations. The oviduct itself was equal in size to that of normally laying hens, indicating the continued secretion of estrogen. In other hens, the injection of LH or of progesterone was followed by ovulation and lay of normal eggs.

These observations were confirmed and extended by van Tienhoven (63), who noted an increasing effectiveness of thread loops in the magnum with increasing distance from the infundibulum, and more regular suppression of ovulation by loops placed in the isthmus. Loops similarly placed in the uterus, where the shell of the egg is deposited, were without effect on the course of ovulation.

Huston and Nalbandov (35) believed the oviducal irritant to operate over neurogenic pathways to block the usual activation of the pituitary for release of OIH (or LH). Since either LH or progesterone will induce ovulation of the mature follicle or follicles, the induced condition is apparently comparable with that existing during the period of lapse, and nervous blockade of the usual stimulus for OIH release might reasonably be postulated. The mechanism by which such a blockade might be accomplished in the experimental birds and the possible role of the oviducal egg will be discussed later.

Brain Lesions and Injections

The effects of electrolytic lesions in the hypothalamus have recently been investigated in the normally ovulating hen (48). Exploratory experiments soon indicated that lesions in a medial region in the ventral preoptic hypothalamus caused an immediate and prolonged interruption of ovulation. Lesions elsewhere in the hypothalamus also, as a rule, interrupted ovulation, but not regularly nor immediately, nor generally for more than about 15 days. Subsequently, lesions in the median eminence were often found to be effective in the immediate interruption of ovulation, but this region was not adequately investigated.

In view of the consistent interruption of ovulation following placement of lesions in the ventral preoptic region, experiments were undertaken toward further delimitation of the effective locus. This, as described by Ralph, "is just dorsal to the optic chiasma, at the extreme rostral end of the hypothalamus, lies laterally less than 2 mm from the midline, and within a ventral portion of the nucleus praeopticus paraventricularis". Lesions of 1 to 2 mm diameter, placed within this region 0.5 to 1 mm on each side of the midline, regularly prevented ovulation, while the response to smaller lesions so placed was irregular.

The effects of hypothalamic lesions on progesterone-induced ovulation of the C_1 follicle were also investigated (51, 52). Progesterone was administered

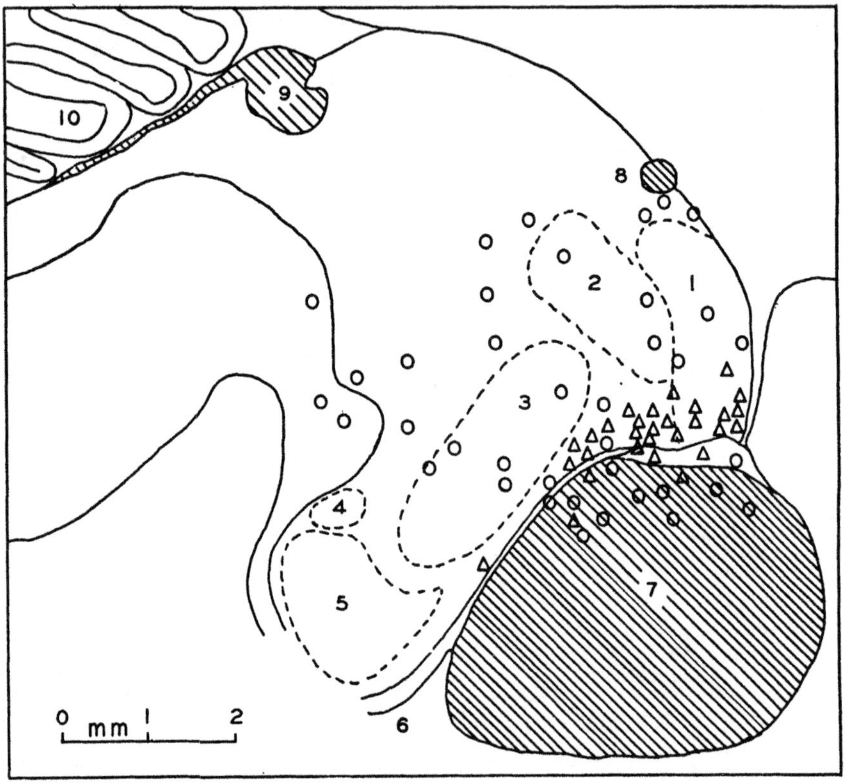

FIG. 3. Mid-sagittal plane of chicken diencephalon on which certain hypothalamic nuclei and the sites of all lesions made within 2 hr following administration of progesterone are projected. Symbols indicate the approximate center of each lesion: O—ovulation; Δ—failure of ovulation. 1 and 2—principal and accessory parts of preoptic paraventricular nucleus, 3—lateral hypothalamic nucleus, 4—mammillary nucleus, 5—tuberal nucleus, 6—median eminence, 7—optic chiasma, 8—anterior commissure, 9—posterior commissure, 10—cerebellum. Fiber tracts not shown. Limits of nuclei are somewhat arbitrary. From Ralph and Fraps (52).

subcutaneously, 1 mg/hen, at about 4.00 p.m. for effect on the C_1 follicle. Lesions varying in size and position were placed at known times thereafter. Progesterone-induced ovulation was regularly prevented only by lesions placed in the anterior region of the ventro-median hypothalamus—the region shown to be involved in normal ovulation—or along fiber tracts originating in this region and directed caudally toward the median eminence (Fig. 3). Ovulation was not regularly prevented by lesions placed elsewhere. In view of these observations, it was suggested that certain neurones of the paraventricular nucleus may be the site of progesterone "excitation", although the possibility that these neurones and their associated fibers are only elements in a structural complex was not excluded.

Participation of the preoptic hypothalamus in the normal processes of ovulation of the C_1 follicle was found not to be essential beyond about 6 hr before the event, since lesions placed at less than about 6 hr before expected ovulation did not prevent its occurrence (48). Following the systemic injection of progesterone, the integrity of the preoptic hypothalamus must be maintained for about 2 hr, that is, to within about 6 hr before the time of expected ovulation (52). Observations based on the effects of lesions cannot define the time of onset of hypothalamic activity in normally timed processes. But since the same highly essential hypothalamic region becomes dispensable at about the same hour before normal and progesterone-induced ovulation, onset of activity may be inferred to occur by the same interval prior to normal ovulation as does onset of activity associated with progesterone-induced ovulation. As has been noted elsewhere (16, 17), ovulation of the C_1 follicle follows systemic administration of progesterone by not more than 8 hr, and thus "activation" of the hypothalamic region cannot occur at a greater interval prior to ovulation. In these terms, the minimal duration of hypothalamic participation in the ovulatory process, normally incident or progesterone-induced, is of the order of 2 hr.

According to Rothchild and Fraps (58), the anterior pituitary must remain *in situ* until some 4 to 6 hr before expected normal ovulation if ovulation is to occur. The same authors (59) observed that removal of the pituitary within 2 hr following progesterone injection prevented all expected ovulations, and that the gland must remain *in situ* for 4 hr to assure maximal incidence of progesterone-induced ovulation. The duration of pituitary participation in the processes of ovulation, again either normal or induced ovulation, would thus appear to vary between 2 and 4 hr. The lesser estimate of pituitary participation, 2 hr, is clearly in good agreement with estimated duration of hypothalamic participation in ovulatory processes, and may indicate concurrent "excitation" and OIH release, as was surmised by van Tienhoven (64) on other grounds. In some hens, however, ovulation apparently required an intact pituitary over somewhat longer intervals from the assumed onset of OIH release. It is difficult to say just how much of the greater range in apparent duration of OIH release in the hypophysectomy experiments can be attributed to differences in techniques, birds, or inaccuracies in estimating times of expected or actual ovulation. It seems possible also, however, that an intact pituitary may be required beyond the interim required for OIH release.

Progesterone is known to disappear rapidly from the blood stream. Taking this fact into account, Rothchild and Fraps (59) thought it improbable that progesterone could act for 2 to 4 hr to assure the release of OIH in adequate quantities. Progesterone, they suggested, may act promptly and

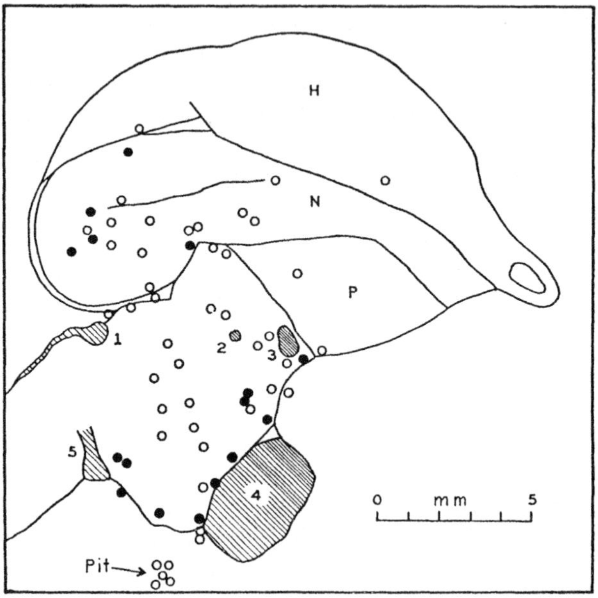

FIG. 4. A parasagittal view of the hen's diencephalon and forebrain, showing the sites of injections of progesterone made bilaterally at 1 mm. Solid circles, induced premature ovulation; open circles, no premature ovulation; 1, posterior commissure; 2, anterior commissure; 3, tractus septo-mesencephalicus; 4, optic chiasma; 5, oculomotor nerve; Pit, pituitary; H, hyperstriatum; N, neostriatum; P, paleostriatum. From Ralph and Fraps (54).

over a limited time in effecting the release of OIH, the intact pituitary being essential for some time thereafter for secretion of a hormone required for maintenance of the ovulable follicle.

In further experiments, the ovulation-inducing effects of small quantities of progesterone injected directly into various regions of the brain were ascertained (54). Stereotaxic procedures used in placing lesions were followed except for replacement of the electrode carrier by a microinjector with a 26 gauge needle. All injections into the brain were placed bilaterally, 5 μg progesterone in propylene glycol at each site in the definitive experiments. Probably no more than half the quantity injected, or about 5 μg/hen, remained at injection sites, as some always followed the needle track and appeared on the surface as the needle was withdrawn. All injections were timed for effect on ovulation of the C_1 follicle, and results were established by usual palpation procedures.

Ovulation was induced following injections, 1 mm bilaterally, in the anterior and ventral hypothalamus, and in the caudal neostriatum (Fig. 4). The more anterior and dorsal effective sites in the hypothalamus are found within the preoptic paraventricular nucleus. Those along the dorso-caudal surface of the optic chiasma lie in the anterior hypophysial tract, and the four most posterior sites are within the tubero-mammillary region.

The stimulatory action of progesterone in the paraventricular nucleus and in the anterior hypophysial tract might have been expected in view of the earlier finding that lesions in these regions, placed within 2 hr following the systemic administration of progesterone, regularly prevent the expected ovulation. Such lesions, however, destroy only a part of the progesterone-sensitive structures, and raise the question as to the effectiveness of lesions in these structures. Exploratory probings indicated no interruption of progesterone-induced ovulation following the placement of lesions of about 2 mm diameter in the neostriatum. The effect of lesions in the tubero-mammillary region has not been investigated.

Two other investigations in this series may be mentioned briefly. Small lesions in the median diencephalon of regularly ovulating hens interrupted ovulation in most hens (53). Lesions in the preoptic hypothalamus, anterior hypophysial tract or dorso-caudal thalamus resulted in lengthier interruptions than did lesions in the central diencephalon, but there was much variability. All lesions were placed 12 hr or more before next-expected ovulation, and comparisons of relative immediacy of interruption of OIH release are not possible. A selective effect on OIH release could not have been detected in hens which resumed ovulation before termination of the observation period (42 days), but the regressed condition of ovaries and oviducts in some hens sacrificed at the close of this period points to a more general interference with gonadotropin secretion.

Destruction of the supraoptic region of the hypothalamus of the hen was shown by Ralph (50) to result, as a rule, in polydipsia. Most of the birds were out of lay when selected for test, but a number resumed ovulation and lay while under observation. Follicular maturation, ovulation and oviposition thus proceeded, apparently normally, in some birds bearing extensive lesions and exhibiting polydipsia. The supraoptic nucleus would therefore appear not to be essential for reproduction in the hen, at least not under the conditions of these experiments. It is of some interest that the lesions causing polydipsia were located, in all instances, lateral to the paraventricular region shown to be essential for maintenance of gonadotropin secretion and for OIH release (48, 52).

Assenmacher (1) described testicular atrophy and failure to respond to artificial illumination in ducks bearing extensive lesions in the supraoptic and paraventricular region of the anterior hypothalamus. These lesions were hand placed, and possibly always damaged the paraventricular nucleus, in which event there need be no incompatibility with the results described by Ralph (50). Nor do Ralph's findings necessarily exclude participation of the supraoptic region in the accelerated response which might be expected under lengthened photoperiod.

Considering the results of these several investigations insofar as they bear on gonadotropic functions of the anterior pituitary, Ralph (49) suggested that afferent neural stimuli and the effects of hormones "are in some manner mediated, in large part or entirely, by neurosecretory cells of the hypothalamus, particularly those of the paraventricular nucleus, and it is the activities of these cells which are responsible for regulation of gonadotropin release in the hen". This summary view of hypothalamic function and indispensability in the hen is in accord with conclusions arrived at by others (see (60)).

While the central role of neurosecretory cells in regulation of pituitary gonadotropin function seems thus to have been established, we should emphasize again that we do not know the duration of the stimulus which effects OIH release specifically. This may be brief, as was noted earlier. If so, it is conceivable that the stimulus effecting "release" may act at the level of the median eminence to cause or to permit an abrupt outpouring of accumulated neurosecretory material into the portal vessels. In the male white-crowned sparrow, Oksche *et al.* (46) state that the median eminence can be regarded as a depot of neurosecretory material, exceeded only by the neurohypophysis. They remark also on the reduced quantity of the substance seen in the median eminence of birds on a 20-hr photoperiod during the second half of the daily photoperiod and on its reaccumulation during the dark period. It would obviously be of great interest to know whether such a depletion of neurosecretory materials does or does not take place in the hen in association with OIH release from the pituitary, not only in the median eminence, but also in the paraventricular nucleus. Legait (40) observed an association between reproductive condition of the hen and apparent neurosecretory activity of cells of paraventricular and supraoptic nuclei, but these observations were not related to presumed time of OIH release.

HYPOTHESES OF THE OVULATION CYCLE

Several hypotheses have been proposed to account for lag, or for lag and the period of lapse, in the hen's ovulation cycle (3, 15, 42–44). It is assumed that external stimuli, and more particularly light, act through the central nervous system to regulate, over neuroendocrine pathways, the output of pituitary gonadotropin (whether FSH mainly, or the gonadotropic complex) responsible for follicular growth and development. The frequency with which follicles become available for the ovulatory process determines the quantitative aspects of the cycle, viz., sequence length (n), cycle length ($n+1$) and ovulation frequency $n/(n+1)$.

The hypothesis of the cycle proper proposed several years ago (15) was essentially a statement of possible relationships between diurnally varying thresholds of response in a neural component of the OIH release mechanism and excitation hormone (progestagen?) concentrations associated with

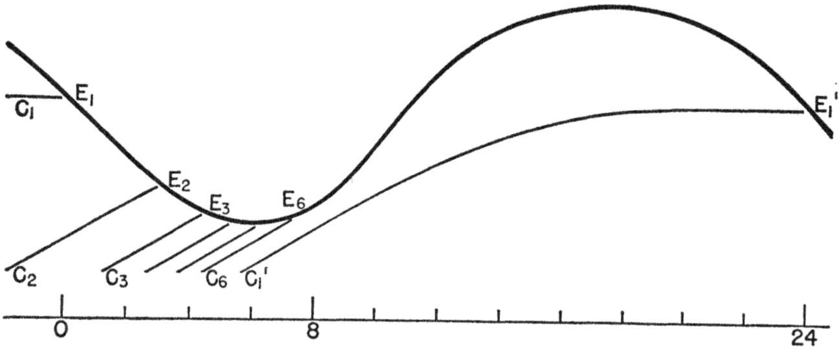

FIG. 5. Diagrammatic representation of possible relationships between diurnal rhythmicity in thresholds of response in a neural component of the OIH release mechanism (the curve through E_1, E_2 . . . E_6 and E_1') and excitation hormone concentrations associated with the follicles C_1, C_2 . . . C_6 and C_1' in a 7-day cycle ($n=6$). Zero hour corresponds to about 10.00 p.m. in hens under lights from 6.00 a.m. through 8.00 p.m. Based on Fraps (15).

follicular maturation. These relationships are shown for a 7-day cycle ($n = 6$) in Fig. 5. Thresholds of response (the inverse of sensitivity) are described by the curve passing through E_1, E_2 ... E_6 and E_1'. Excitation hormone concentrations associated with successive follicles of the sequence, assumed to increase by substantially the same course with respect to the preceding OIH release (or ovulation), are represented by C_1, C_2 ... C_6 and C_1'. The first excitation, E_1, takes place on day 1 of the cycle at zero hour in the figure (e.g. 10.00 p.m.), initiating the release of OIH which causes ovulation of the C_1 follicle. The second excitation, E_2, occurs on day 2, some several hours later than did E_1 on day 1, the third somewhat later on day 3, and so on through E_6, which takes place about 8 hr later on day 6 than did E_1 on day 1 and completes the sequence. In this scheme, it is to be observed that each excitation hormone curve beyond the second (C_2) is displaced, in time of day, by the extent of lag associated with the previous excitation. If this is true also of the C_1' curve, excitation cannot occur on day 7 because of the relatively high nervous thresholds existing at the time of day at which usually effective concentrations are attained. The period of lapse (hours 8–16) thus intervenes, but since excitation hormone concentrations are assumed to continue to increase during this period, the first excitation of the cycle, E_1 or E_1', takes place at relatively high threshold values. It is this circumstance which, presumably, accounts for the relatively great extent of lag associated with E_2 and thus with lag in ovulation of the second follicle of the sequence (Fig. 1).

In this formulation of cyclic relationships, considerable emphasis has been placed on the role of diurnal periodicity (or rhythmicity) in thresholds of response in the neural component of the system (15–17). There can be little doubt that some phase or phases of the prevailing photoperiod determine in large measure the hours of the 24 within which nervous activation of the pituitary for OIH release may normally occur. In this sense the meaning of diurnal periodicity is reasonably clear. The supposition that, within this period, thresholds of response vary with *time of day* introduces, however, a notion of rhythmicity rather than of simple periodicity. The postulated rhythmicity may be considered in part at least a characteristic of the "center" exhibiting diurnal periodicity, or an expression mainly of ovarian (and perhaps other) hormone actions on such a center. While in one form or another it does seem necessary to postulate varying parameters of nervous response to an excitation hormone, it is not supposed that the relationships represented in Fig. 5 are the only ones possible.

Estrogen

Although the nature of the delaying action of exogenous estrogen on ovulation of the C_2 follicle contributed to formulation of the hypothesis discussed above, it was not until the observation of a similar gonadotropin-induced delay, presumably mediated through increased levels of endogenous estrogen acting at a neural level, that the substance was seriously thought to play a part in the appearance of lag (25). The normal OIH release represents certainly an increase in circulating gonadotropin levels, whether of LH alone or of the gonadotropic complex. We might reasonably expect such a release to effect, as presumably did the injection of LH or of LH+FSH, an increase in levels of circulating estrogen. There are also grounds, to be discussed later, for believing that the oviducal egg may stimulate estrogen production during some 4 to 5 hr following its ovulation. However this may be, estrogen levels in the regularly ovulating hen would appear to vary in a pattern which is closely associated with the occurrence of OIH release. It may be suggested then that relatively high estrogen levels so generated act to suppress the appearance of low thresholds (or high sensitivity) in the neural component of the OIH release mechanism. With subsequently decreasing estrogen levels, at a time related to time of preceding OIH release (and possibly the early oviducal egg), thresholds in the neural component would be expected to fall and excitation to become possible. Each OIH release (and egg) except the last of the sequence would thus become a factor in determination of time of the succeeding excitation and therefore of the extent of lag. The last OIH release, by delaying onset of low thresholds to or beyond the time of day at which the period of lapse intervened, would thereby terminate the sequence. Estrogen levels presumably would be low at the hour of excitation and OIH release for the first follicle of the succeeding cycle or sequence, and excitation would occur in response to the appropriate phase of photoperiod at the onset of the "open" period, which by definition is the case.

This schematic statement of presumed periodicity in estrogen levels and effects is no doubt overly simple. We do not know, for example, when inhibitory levels may be attained, although gonadotropin injected as much as 13 hr before estimated hour of expected OIH release for ovulation of C_2 follicles effectively blocked the release (25). The considerable interval (24 to 29 hr) between a given OIH release and an effect on the succeeding OIH release thus would seem to present no problem.

Progesterone

Since progesterone has been shown to effect OIH release over the same hypothalamic structures involved in the normal release and, in addition, in similar relationships insofar as these have been determined, it has been suggested that progesterone (or a progestagen) might be the natural ovarian hormone eliciting nervous "excitation". If this were so, we should be able to adduce some evidence that progesterone is produced by the hen's ovary and is found in the blood stream.

Using the bioassay of Hooker and Forbes (34), progestogenic activity was demonstrated in the blood of actively ovulating hens (27). In other tests, the same authors found blood levels of what then was believed to be progesterone to exceed 5 μg/ml (unpublished results). Although the Hooker–Forbes test is now known not to be specific for progesterone, the inference based on this test apparently was confirmed when the substance was identified on chromatograms of extracts of ovaries of regularly laying hens (39). Progesterone was found in extracts of maturing as well as of ruptured follicles, but these authors failed to detect the substance in the blood of ovulating hens. This was accomplished, however, by Lytle and Lorenz (41) in extracts of samples consisting largely of blood from the ovary "prior to contact with the liver or any capillary bed". Their extracts were estimated to contain an average of about 0.05 μg/ml blood. In comparison with values yielded by the Hooker–Forbes test, this may seem a very low concentration, but physicochemical determinations of progesterone in the systemic blood of pregnant women have likewise failed to yield values comparable with those indicated by the bioassay of Hooker and Forbes (68). Other naturally occurring compounds, metabolites of progesterone, now are known to exhibit progestational activity by the Hooker–Forbes and Clauberg tests and are therefore considered to be gestagens (69). While such compounds have not been demonstrated in the blood of hens, it seems not improbable that the Hooker–Forbes test measures "the circulating form or forms of the luteal hormone" (12) in the hen as in other species. It is of some interest in this connection that Lytle and Lorenz (41), referring to earlier work by Lytle, state that chemical analysis failed to identify progesterone in blood drawn by heart puncture, although this blood yielded positive responses by the Hooker–Forbes test. Lytle and Lorenz note also that relatively large samples, drawn to circumvent loss in peripheral tissues but less completely defatted than were their definitive samples, uniformly failed in chemical tests to yield measurable quantities of progesterone while eliciting positive responses in the Hooker–Forbes bioassay.

The demonstration that progesterone is formed in the hen's ovary, is secreted as progesterone into the systemic blood, and is associated with progestogenic activity as measured by the Hooker–Forbes test, would appear to support the conclusion that the naturally occurring "excitation" hormone is a progestagen if not progesterone itself.

The stimulus for the postulated formation of progesterone in the maturing follicle must remain a matter of conjecture. It seems possible that the same gonadotropin release causing ovulation of the mature follicle may initiate in the succeeding follicle the processes leading to the elaboration of progesterone. Theoretically, at least, prolactin may be involved in the maintenance of progesterone production, or the "basal level" of LH may be a factor. The subject obviously calls for more attention than has been accorded it in the past.

A not unrelated question concerns possible functions of the hen's ruptured ovarian follicle which, as van Tienhoven (65) has recently emphasized again, is not to be confused with the mammalian corpus luteum. The ruptured follicle is essential for oviposition (57), and it contains progesterone (39). Practically nothing else seems to be known about the structure. Its rapid resorption following ovulation need not exclude some important short-term role in the cycle, but one could only speculate on what this might be.

The Nalbandov Hypotheses

Two explanations of the ovulation cycle have been developed by Nalbandov (42, 44). Both stem from the results of experiments, described earlier, demonstrating the suppression of LH release for ovulation, but not of other gonadotropic-dependent functions, by irritants in the magnum or isthmus of the oviduct (35, 63). In accounting for their observations, Huston and Nalbandov (35) postulated that the pituitary of the ovulating hen secretes FSH and LH at a continuing and relatively steady basal level; periodically, LH is released in greater quantities to effect ovulation. The oviducal irritant was believed to suppress, over neurogenic pathways, only the periodic LH releases required for ovulation. These authors, and Nalbandov (42), considered also the possibility that the presence of an egg in the magnum might likewise suppress the periodic LH release required for ovulation. On this view, neurogenic inhibition of the ovulatory LH release mechanism ceases when the egg clears the magnum (or isthmus) and "LH is secreted in sufficient quantities to cause the next ovulation" (42).

In a recent reconsideration of the problem, Nalbandov (44) points out that the period during which the neurogenic stimulus may act is no more than about 5 hr following ovulation. In the two-member sequence, the 5-hr period following ovulation of the C_1 follicle would thus end 15–16 hr before OIH release for ovulation of the second follicle, assuming 8 hr to elapse between OIH release and ovulation. Even supposing an improbable 14-hr interval between OIH release and ovulation, the neurogenic stimulus would cease 9–10 hr before the second release of OIH in the 2-member sequence. In the light of such considerations and, in addition, the failure of the earlier hypothesis to account for the period of lapse, Nalbandov (44) recently proposed a different interpretation of effects of the neurogenic stimulus (or inhibition) from the oviduct.

The hypothesis now proposed rests on several related propositions. Light is believed not to regulate "rhythmicity of the laying cycle of birds", although it does determine rate of pituitary function and thus has a "permissive effect" on reproductive performance. The bird's pituitary is assumed to secrete a single gonadotropic complex with FSH- and LH-like properties rather than the two separate entities usually assumed. Secretion of this complex is suppressed during passage of the egg through the magnum and isthmus of the oviduct, a period of some 4–5 hr. Secretion of the gonadotropic complex is resumed when the egg clears the isthmus and circulating gonadotropin slowly returns to pre-inhibition levels; with attainment of these levels, ovulation is induced.

Of these several assumptions, the crucial one with respect to the timing of ovulation is clearly that of pituitary recovery following the 5-hr period of inhibition. As stated by Nalbandov, sequence length "would be determined by the rate at which the pituitary gland could recover from each episode of neural inhibition. Thus, rapid recovery would permit long clutches, while slow recovery would result in short clutches." The period of lapse is accounted for similarly: "With each succeeding cycle of inhibition and release hypophysial recovery rate becomes slower until at the end of the clutch the pituitary gland does not recover in time to cause the ovulation of the next egg, and the clutch is interrupted."

Several implications of the concept of pituitary recovery following episodes of inhibition may be noted. Rate of recovery would plainly have to be very finely adjusted to account for lag relationships seen in the ordinary ovulation sequence, an improbable demand upon "recovery" in any guise. In sequences of three or more members, rate of recovery would actually increase, not decrease, with the several successive episodes of inhibition following the first, since the intervals between successive ovulations are decreasing. In lengthy sequences, recovery would proceed at the same, and at a relatively rapid rate, not at onset of the sequence but during those phases in which lag approaches or equals zero (Fig. 1). But supposing these and other aspects of recovery within the sequence to be accounted for, there remains the formidable period of lapse. We have seen earlier that through most or all of this period there coexist an ovulable follicle and an apparently competent pituitary. If recovery were indeed a decisive factor in pituitary function it would thus appear to have been completed by about the same course as is assumed following episodes of inhibition within the sequence. Yet the first ovulation of the oncoming sequence occurs in association with the prevailing photoperiod, many hours later than would be expected in terms of pituitary recovery. The simple fact that ovulation of the C_1 follicle does occur in close association with some phase of photoperiod over a wide range of photoperiods (38) would seem to cast doubt, apart from any other consideration, on the postulated role of pituitary recovery during the period of lapse.

One is certainly inclined to agree with Nalbandov that the oviducal egg most probably does play a role in some aspect of the ovulation cycle. If the hypotheses proposed by Nalbandov (42, 44) in this connection seem unsatisfactory, we should perhaps inquire whether the experimental observations on which these proposals are based have in fact been accounted for adequately, or if not, whether more likely explanations can be suggested.

The experimental oviducal irritant appears to maintain a gonadotropic hormone balance similar in some important respects to that imposed by the continuing administration of FSH or PMS (4). The daily injection of such preparations in adequate quantities maintains follicular growth but invariably interrupts ovulation after a day or two, thus resulting in a gradual accumulation of ovulable follicles (28). Small follicles may also be caused to grow more rapidly than usual, further increasing the mass of follicular tissue. Under these conditions we should certainly expect higher than normal estrogen levels, and it is not likely that these would show much diurnal variation, certainly not under the pressure of daily PMS injections. On the basis of evidence advanced earlier, the total suppression of OIH release can be attributed to these continuing high estrogen levels, and the site of estrogen action would be in some neural component of the OIH release mechanism (25).

In view of the fact that oviducal irritants and continuing gonadotropin administration are similarly effective in suppressing OIH release, it may be suggested that the oviducal irritant acts over neurogenic pathways to stimulate or to maintain those nervous activities, ordinarily periodic, which are associated with the output of gonadotropins at a level favoring the secretion of estrogen into the blood stream at concentrations capable of blocking excitation for OIH release. In these terms, the oviducal irritant acts as a stimulus at the neural level, and only secondarily in an inhibitory capacity.

It may be objected that the follicular aggregates resulting from the oviducal thread and continuing gonadotropin administration are not comparable, the former representing over long periods an essentially normal hierarchy, whereas the latter comes to include a number of ovulable follicles as well as rapidly growing smaller follicles. The differing ovarian complements may simply reflect quantitative differences in stimulation, since Huston and Nalbandov (35) note that in some of their early experiments, in which key chains and other large irritants were employed, the ovary sometimes carried "six or more follicles of ovulatory size". They observed also, in hens carrying only the oviducal thread, "a few sporadic ovulations which were widely spaced", suggesting a relatively moderate stimulation (and moderate estrogen inhibition) under these conditions. On the other hand, most if not all descriptions of the ovary following gonadotropin administration have been based on manifestly heavy stimulation.

If a continuing oviducal irritant may act in the manner suggested, the oviducal egg during its passage to the uterus may likewise stimulate the elaboration and secretion of estrogen. We have considered already a possible role of varying estrogen concentrations in the ovulation cycle, namely, their participation in timing of successive excitations in a manner which may account, in part at least, for lag and termination of the sequence. Possibly the oviducal egg is of greater importance in this respect than is the release of OIH. Perhaps the actions of OIH and the oviducal egg are related in some fashion not presently suspected. Whatever the facts may finally turn out to be, the role suggested here for the oviducal egg seems in accord with experimental evidence concerning the action of estrogen in the hen's ovulation cycle, as well as with a plausible interpretation of the effects of the continuing oviducal irritant.

It is well known that ovulation may occur in hens whose oviducts are incapable of engulfing the ovulated yolk, either as a result of surgical operations on the oviduct (47) or of naturally occurring conditions (36). The timing of successive ovulations in such hens, not presently known, might tell us much concerning the possible participation of the oviduct in the ovulation cycle. By X-ray or other techniques it should be possible to establish this obviously important datum.

The Hypothesis of Bastian and Zarrow

These authors (3) based their hypothesis of the ovulation cycle on the postulation of "two separate and independent cycles" which "interact in such a way as to result in the typical ovulatory cycle of the hen", to result, that is, in the appearance of what we have called lag, and the period of lapse. One of their concepts is that there is present an effective ovulatory stimulus (LH or OIH) over an extended period, e.g. 8 hr, each night, including the night preceding the day during which ovulation fails to occur. According to the second concept, follicles attain to maturity or ovulability at fairly regular intervals in cycles or sequences of given length. It is recognized that follicular maturation is a gradual process, and ovulability therefore a relative condition.

The interaction of these two "cycles" means essentially that if a follicle attains to ovulability at a sufficiently early time within the diurnally recurrent period of elevated LH levels, it is ovulated. But if a follicle, i.e. the oncoming C_1 follicle, comes to high sensitivity too late in a given LH release period, its ovulation is carried over to the following period, by which time it has become highly responsive, presumably in part because of the maturation promoting action of LH during the preceding night when this follicle approached but did not quite achieve response to prevailing LH levels. With some minor qualifications concerning follicular maturation, Bastian and Zarrow believed their hypothesis capable of accounting also for lag in the sequence, and thus for the "asynchronous ovulation rhythm of the hen".

Bastian and Zarrow advanced no direct evidence in support of their main premise, the recurrent and prolonged secretion of LH during the same hours of each 24. This concept appears to have had its origin in recognition of the synchronization with photoperiod of the hours of the 24 within which OIH release occurred, together with participation of the central nervous system in control of pituitary gonadotropin secretion. If some phase of photoperiod, such as onset of darkness, invariably activated the nervous component of the system and thus caused the pituitary to release LH, such release would of course be expected on the night preceding the day of no ovulation. As we have seen earlier, release of LH during this night appears to be unnecessary to account for the subsequent high terminal ovulability of the C_1 follicle, a conclusion which of itself need not disprove the postulated release. But if LH is actually so released, the oncoming C_1 follicle would be subjected, through at least a part of the night preceding LH release for its ovulation, to what in effect would appear to be subovulatory levels of the gonadotropin, a condition which often results in atresia, as Bastian and Zarrow (3) themselves and others (21, 22, 64) have found experimentally. Atresia might also be expected to intervene at or near the termination of the ovulating sequence if in fact the ovarian follicles mature at fairly regular intervals, as is postulated by Bastian and Zarrow. The grounds for questioning the validity of this second postulate have been discussed in connection with follicular maturation and need not be repeated here. It is of some interest to observe, however, that even though the order of follicular maturation described earlier and represented in Fig. 2 be accepted, the release of LH during the night preceding the release actually effecting ovulation of the C_1 follicle—during the period, *p*, of the figure—might also be expected to result not infrequently in atresia.

As has been noted elsewhere (18), Bastian and Zarrow and this author are in agreement in assigning to photoperiod the basic role of timing the appearance and termination of the "open" period of low thresholds in the neural component of the OIH (or LH) release mechanism. But while Bastian and Zarrow conceive of an immediate and constant functional relationship between the appearance of the open period and OIH release, much evidence reviewed in this paper impresses the conviction that timing of the specific nervous activity resulting in OIH release is conditioned largely by the ovarian hormones and the order of follicular maturation.

REFERENCES

1. Assenmacher, I., *Arch. Anat. microsc. et Morphol. exp.* **47**, 447–572, 1958.
2. Bastian, J. W. and M. X. Zarrow, *Proc. Soc. Exp. Biol. and Med.* **79**, 249–252, 1952.
3. Bastian, J. W. and M. X. Zarrow, *Poul. Sci.* **34**, 776–788, 1955.
4. Bates, R. W., E. L. Lahr and O. Riddle, *Amer. J. Physiol.* **111**, 361–368, 1935.
5. Benoit, J. and I. Assenmacher, *Arch. Anat. microsc. et Morphol. exp.* **42**, 334–386, 1953.
6. Benoit, J. and I. Assenmacher, *J. Physiol. (Paris)* **47**, 427–567, 1955.
7. Benoit, J. and I. Assenmacher, *Recent Prog. Hormone Res.* **15**, 143–164, 1959.
8. Donovan, B. T. and J. J. van der Werff ten Bosch, *J. Physiol.* **147**, 78–92, 1959.
9. Donovan, B. T. and J. J. van der Werff ten Bosch, *J. Physiol.* **147**, 93–108, 1959.
10. Everett, J. W., *Anat. Rec.* **109**, 291, 1951.
11. Everett, J. W. and C. H. Sawyer, *Endocrinology* **47**, 198–218, 1950.
12. Forbes, T. R. and C. W. Hooker, *Endocrinology* **61**, 281–286, 1957.
13. Fraps, R. M., *Anat. Rec.* **87**, 443, 1943.
14. Fraps, R. M., *Anat. Rec.* **96**, 573–574, 1946.
15. Fraps, R. M., *Proc. Natl. Acad. Sci. U.S.* **40**, 348–356, 1954.
16. Fraps, R. M., *Memoirs Soc. Endocrinol.* No. **4**, 205–219, 1955.
17. Fraps, R. M., in *Progress in the Physiology of Farm Animals*, vol. **2** (Edited by John Hammond), pp. 661–740. Butterworths Scientific Publications, London, 1955.
18. Fraps, R. M., in *Photoperiodism and Related Phenomena in Plants and Animals* (Edited by R. B. Withrow), pp. 767–785, Publ. No. 55, Am. Assoc. Adv. Sci., Washington, D.C., 1959.
19. Fraps, R. M. and J. F. Case., *Proc. Soc. Exp. Biol. and Med.* **82**, 167–171, 1953
20. Fraps, R. M. and M. H. Conner, *Nature* **174**, 1148–1149, 1954.
21. Fraps, R. M. and A. Dury, *Anat. Rec.* **84**, 453, 1942.
22. Fraps, R. M. and A. Dury, *Anat. Rec.* **84**, 521–522, 1942.
23. Fraps, R. M. and A. Dury, *Anat. Rec.* **87**, 442–443, 1943.
24. Fraps, R. M. and A. Dury, *Proc. Soc. Exp. Biol. and Med.* **52**, 140–142, 1943.
25. Fraps, R. M. and H. L. Fevold, *Proc. Soc. Exp. Biol. and Med.* **90**, 440–446, 1955
26. Fraps, R. M., H. L. Fevold and B. H. Neher, *Anat. Rec.* **99**, 571–572, 1947.
27. Fraps, R. M., C. W. Hooker and T. R. Forbes, *Science* **108**, 86–87, 1948.
28. Fraps, R. M. and G. M. Riley, *Proc. Soc. Exp. Biol. and Med.* **49**, 253–257, 1942.
29. Green, J. D., *Amer. J. Anat.* **88**, 225–312, 1951.
30. Green, J. D. and G. W. Harris, *J. Endocrinol.* **5(3)**, 136–146, 1947.
31. Harris, G. W., *Physiol. Rev.* **28**, 139–179, 1948.
32. Harris, G. W., Monographs Physiol. Soc., No. 3. Edward Arnold, London, 1955.
33. Heywang, B. W., *Poul. Sci.* **17**, 240–247, 1938.
34. Hooker, C. W. and T. R. Forbes, *Endocrinology* **41**, 158–159, 1947.
35. Huston, T. M. and A. V. Nalbandov, *Endocrinology* **52**, 149–156, 1953.
36. Hutt, F. B., K. Goodwin and W. D. Urban, *Cornell Vet.* **46**, 257–273, 1956.
37. Lacassagne, L., *Annales de Zootech.* **5**, 335–362, 1956.
38. Lanson, R. K., Unpublished Ph.D. thesis. Rutgers University, New Brunswick New Jersey, 1959.

39. LAYNE, D. S., R. H. COMMON, W. A. MAW and R. M. FRAPS, *Proc. Soc. Exp. Biol. and Med.* **94**, 528–529, 1957.
40. LEGAIT, H., *Arch. Anat. microsc. et Morphol. exp.* **44**, 323–343, 1955.
41. LYTLE, I. M. and F. W. LORENZ, *Nature* **182**, 1681, 1958.
42. NALBANDOV, A. V., *Poul. Sci.* **32**, 88–103, 1953.
43. NALBANDOV, A. V., *Reproductive Physiology*, W. H. Freeman, San Francisco, 1958.
44. NALBANDOV, A. V., in *Comparative Endocrinology* (Edited by A. Gorbman), pp. 161–173, John Wiley, New York, 1959.
45. NEHER, B. H. and R. M. FRAPS, *Endocrinology* **46**, 482–488, 1950.
46. OKSCHE, A., D. F. LAWS, F. I. KAMEMOTO and D. S. FARNER, *Z. Zellforsch.* **51**, 1–42, 1959.
47. PEARL, R. and M. CURTIS, *J. Exp. Zool.* **17**, 395–424, 1914.
48. RALPH, C. L., *Anat. Rec.* **134**, 411–431, 1959.
49. RALPH, C. L., *Chicago Acad. Sci., Special Publ.* No. **14**, 4–5, 1959.
50. RALPH, C. L., *Am. J. Physiol.* **198**, 528–530, 1960.
51. RALPH, C. L. and R. M. FRAPS, *Anat. Rec.* **130**, 360–361, 1958.
52. RALPH, C. L. and R. M. FRAPS, *Endocrinology* **65**, 819–824, 1959.
53. RALPH, C. L. and R. M. FRAPS, *Am. J. Physiol.* **197**, 1279–1283, 1959.
54. RALPH, C. L. and R. M. FRAPS, *Endocrinology* **66**, 269–272, 1960.
55. RILEY, G. M. and R. M. FRAPS, *Endocrinology* **30**, 537–541, 1942.
56. ROTHCHILD, I., *Fed. Proc.* **8**, 135, 1949.
57. ROTHCHILD, I. and R. M. FRAPS, *Proc. Soc. Exp. Biol. and Med.* **56**, 79–82, 1944.
58. ROTHCHILD, I. and R. M. FRAPS, *Endocrinology* **44**, 134–140, 1949.
59. ROTHCHILD, I. and R. M. FRAPS, *Endocrinology* **44**, 141–149, 1949.
60. SCHARRER, E., in *Comparative Endocrinology* (Edited by A. Gorbman), pp. 233–249, John Wiley, New York, 1959.
61. SHIRLEY, H. V. and A. V. NALBANDOV, *Endocrinology* **58**, 477–483, 1956.
62. SHIRLEY, H. V. and A. V. NALBANDOV, *Endocrinology* **58**, 694–700, 1956.
63. VAN TIENHOVEN, A., *Anat. Rec.* **115**, 374–375, 1953.
64. VAN TIENHOVEN, A., *Endocrinology* **56**, 667–674, 1955.
65. VAN TIENHOVEN, A., in *Reproduction in Domestic Animals*, vol. II (Edited by H. H. Cole and P. T. Cupps), pp. 305–342, Academic Press, New York, 1959.
66. VAN TIENHOVEN, A., A. V. NALBANDOV and H. W. NORTON, *Endocrinology* **54**, 605–611, 1954.
67. WINGSTRAND, K. G., *The Structure and Development of the Avian Pituitary*, C. W. K. Gleerup, Lund, Sweden, 1951.
68. ZANDER, J., *Nature* **174**, 406–407, 1954.
69. ZANDER, J., T. R. FORBES, A. M. VON MÜNSTERMANN and R. NEHER, *J. Clin. Endocrinol. and Metab.* **18**, 337–353, 1958.
70. ZARROW, M. X. and J. W. BASTIAN, *Proc. Soc. Exp. Biol. and Med.* **84**, 457–459, 1953.

HORMONAL AUGMENTATION OF FERTILITY IN SHEEP AND CATTLE

JOHN HAMMOND, JR.
Cambridge University School of Agriculture

INTRODUCTION

A QUARTER of a century has passed since Cole and Miller (18) used gonadotropin to obtain fertility in anestrous sheep. In reviewing the progress which has been made since then, I intend to deal principally with the control of ovulation and estrous behavior, largely neglecting the many other factors—including fertilization and fetal loss—that intervene between mating and weaning.

Hormonal control of ovulation has potential agricultural uses in two main fields. Given a satisfactory technique of transplantation, there will be genetic applications such as the multiplication of offspring from particular dams, and the acceleration of a breeding program by production of young from immature females. This might find wide application, but yet could be worthwhile on a small scale. The other type of application, increasing the number of young born, is only likely to be worthwhile if it can be carried out widely and cheaply.

For this reason most investigators have used the gonadotropins of pregnant mare serum (PMS) and human pregnancy urine (PU). Those workers who have employed pituitary extracts have generally administered predominantly follicle-stimulating preparations subcutaneously, and given LH-rich extracts intravenously. To avoid cumbersome phraseology, I shall use the (inaccurate) terms "FSH" and "LH" in referring to these pituitary extracts. Unless otherwise specified, it should be understood that PMS and "FSH" have been given subcutaneously and PU and "LH" intravenously.

While PMS hormone circulates in the mare in enormous quantity, a succession of follicles develop and ovulate (70); yet the urinary estrogen is not obviously raised (17) and relatively small amounts of exogenous estrogen given at this time will induce abortion (21). Thus PMS appears to have the properties ascribed by Simpson, Li and Evans (72), in 1951, to purified FSH. In all the work with farm animals one has to allow for endogenous hormone production complicating the response; on the other hand, we may perhaps be allowed the simplification of regarding PMS as a pure type of FSH.

NORMAL REPRODUCTIVE PATTERNS

The sheep has a restricted breeding season which is photoperiodically regulated. Breeds differ in the length of breeding season and also in the degree of ovarian activity during anestrus. There are differences in the normal incidence of twin and multiple ovulations in different breeds. The first ovulation of the breeding season is not accompanied by estrus (36), and the time of this ovulation may be hastened by the introduction of a ram into the ewe flock (73). So-called "silent heats", ovulation unaccompanied by estrus, may also occur during the breeding season, particularly in animals growing under poor nutritive conditions (38). Heat without ovulation may occur at the end of the season (1).

The cow, on the other hand, though probably affected by photoperiod, breeds throughout the year. Silent heats however do occur, and even anestrus has been observed, mostly in heifers under poor winter feeding conditions. The incidence of twinning may be as high as 4% (30), but in general it is very low, especially in beef breeds.

Ignoring considerable seasonal and individual differences, the cycle of the sheep may be said to last 16 or 17 days, with heat lasting about 30 hr and ovulation occurring at about the end of heat. The cycle in the cow lasts 20–21 days, heat lasts about a day, and ovulation occurs 10 hr or so after the end of heat (16).

It is not unusual to speak of "follicular" and "luteal" phases of the ruminant cycle, but there is no event such as menstruation to demarcate the end of the luteal phase. Grant (37) has constructed an average curve for the growth and regression of the sheep corpus luteum, but size does not necessarily parallel activity. Japanese workers (56, 57) consider the corpus luteum to be non-functional if injected estrogen induces estrous behavior. Their results appear to indicate that estrus can be advanced by 2–3 days, possibly by more.

When the corpus luteum is removed from the ovary, follicle growth, estrus and ovulation follow, and the cycle rhythm is rephased. In sheep the interval is 2–4 days (52); in cattle estrus most commonly occurs 4 days later but a 3-day interval is nearly as frequent. If one accepts that this represents the normal rate of follicle development one may conclude that, in the cow, the corpus luteum regresses, and follicle growth starts, about 3 days before the onset of heat and that in the sheep the interval is probably less. Alternatively, normal follicle growth is slower and the two phases of the cycle overlap.

The chances of survival of induced multiple pregnancies seem to differ in the sheep and cow. In the sheep there is a loss of fertilized ova at and before the stage of implantation (11, 62). There seems to be a maternal restriction upon litter size at an average figure of, in general, less than 3. With very large numbers of ovulations, Casida *et al.* (11) noted a tendency to total loss after the stage of implantation.

In the cow there seems to be early partial loss (35), but with only 4 or 5 ovulations total loss has been noted at about half term (42) or earlier (9, 35). In the cow therefore very close control is required over the number of ovulations, but in the sheep this seems of little importance.

OVULATION AND HEAT IN ANESTRUS

Most workers have found that a single injection of FSH or of PMS will induce ovulation in almost all treated sheep. Estimates of the time of ovulation, based upon the time of slaughter and the appearance of the induced corpora, range from 24 to 72 hr after injection, most commonly within 48 hr (44, 61). A group of animals treated by Robinson (61) provide an exception; some failed to ovulate even after two treatments with 800 i.u. PMS and there does not seem to have been very much follicle growth. While some of these animals were of a breed with a more restricted season than those usually treated, all apparently had in common a poor nutritional status.

After a single injection of FSH, PMS or PU the number of ovulations has nearly always been within the normal range for the breed, and the ovulations apparently occurred synchronously (34, 44). Instances have been noted of two series of ovulations following a single injection of PMS: this may account for multiple corpora lutea in some ewes so treated by Robinson (61). Casida and colleagues (4, 54) have obtained multiple ovulations in anestrous sheep with repeated FSH injections followed by LH; it seems unlikely that all the ovulations were synchronous.

Although the number of ovulations has been relatively constant, the extent of follicle development has in general paralleled the dosage of FSH or PMS, but this is by no means always obvious with PMS (44).

Whereas a single gonadotropin treatment induces ovulation, this is rarely accompanied by heat. Furthermore, artificial insemination has usually failed to produce fertilization of the ova shed (41, 44). This has been attributed to failure of sperm transport (58) and there is no reason to doubt the maturity of the ova shed (5).

The few sheep coming on heat have usually been found to have had a corpus luteum regressing at about the time of injection and so have been not anestrous in the strict sense. Two treatments with PMS, a cycle interval apart, have been used to induce ovulation accompanied by fertile mating (18). The success achieved has been very variable: sometimes very different results have been obtained by the same workers in successive seasons (79). There is no obvious reason for doubting that the second treatment also induces ovulation: yet heat is often not shown. Gordon (34) obtained heat in only 4 of 59 ewes treated at 16-day intervals. Failure of proper luteal function has been suggested, but Robinson (61) found no evidence for alteration of the period of luteal function, and modifications of PMS dosage and of the interval between treatments have met with no great success.

In contrast to the frequent failure of heat to attend a second induced ovulation, there is a marked tendency for heat to occur spontaneously at a cycle interval after treatment (44). Furthermore, fertility to service at such heats appears good; Gordon (34) had 11 lactating ewes which came on heat in this way, and 8 of them lambed.

Attempts have been made to obtain heat with ovulation by combined treatment with estrogen and PMS. However, while estrogen alone will sometimes induce ovulation, given with PMS it sometimes prevents the ovulation which might otherwise have been expected. Hammond (41) concluded that estrogen caused a discharge of endogenous gonadotropin and produced ovulation only in those animals which had already a large follicle, while PMS would indirectly cause ovulaton, triggering a pituitary discharge with estrogen from the ripened follicle. In animals whose follicles were small at the time of treatment insufficient pituitary stores would remain to ovulate the follicles when grown. Alternatively, a premature discharge may render the follicles incapable of ovulating. He found cystic follicles far more often with the combined treatment than with either substance given separately.

Besides interference with ovulation, there was the difficulty that heat and ovulation were not synchronized; the latent period between estrogen and heat was greater than that between PMS or estrogen and ovulation. Estrogen induced heat more effectively in animals in which ovulation was blocked. A regressing corpus luteum is normally required for estrus, but secretion from newly formed corpora antagonized the estrogen.

Robinson and colleagues (53, 64, 67, 69) have investigated estrogen progesterone interaction in the spayed ewe. Progesterone pretreatment lowers the threshold dose of estrogen needed to cause estrous behavior and also shortens the latent period before heat is manifested; 50% of treated animals came on heat within 36 hr of estrogen administration. Maximal response to a dose of estrogen (which, given alone, was subthreshold) required more than 6 days' pretreatment with progesterone and an interval of 24–48 hr between the final dose of progesterone and administration of the estrogen. It appears that progesterone produces transitory sensitization to estrogen; the proprioceptor concerned is not in the uterus, as had been suggested, because hysterectomy did not affect response.

Estrus following a single injection of PMS has been obtained by pretreatment either with testosterone (19, 61) or with progesterone (26, 63). Progesterone has usually been given in oil over a period of 3–15 days, followed by PMS 2 or 3 days later. In these circumstances the ovulation rate has been normal (26, 34, 65). There was a tendency to multiple ovulations when a single large dose of progesterone (75 mg) was followed by PMS 2 days later (65). Robinson (65) reported great uniformity in the time of onset of heat, but when Gordon (34) used suspensions of crystalline progesterone time of onset of heat was erratic. Those that came on heat also ovulated and had a normal number of corpora lutea; but many of the others also ovulated, and these had an appreciably higher average ovulation rate.

Testosterone given at the same time as PMS, or one day earlier, tended to block ovulation, and cystic or luteinized follicles were common (61). Testosterone thus appears to share with progesterone the property—more apparent when results in the breeding season are considered—of blocking an ovulating release of endogenous gonadotropin.

When prolonged treatment with progesterone is given, there is a distinct tendency for ovulation and heat to follow cessation of treatment, even though no gonadotropin is administered (23, 26, 65)—just as it may follow regression of an induced corpus luteum. This might be explained by supposing that progesterone, besides blocking pituitary release of hormone, also causes its accumulation and hence a tendency for discharge when progesterone is withdrawn.

Almost without exception, ovulation occurs when PMS is given 2–3 days after a series of progesterone injections (2, 26, 34, 48, 65). Raeside and Lamond (60) got better results with this schedule than with PMS alone. The incidence of estrus, as reported by these workers and by others (22, 66), was generally 80–100%. Fertility, however, is more variable, and it is difficult to know whether this is due to minor differences in method of treatment, differences in the animals treated, or merely in quality of insemination. In non-lactating sheep Dutt (26) found 50% of ova fertilized; Dauzier (22) and Gordon (34) report conception rates near normal (70–80% and 70%) and also definitely low (43%), while Robinson (66) obtained very few pregnancies.

There seems to be a definite difference in response of lactating and of non-lactating ewes, which has been observed both with PMS twice at a cycle interval (49), and also with a single PMS treatment following progesterone (34). Both the incidence of heat in those treated, and the proportion of those served lambing, is lowered by lactation.

When a ewe lambs early in the breeding season there is a lactation anestrus of about 6 weeks (34). When lactation is combined with seasonal anestrus it seems likely there will be a greater degree of ovarian inactivity, and hence possibly a greater average time interval between PMS injection and ovulation. It may be that the time relationship between heat and ovulation is affected, but this has not been investigated, nor have the frequencies of ovulation and of fertilization been determined in the ewe treated while lactating.

OVULATION IN THE BREEDING SEASON

Midcycle and Pregnancy

For a variety of reasons, induction of ovulation during the luteal phase of the cycle has not been widely attempted. Russian workers had found that midcycle ovulation did not affect the length of cycle in sheep or cattle (44). It is thus unlikely that ova so shed could reach implantation and maintain a corpus luteum of pregnancy. The treated animals rarely come on heat; sometimes they show signs of heat but refuse to accept the male. After insemination the ova are usually not fertilized (54, 71, 78), possibly because the sperm are not capacitated (13); furthermore, insemination through the cervix uniformly caused pyometra (78). Poor recovery of the ova shed, once suspected to be due to failure to leave the follicle, is probably due to disturbed ovum transport. Rapid tubal transport under the influence of the corpus luteum (62, 71) would cause the ova to reach the uterus before they were likely to be able to survive in the uterine secretions (12).

Pregnant animals have been treated rarely, and usually inadvertently. Ovulation has occurred after FSH as a single dose (sheep, 44) or repeated doses (cow, 9), after PU following PMS (cow, 43), and after PU alone (sheep, 62). But it does not seem to be induced easily by a single dose of PMS (cow, 43; sheep, 62).

During the luteal phase of the cycle, Casida *et al.* (9) found that repeated subcutaneous pituitary injections caused follicle growth, but did not uniformly produce ovulation. However, similar treatment (or with FSH) when followed by an intravenous injection consistently induced multiple ovulation. Multiple ovulation in sheep has been brought about in the same way (54). Repeated injections of FSH, followed by PU or LH, have also been used to induce multiple ovulation in cattle (78).

After a single dose of FSH to sheep in the luteal phase, ovulation or luteinized follicles were sometimes observed (44), but not after PMS. In cattle Folley and Malpress (31) noted what they called "shock" ovulations of one or two follicles which sometimes occurred within 48 hr of a single dose of FSH but not of PMS.

In the presence of an active corpus luteum, ovulation in cows rarely occurred after PMS (71); it happened more often with a high dose, and more readily after FSH (43). Multiple ovulation was, however, readily induced when PMS was followed by PU (7, 71).

Rowson (71) drew attention to quantitative and qualitative differences in the response of cows to crude and purified PMS. Doses assayed as equipotent in the rat were not so in cows. The purified material produced less follicle growth and furthermore a smaller proportion of the large follicles ovulated when PU was administered. While this might be due to loss of synergistic LH activity during purification it is conceivable that differences in rate of absorption or elimination are responsible.

The effect of a single large dose of gonadotropin may be prolonged (31). Brock and Rowson (7) found the number of follicles ovulated by PU after PMS increased until the interval between the two treatments was at least 7 days. Abnormal, cystic looking, and partly luteinized follicles may be seen after massive or prolonged treatment (9, 29), but Folley and Malpress (31) found this condition transitory; a persistent cystic condition, such as sometimes occurs in infertile cows, was not produced.

Follicles developed by PMS or FSH in the presence of a corpus luteum do not in general ovulate spontaneously; one may suppose that progesterone blocks an endogenous ovulating release of hormone. The blockage is probably not absolute, for estrogen can induce midcycle ovulation (sheep, 44). Conceivably a partial pituitary "escape" might cause ovulation, or, being inadequate for that, be enough to luteinize a follicle or make it cystic. However, "shock" ovulations (or abortive attempts at ovulation) might also be due to a sudden rise in the level of gonadotropin circulating; and would then presumably be more likely with larger doses, greater ease of absorption (or intravenous administration), and with greater luteinizing activity of the material used—with FSH rather than with PMS.

AFTER REMOVAL OF THE CORPUS LUTEUM

Hammond and Bhattacharya (43) found that, when given to cows at or after the time of corpus luteum removal, PMS and FSH could induce twin or multiple ovulations, but in about 50% only one egg was shed. They found that the times of heat and of ovulation were advanced. Rowson (71), however, often found delay or failure to ovulate when he gave purified PMS at expression of the corpus luteum, and subsequent treatment with PU often did not induce ovulation. Umbaugh (75) reports that FSH in subcutaneous waxy implants, made when the corpus luteum was removed, did not produce multiple ovulation; but many follicles were observed to ovulate within about 30 hr when the same material was given again four days later, this time intravenously.

From small series of cows given PMS at two dose levels 0–5 days before expression of the corpus luteum Hammond and Bhattacharya (43) concluded that, in general, the longer the interval between doses and the larger the dose, the greater was the number of ovulations and the shorter the interval to ovulation after expression of the corpus luteum. However, they noted on the one hand animals in which a large dose produced little follicle growth, and on the other, multiple ovulations from a small dose. Modification of dosage and interval failed to yield twin ovulations consistently (42).

This procedure was also technically unsatisfactory for producing multiple ovulations because of the risk of damaging follicles when expressing the corpus luteum. Follicles which were ruptured or bruised sometimes luteinized and then might block further ovulation.

Dowling (25) used this same procedure to produce multiple ovulations both with FSH and with purified PMS. He found the interval to heat was in most cases decreased. Whereas most ova were fertilized after FSH, very few were cleaved in PMS-treated animals. This may be related to greater follicle development, and larger numbers of corpora, in the latter group, and to accelerated tubal transport. An association between multiple corpora and degenerate ova was noted by Brock and Rowson (7) in cows in which estrus was delayed following PMS administration at the time of corpus luteum removal.

The number of ovulations was greater as the interval between injection and heat increased (7); one may suppose that the longer the PMS has to act, the larger will be the number of follicles mature enough to respond either to an endogenous ovulating release of hormone or to administered PU.

This factor of timing may have affected the observations of Rowson (71) regarding the influence of preliminary removal of the corpus luteum on the ovulating effectiveness of PU following PMS treatment. But other data (7) support the finding that, with PMS followed by PU, fewer follicles, and a smaller proportion of those reaching a large size, ovulate if the corpus luteum has been removed. A similar difference (71) existed between the response to whole serum and to processed PMS given at the time of corpus luteum removal (with no subsequent PU). There were fewer ovulations with processed PMS; indeed many cows so treated failed to ovulate within a period of about a week.

The papers quoted all agree on individual variation in the follicle growth produced, but there are divergent opinions as to whether the general effects to be expected from PMS given at the time of corpus luteum removal are acceleration or delay of heat and ovulation, and ovulation of one or of many follicles. Factors possibly responsible for these differences include not only the different forms in which PMS was given, but also different dose levels, those of Rowson being generally higher.

Dowling points out that the cow can produce enough hormone to ovulate many artificially stimulated follicles, and scanty data provided by Brock and Rowson suggest that PU given at heat, following PMS given when the corpus luteum was removed, does not increase the number of ovulations.

The finding of many large follicles and few corpora after a dose of PU which is known to be effective in ovulating a large proportion of a similar number of follicles would appear to indicate that when the PU was given the follicles were either too immature to respond or else were already cystic.

It seems possible that a small dose of PMS might speed follicle growth after corpus luteum removal, and so, indirectly, hasten ovulation; but a large dose, rapidly absorbed, might provide a premature or subthreshold stimulus to ovulation and thus abort the larger follicles. Ovulation would then be delayed until a fresh generation of follicles matured.

AFTER REGRESSION OF THE CORPUS LUTEUM

The aims and methods of investigation differ with sheep and cattle and it is therefore convenient to consider the species separately.

Treatment of cattle towards the end of the cycle, either with FSH or PMS, has consistently induced multiple ovulation (9, 10, 25, 29, 31, 78), though there is a tendency to reduced response with repeated treatments (77). Though multiple ovulations may be readily obtained, it would appear that the actual number is not easily predictable. Sometimes poor recovery of ova and apparent failure of fertilization have been reported (25, 29). It has sometimes been the practice to give an intravenous injection at the time, or predicted time, of heat (9, 29, 78), but there does not seem to be any definite indication that this procedure results in a larger number of ovulations or better fertility.

With a standard dose of PMS, Hammond and Bhattacharya (43) considered that the ovulatory response was less erratic when given 3 days before the time, or presumed time, of heat than when given at the time of corpus luteum removal. Twin ovulations were general under the former conditions. However, similar treatment of animals allowed to calve gave less good results (42). There was, in practice, considerable difficulty in timing the injection so that heat followed 3 days later. Ovulation counts by rectal palpation of corpora (which were not entirely accurate; on occasion there were more calves born than corpora counted) revealed twin ovulations in a minority and occasional animals with 4 or 5 corpora lutea. Contributory to these results are probably individual variation of cycle length and individual breed and perhaps seasonal differences in sensitivity.

Recently Gordon (35) has been trying similar treatment on a larger scale, and has had better success both in timing of the injection and in choice of dosage level. Preliminary results based on rectal palpation (and which await the tests of parturition and of further experience) indicate a considerable discrepancy between number of corpora lutea and number of fetuses.

In the cow (8) with good quality insemination the ovum is nearly always fertilized but about 30% fail to survive, so that there is only about 70% conception to service at a given heat period. Gordon's figures suggest that with twin ovulations the conception rate is greater than this, but the chances of both ova surviving are rather poor. This contrasts with Dutt's (27) finding in the sheep of 143% lambing in sheep with estimated 147% ovulation.

A single FSH injection to sheep, given towards the end of the cycle, has been noted to produce luteinization of unovulated follicles as well as multiple ovulation (44); but luteinized follicles were detected only in sheep killed several days after ovulation. It is thus conceivable that Gordon may have been misled about the number of twin ovulations—as opposed to twin corpora —in his animals.

In sheep, PMS given on the 12th or 13th day of the cycle increases the ovulation rate, and there is a general parallelism between dose and ovulation rate (2, 62, 76). There is general agreement that the range of response increases with dosage, single ovulations occurring even with the higher dose levels. This treatment has the effect of shortening the cycle slightly (2, 62, 76), but does not appear to affect the length of estrus (62).

Treatment with a large dose, repeated at heat, reduced the fertility of a flock allowed to lamb (62), but smaller doses have raised the lambing percentage, without at all affecting the conception rate, in a series of 1200 treated ewes (33). However, a small dose can seriously affect conception rate (76).

Ewes injected between the 12th and 14th day of the cycle had a high conception rate, but those treated on the 10th and 11th day did not. Wallace notes that the effect was even more marked if expressed in terms of interval between treatment and heat: for intervals of over 5 days conception was very poor. It should be stressed that any effect of treatment on cycle length was very slight. Though the effect of treatment on the non-pregnant animals is unknown it may reasonably be presumed that they did not have multiple ovulations, because in those pregnant (which includes the great majority of those served within 5 days) the maximal average ovulation rate, of just over 2, was found in those on heat at no more than 2 or 3 days after treatment.

Thus there is no obvious ground for assuming disturbance either of the time relationship between heat and ovulation, or of fertilization or tubal transport associated with multiple corpora lutea. With these excluded, there remain failure of ovulation or ovulation of defective ova. If the latter be accepted for the sheep, it may well apply also to the cattle results already quoted (7, 25).

AFTER PROGESTERONE TREATMENT

In the absence of the bull, heat is not easily detected in beef cattle suckling calves. Treatment by injection at a known stage of cycle is therefore not easily practicable. Even when heat is detected, individual variability hampers accurate prediction of the next estrus. Prolongation of the cycle by progesterone treatment therefore may be of advantage to ensure more precise timing of the endogenous ovulatory discharge. Casida and colleagues have prolonged the cycle by daily injections of progesterone in oil (sheep, 28; cow, 14). With high enough dosage ovulation is inhibited, but follows cessation of treatment. With lower dosage there may be formation of cystic follicles. After a single treatment with crystalline suspensions there has been irregularity about the time of onset of heat, silent heats, low fertility after mating, and a marked tendency to formation of cystic follicles (22, 24, 55). Even with daily injections in oil there has been some abnormality, principally increased incidence of silent heats (29, 46, 74). Clearly careful control of dose level and of the decrease in blood concentration are necessary to achieve normal heat and ovulation.

Robinson (68) got very good synchronization of estrus and ovulation (90% estrus within 24 hr) with daily progesterone followed by PMS. In this experiment the lambing percentage was not significantly raised, but there was no reduction of conception rate. Rowson (71) found that progesterone given after removal of the corpus luteum protected follicles stimulated by PMS from loss of capacity to ovulate. It seems therefore that this type of treatment offers considerable prospects of success.

OVULATION BEFORE PUBERTY

The ruminant ovary contains Graafian follicles at birth. Mansour (50) gave a single dose of PMS to lambs at different ages and observed increasing response with increase of age and of body weight. One-week-old animals showed no obvious follicle growth, later there were luteinized follicles, and later still ovulations. Progesterone treatment preceding PMS enhanced the response.

Ovulation in calves, sometimes multiple, has been obtained with repeated FSH followed by LH (9, 10). Marden (51) noted greater frequency of multiple ovulations after two treatments, and seems to have had some success with a single series preceded by progesterone. Similar treatment by Black *et al.* (6) did not noticeably enhance the ovulation rate.

So far as one can tell, the response before puberty does not differ from the extremes of response found in anestrus.

OTHER POSSIBILITIES

So far administration of gonadotropins has mainly been considered. Steroid, or other, stimulation of endogenous gonadotropin secretion might, if practicable, well prove cheaper than administration of PMS.

Induction of ovulation in anestrous sheep by progesterone has already been mentioned. In sheep in which the cycle was prolonged with progesterone the ovulation rate tended to be decreased (28), though in the sow (3) an increase has been noted.

Estrogen implants given to induce lactation in cattle (20) inhibited the ovarian cycle, which was not immediately resumed upon cessation of treatment. There was a period of cystic follicle formation followed by one in which twin ovulations, and calvings, were more frequent than normally.

The cyst formation one may attribute to failure of pituitary hormone reserves for ovulation to be accumulated in the absence of a corpus luteum. In the treatment of chronic cysts in cattle (39) the cyst is ruptured and a fresh follicle develops which is itself liable to become cystic. But this follicle may be induced to ovulate by PU (43) or to luteinize by manual rupture before the granulosa degenerates. Thereafter a normal cycle is resumed. It is not easy to see how altered pituitary reserves could also account for the occurrence of twin ovulations. It might be that the normal extent of stimulation of follicle growth is limited by estrogen, and that heavy and prolonged estrogen treatment desensitized the regulating mechanism.

DISCUSSION

Both in immaturity and with poor nutritive conditions it seems that there may be impaired follicle growth and ovulation in response to PMS. It also seems that pituitary extracts are then more effective than is PMS. If this is because PMS requires the synergism of endogenous LH, one might suppose that immaturity and low plane of nutrition depress LH secretion.

It is an accepted belief with sheep that "flushing"—raising the plane of nutrition shortly before mating—increases the ovulation rate. Wisconsin workers (32) would revise this, and say that flushing raises the rate to normal. However that may be, Wallace (76) found that both PMS treatment and flushing raise the ovulation rate, and that both also shorten the cycle length. This evidence might be taken to suggest that poor nutrition depresses FSH secretion.

However, one thing that seems well established is that the ovulation rate depends not only on the amount of hormone available for follicle growth but also on the time available for its action. A change in ovulation rate is not necessarily due to an altered quantity of secretion.

There is a seasonal change in ovulation rate (1, 40, 47, 52) and this is not of nutritional origin (59). The ovulation rate rises to a maximum at a time when estrus is most intense and conception rate highest (1). The cycle length, however, is not then at a minimum; on the contrary, there is a tendency for the length to increase in the first part of the season (2, 40).

Work at Cornell (45) shows the ovulatory release of hormone to be neurogenic and, in the cow, that it occurs after the start of heat. Either delay in this release or advancement of the stimulus to follicle growth relative to luteal regression might alter ovulation rate.

There seems no reason to doubt that steroids act centrally in the induction both of heat and of the ovulatory discharge from the pituitary. Quite apart from the results of Clegg *et al.* (15) with hypothalamic lesions, the hormone work on sheep would seem to indicate the points of action differ for the two effects. Progesterone appears to antagonize estrogen at each, but possibly the steroids interact differently at the two sites.

The occurrence of silent heats after hormone treatment, or under poor nutrition, might be due to factors of timing, or of level of estrogen secretion under altered FSH : LH balance, or even of some adrenal corticoid antagonism to heat but not to ovulation.

Estrogen appears to provoke an explosive ovulatory discharge. The discharge of hormone on progesterone withdrawal—which leads eventually in some anestrous sheep to ovulation—initially must cause follicle growth and is probably not similarly explosive. A sudden rise in hormone level seems likely to impair the capacity of follicles to ovulate. If one considers how one or two follicles gain an advantage over the rest, an initially slow, continuous and increasing release of hormone would appear probable, such as might occur if its secretion rate were inversely related to the level of circulating progesterone.

Consistently to obtain multiple ovulation artificially one depends upon luteal—or progesterone—restraint of the ovulating discharge. In the normal breeding season of the sheep, lengthening of the cycle—and so, perhaps, of luteal function—is associated with increased ovulation rate. In ruminants at least, the factors regulating follicle growth seem at the present time scarcely separable from those governing luteal function.

REFERENCES

1. AVERILL, R. L. W., *Studies on Fertility* **7**, 139, Oxford, 1955.
2. AVERILL, R. L. W., *J. Agric. Sci.* **50**, 17, 1958.
3. BAKER, L. N., L. C. ULBERG, R. H. GRUMMER and L. E. CASIDA, *J. Animal Sci.* **13**, 648, 1954.
4. BELL, T. D., L. E. CASIDA, G. BOHSTEDT and A. E. DARLOW, *J. Agric. Res.* **62**, 573, 1941.
5. BERRY, R. O. and H. P. SAVERY, in *Reproduction and Infertility*, III, Symposium (Edited by F. X. Gassner), p. 75, Pergamon Press, London, 1958.
6. BLACK, W. G., L. C. ULBERG, R. E. CHRISTIAN and L. E. CASIDA, *J. Dairy Sci.* **36**, 274, 1953.
7. BROCK, H. and L. E. ROWSON, *J. Agric. Sci.* **42**, 479, 1952.
8. CASIDA, L. E., *Iowa State Coll. J. Sci.* **28**, 119, 1953.
9. CASIDA, L. E., R. K. MEYER, W. H. MCSHAN and W. WISNICKY, *Amer. J. Vet. Res.* **4**, 76, 1943.
10. CASIDA, L. E., A. NALBANDOV, W. H. MCSHAN, R. K. MEYER and W. WISNICKY, *Amer. Soc. Animal Prod.* **33**, 302, 1940.
11. CASIDA, L. E., E. J. WARWICK and R. K. MEYER, *J. Animal Sci.* **3**, 22, 1944.
12. CHANG, M. C., *Nature, Lond.* **161**, 978, 1948.
13. CHANG, M. C., *Endocrinology* **63**, 619, 1958.
14. CHRISTIAN, R. E. and L. E. CASIDA, *J. Animal Sci.* **7**, 540, 1948.
15. CLEGG, M. T., J. A. SANTOLUCITO, J. D. SMITH and W. F. GANONG, *Endocrinology* **62**, 790, 1958.
16. COLE, H. H. and P. T. CUPPS, *Reproduction in Domestic Animals*, New York, 1959.
17. COLE, H. H. and G. H. HART, *J. Amer. Vet. Med. Ass.* **101**, 124, 1942.
18. COLE, H. H. and R. F. MILLER, *Amer. J. Physiol.* **104**, 165, 1933.
19. COLE, H. H., G. H. HART and R. F. MILLER, *Endocrinology* **36**, 370, 1945.
20. DAY, F. T. and J. HAMMOND, JR., *J. Endocrinol.* **4**, 53, 1944.
21. DAY, F. T. and I. W. ROWLANDS, *J. Endocrinol.* **5**, 1, 1946.
22. DAUZIER, L., *Ann. Zootech.* **7**, 341, 1958.
23. DAUZIER, L. and S. WINTENBERGER, *Ann. Zootech.* **6**, 49, 1957.
24. DONKER, J. D., J. R. NICHOLS, E. F. GRAHAM and W. E. PETERSEN, in *Reproduction and Infertility*, III, Symposium (Edited by F. X. Gassner), p. 171, Pergamon Press, London, 1958.
25. DOWLING, D. F., *J. Agric. Sci.* **39**, 374, 1949.
26. DUTT, R. H., *J. Animal Sci.* **12**, 513, 1953.
27. DUTT, R. H., *J. Animal Sci.* **13**, 464, 1954.
28. DUTT, R. H. and L. E. CASIDA, *Endocrinology* **43**, 208, 1948.
29. DZUIK, P. J., J. D. DONKER, J. R. NICHOLS and W. E. PETERSEN, *Minn. Agric. Exp. Sta. Tech. Bull.* **222**, 1958.
30. ERB, R. E. and R. A. MORRISON, *J. Dairy Sci.* **42**, 512, 1959.
31. FOLLEY, S. J. and F. H. MALPRESS, *Proc. Roy. Soc.* **B132**, 164, 1944.
32. FOOTE, W. C., A. L. POPE, A. B. CHAPMAN and L. E. CASIDA, *J. Animal Sci.* **18**, 453, 1959.

33. GORDON, I., *J. Agric. Sci.* **50**, 123, 1958.
34. GORDON, I., *J. Agric. Sci.* **50**, 152, 1958.
35. GORDON, I., Personal communication, 1959.
36. GRANT, R., *Nature, Lond.* **131**, 802, 1933.
37. GRANT, R., *Trans. Roy. Soc. Edinb.* **58**, 1, 1934.
38. HAFEZ, E. S. E., *J. Agric. Sci.* **42**, 199, 1952.
39. HAMMOND, J., *Vet. Med.* **34**, 638, 1939.
40. HAMMOND, J., JR., *J. Agric. Sci.* **34**, 97, 1944.
41. HAMMOND, J., JR., *J. Endocrinol.* **4**, 169, 1945.
42. HAMMOND, J., JR., *J. Agric. Sci.* **39**, 222, 1949.
43. HAMMOND, J., JR. and P. BHATTACHARYA, *J. Agric. Sci.* **34**, 1, 1944.
44. HAMMOND, J., J. HAMMOND, JR. and A. S. PARKES, *J. Agric. Sci.* **32**, 308, 1942.
45. HANSEL, W. and G. W. TRIMBERGER, *J. Animal Sci.* **10**, 719, 1951.
46. HUNTER, G. L., *J. Endocrinol.* **10**, 13 *P*, 1954.
47. HUNTER, G. L., *J. Agric. Sci.* **52**, 282, 1959.
48. HUNTER, G. L., G. P. BISHOP and D. L. BROWN, *J. Agric. Sci.* **51**, 129, 1958.
49. JUDOVITCH, S. S. and M. V. FOMENKO, *Trans. All Union Sov. Res. Inst.* **10**, 65, 1939.
50. MANSOUR, A. M., *J. Agric. Sci.* **52**, 87, 1959.
51. MARDEN, W. G. R., *J. Agric. Sci.* **43**, 381, 1953.
52. MCKENZIE, F. F. and C. E. TERRILL, *Mo. Agric. Exp. Sta. Res. Bull.* **264**, 1937.
53. MOORE, N. W. and T. J. ROBINSON, *J. Endocrinol.* **15**, 360, 1957.
54. MURPHREE, R. L., E. J. WARWICK, L. E. CASIDA and W. H. MCSHAN, *J. Animal Sci.* **3**, 13, 1944.
55. NELLOR, J. E. and H. H. COLE, *J. Animal Sci.* **15**, 650, 1956.
56. NISHIKAWA, Y., N. KURODA and Y. AWAI, *Bull. Nat. Inst. Agric. Sci. (Chiba)* **G10**, 165, 1955.
57. NISHIKAWA, Y., N. KURODA and Y. AWAI, *Bull. Nat. Inst. Agric. Sci. (Chiba)* **G10**, 209, 1955.
58. POLOVTZOVA, V. V. and S. S. JUDOVITCH, *Trans. All-Union Sov. Res. Inst.* **10**, 127, 1939.
59. RADFORD, H. M., *Austr. J. Agric. Res.* **10**, 377, 1959.
60. RAESIDE, J. I. and D. R. LAMOND, *Austr. J. Agric. Res.* **7**, 591, 1956.
61. ROBINSON, T. J., *J. Agric. Sci.* **40**, 275, 1950.
62. ROBINSON, T. J., *J. Agric. Sci.* **41**, 6, 1951.
63. ROBINSON, T. J., *Nature, Lond.* **170**, 373, 1952.
64. ROBINSON, T. J., *Endocrinology* **55**, 403, 1954.
65. ROBINSON, T. J., *J. Endocrinol.* **10**, 117, 1954.
66. ROBINSON, T. J., *J. Agric. Sci.* **46**, 37, 1955.
67. ROBINSON, T. J., *J. Endocrinol.* **12**, 163, 1955.
68. ROBINSON, T. J., *Austr. J. Agric. Res.* **7**, 194, 1956.
69. ROBINSON, T. J., N. W. MOORE and F. E. BINET, *J. Endocrinol.* **14**, 1, 1956.
70. ROWLANDS, I. W., *J. Endocrinol.* **6**, 184, 1950.
71. ROWSON, L. E., *J. Endocrinol.* **7**, 260, 1951.
72. SIMPSON, M. E., C. H. LI and H. M. EVANS, *Endocrinology* **48**, 370, 1951.
73. THOMPSON, D. S. and P. G. SCHINCKEL, *Emp. J. Exp. Agric.* **20**, 77, 1952.
74. TRIMBERGER, G. W. and W. HANSEL, *J. Animal Sci.* **14**, 224, 1955.
75. UMBAUGH, R. E., *Amer. J. Vet. Res.* **10**, 295, 1949.
76. WALLACE, L. R., *J. Agric. Sci.* **45**, 60, 1955.
77. WILLETT, E. L., P. J. BUCKNER and W. H. MCSHAN, *J. Dairy Sci.* **36**, 1083, 1953.
78. WILLETT, E. L., W. H. MCSHAN and R. K. MEYER, *Proc. Soc. Exp. Biol. and Med.* **79**, 396, 1952.
79. ZAWADOWSKY, M. M. and Z. S. MARGULIS, *Trans. Dyn. Dev.* **11**, 80, 1939.

DISCUSSIONS

Chairman: FREDERICK HISAW

DR. WILLIAM F. GANONG: I asked previously that I be excused from the discussion until Mr. Hammond's paper had been given because my experience has not included any work related to avian ovulation. From the point of view of the neuroendocrinologist, there is one point that might be made relative to Dr. Nalbandov's paper. I appreciate the fact that he is not yet ready to extend his hypothesis to mammals, but there are situations in the rat in which there is a good deal of FSH secretion, and still ovulation can be brought about. There are a number of reports, the most recent being that of Van Dyke, Simpson and co-workers (*Proc. Soc. Exp. Biol. and Med.* **95**, 1, 1957), of persistent estrus following anterior hypothalamic lesions. The ovaries of these

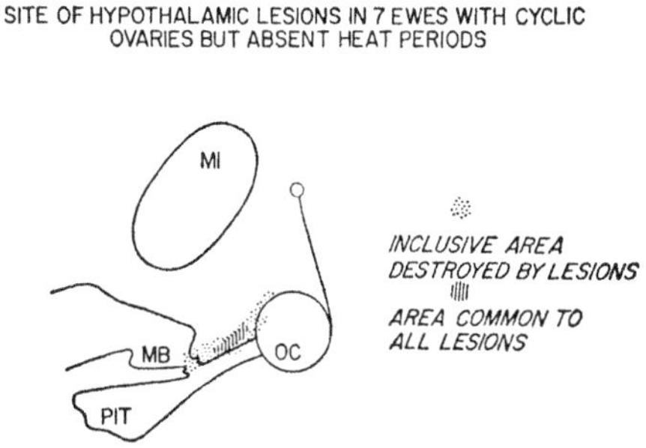

FIG. 1. Reconstruction of lesions on midsagittal section of the hypothalamus. MI, massa intermedia; MB, mammillary body; OC, optic chiasm; PIT, pituitary.

animals contain many follicles and the uteri are enlarged, so presumably a high level of FSH secretion is present continuously. Injection of purified LH leads to prompt ovulation of many of the ovarian follicles.

Mr. Hammond has raised a number of questions about the interrelations in the sheep and the cow between the mechanisms responsible for the production of heat and those responsible for ovulation. Certainly, there seems to be little doubt that heat and ovulation can be separated by appropriate brain lesions in experimental animals.

Dr. Clegg and I have been interested in the role of the hypothalamus in the regulation of the sexual cycle of the sheep. We have now examined the brains of 39 ewes in which localized destruction of various parts of the hypothalamus has been produced stereotaxically (Clegg, M. T., J. A. Santolucito, J. D. Smith and W. F. Ganong, *Endocrinology* **62**, 790, 1958). Lesions were made during the breeding season in all these animals. Twenty-two unoperated animals served as controls. We have observed an absence of heat periods after production of the lesions in 22 of the 39 operated animals. Five of these ewes were killed after the normal controls entered the anestrus season, so it was impossible to say whether or not pituitary stimulation of the ovaries had been inhibited. The ovaries of the remaining 17 were examined while the normal control animals were still cycling regularly. Nine of them showed acyclic ovaries, i.e. corpora lutea were absent and all ovarian follicles were small. In eight ewes, corpora lutea and/or large ovarian follicles were present. Since regression of the corpus luteum is normally complete a day or two after the next heat, the presence of a corpus luteum indicates that ovulation has occurred in the past three weeks. The possibility of a persistent corpus in these animals was ruled out by examining the ovaries at laparotomy and later, at autopsy. Accordingly, in eight ewes the behavioral manifestations of heat were abolished by hypothalamic lesions, presumably without affecting pituitary gonadotropin secretion. The area destroyed by the lesions in seven of these animals is shown in Fig. 1. Part of the brain of the other sheep was inadvertently destroyed, so detailed localization was not possible. The seven lesions were in the basal portion of the hypothalamus, sharing in common an area of destruction just in front of the infundibulum and above the median eminence.

Lesions in other parts of the hypothalamus in 17 animals had no effect on either ovarian cycling or heat. The areas of destruction in these sheep are shown in Fig. 2. It is apparent that extensive lesions in the diencephalon did not affect sexual behavior.

SITES OF HYPOTHALAMIC LESIONS IN 17 EWES WITH NORMAL HEAT PERIODS AND CYCLIC OVARIES

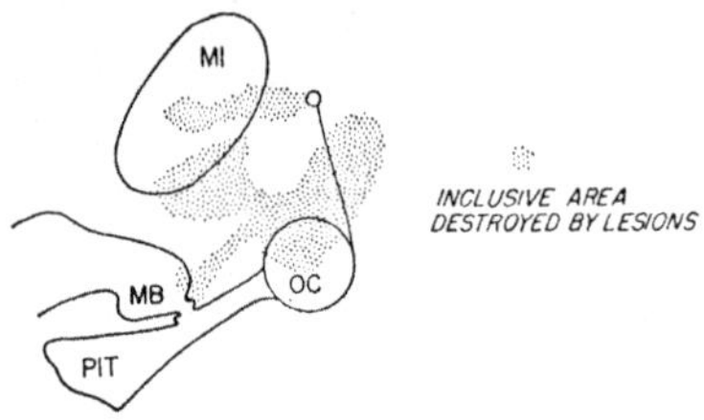

FIG. 2.

Indeed, in a number of instances, ewes with control lesions accepted the male less than 24 hr postoperatively, while still staggering from the effects of the pentobarbital anesthesia. Therefore, the data indicate that the effect of lesions on sexual behavior is specific, and depends on a reasonably discrete area in the anterior hypothalamus.

The idea of a diencephalic centre concerned with sexual behavior is, of course, not new. Dempsey and Rioch (*J. Neurophysiol.* **2**, 9, 1939) and Bard (*Res. Publ. Assn. Nerv. Ment. Dis.* **20**, 551, 1940) originally presented evidence for such a centre by comparing the sexual responses of decorticate and decerebrate guinea-pigs and cats. Subsequently, Brookhart and his associates (*Endocrinology* **28**, 561, 1941) observed absence of mating behavior in female guinea-pigs with anterior hypothalamic lesions, in some cases without ovarian atrophy. Sawyer and Robison (*J. Clin. Endocrinol. and Metab.* **16**, 914, 1956) reported similar results following lesions of the anterior hypothalamus in cats, as Dr. Sawyer mentioned this morning. The exact role played by this "centre" in heat is not clear. Harris, Michael and Scott (Ciba Symposium on *Neurological Basis of Behavior*, p. 236, London, 1958) were able to produce heat in ovariectomized cats by the implantation of minute amounts of estrogen in the posterior hypothalamus, while implantations in the anterior hypothalamus, other parts of the brain, and the periphery were ineffective. An interesting feature of these experiments was the seemingly fixed latent period of three days between hormone implantation and the onset of heat. Somewhat similar results but with a shorter latent period have been obtained in rats by Fisher (*Reticular Formation of the Brain*, p. 251, Boston, 1958). Delgado (*Abstr. 21st Inter. Congr. Physiol.*, p. 29, 1959) has reported "increased sexual activity" in monkeys following remote control stimulation of the hypothalamus, but except for this observation, there is little data on whether or not sexual receptivity can be induced by electrical stimulation of appropriate diencephalic centres. An indirect connection between the hypothalamic centre and the behavioral events has also not been ruled out. As Mr. Hammond said, his original suggestion that tonic contractions of the uterus play a role in heat (Hammond, Jun., *J. Endocrinol.* **4**, 169, 1945) is probably not true for sheep, since Robinson (*Endocrinology* **55**, 403, 1955) was able to produce heat in hysterectomized ewes. However, the cow is apparently different. The cow becomes anestrus after hysterectomy, and Dr. Hansel pointed out that even when ovulation is induced by administration of exogenous gonadotropins, the hysterectomized cow does not show behavioral estrus. This apparent species difference certainly invites further investigation.

Our studies in the sheep therefore add this species to the list of animals in which a hypothalamic centre must be intact for heat to occur. This centre is probably stimulated directly by estrogens, and it is an inviting hypothesis that the action of progesterone in potentiating the heat-producing action of estrogen rests in some sort of a priming action on this brain centre. Certainly, there is ample precedent for an action of progesterone on the brain in the data presented by Dr. Sawyer this morning, and

SITE OF HYPOTHALAMIC LESIONS IN 9 EWES WITH NO HEAT PERIODS AND ACYCLIC OVARIES

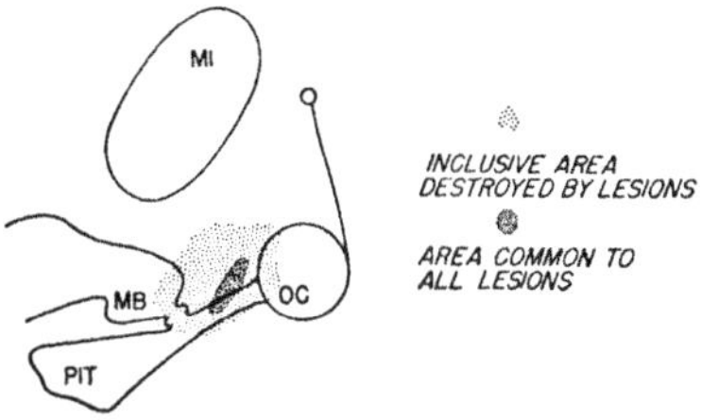

FIG. 3.

progesterone therapy not only lowers the heat-producing threshold for estrogen, but is essential if heat periods are to recur cyclically (Robinson, *Endocrinology* **55**, 403, 1955).

The brain also appears to be involved in the control of anterior pituitary secretion of gonadotropins in the ewe, as in other species. As indicated above, nine of the ewes in our series showed in addition to absence of behavioral estrus, only small follicles and no corpora lutea in their ovaries. This fact indicates that periodic stimulation of the ovary was no longer present after the lesions were made. The sites of these lesions are shown in Fig. 3. These animals also had ventral hypothalamic lesions, but the common area of destruction in these sheep was more ventrally and caudally located than the common area in the sheep with the absent heat only. All these animals had some pituitary stalk damage, but the lesions probably did not produce their effect by damaging the pituitary blood supply because in those animals in which they were studied, thyroid function and adrenal size and morphology were normal. In two of the animals, 17-hydroxycorticoid levels in the peripheral blood following surgical stress were abnormally low, but in the remaining animals they were normal (Clegg and Ganong, *Endocrinology*, in press, 1960).

We have been interested in correlating the physiological effects of these hypothalamic lesions with changes in the gonadotropic potency of the anterior pituitary. The LH potency of the pituitaries from the animals with lesions has been measured by the ventral prostate response in hypophysectomized assay rats, and the follicle-stimulating potency by the effect on ovarian weight in immature rats receiving chorionic gonadotropin (Clegg *et al.*, *Endocrinology* **62**, 790, 1958). The values found in normal ewes, ewes with lesions that did not affect the sexual cycle, and ewes with cyclic ovaries but absent heat periods are summarized in Table 1. The differences between the latter two groups of animals and the normal controls are not statistically significant, an additional piece of evidence in favour of the concept of a hypothalamic centre concerned with sexual behaviour which is independent of the areas concerned with regulation of gonadotropin secretion by the pituitary. We do not as yet have sufficient data for statistical analysis of pituitary gonadotropin content in sheep with lesions and acyclic ovaries. However, it is interesting that in the two ewes assayed to date, a slight depression of LH activity and a relatively marked depression of FSH potency was present. There is no comparable data on sheep and very little information on other species in the literature. Bogdanove, Spiritos and Halmi (*Endocrinology* **57**, 302, 1955) found that total gonadotropin content was low in the pituitaries of rats with hypothalamic lesions and testicular atrophy. Davidson, Contopoulos and Ganong

TABLE 1. PITUITARY GONADOTROPIN CONTENT OF SHEEP

Values are means ± standard error of the mean. Assayed against Armour FSH and LH.

	FSH Armour units per ant. lobe	LH mg equiv. per ant. lobe
12 unoperated ewes; cycling normally	1.84±0.24	20.8±1.3
11 ewes with lesions; cyclic ovaries, normal heat periods	1.57±0.27	23.0±6.4
6 ewes with lesions; cyclic ovaries, heat absent	1.42±0.25	23.1±7.8

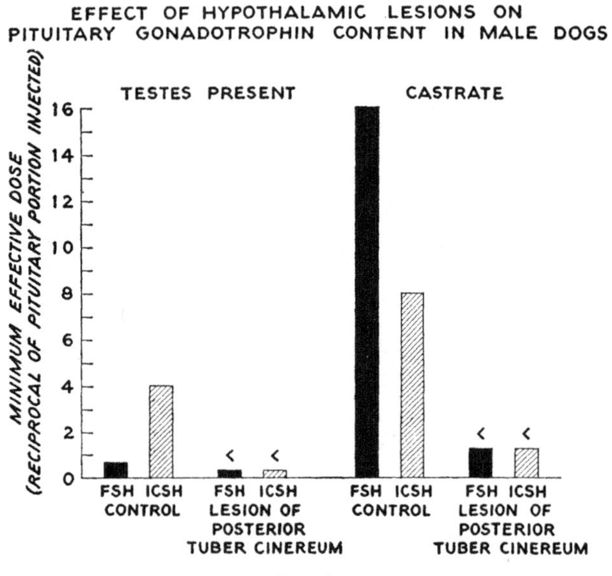

FIG. 4.

(*Endocrinology*, in press, 1960) found depression of both FSH and LH activity in dogs with posterior median eminence lesions and testicular atrophy. In the rat and the dog, lesions which led to testicular atrophy were generally more posterior than those in the ewes with acyclic ovaries, but the significance of this point is difficult to assess.

There was some discussion this morning about the locus of the feedback of gonadal hormones in regulating gonadotropin secretion. I noticed that most of the speakers were noncommittal, indicating the site of feedback in their diagrams by arrows pointing both to the pituitary and hypothalamus. It is interesting in this regard that while castration causes a sharp rise in the pituitary content of both FSH and LH

(ICSH) in the male dog, the castrate dog with a hypothalamic lesion shows approximately the same low level of gonadotropin as the non-castrate lesion dog. This is shown in Fig. 4, which summarizes data obtained using Dr. Simpson's assay method for the

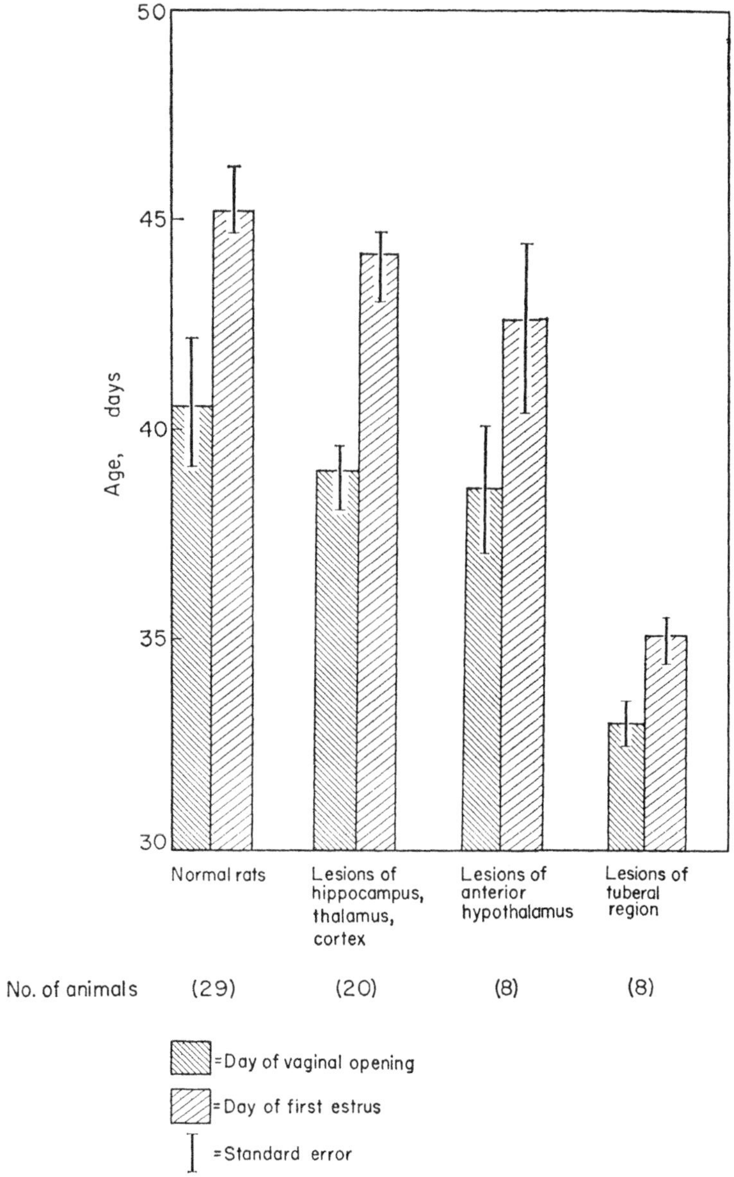

FIG. 5. Effect of brain lesions on the onset of puberty.

gonadotropins (Davidson, Contopoulos and Ganong, *Endocrinology*, in press, 1960). This suggests that the feedback mechanism regulating gonadotropin secretion in the male dog is primarily at the hypothalamic rather than the pituitary level. In the case of ACTH and TSH, there is considerable evidence that the feedback is at the level of the pituitary, so apparently the mechanism involved in gonadotropin secretion is different.

Dr. Harris and Dr. Critchlow have presented data from their laboratories indicating that certain hypothalamic and limbic lesions are associated with precocious puberty in female rats. The data are quite striking and consistent, but I must admit that I am somewhat surprised at their inability to localize this response to a single

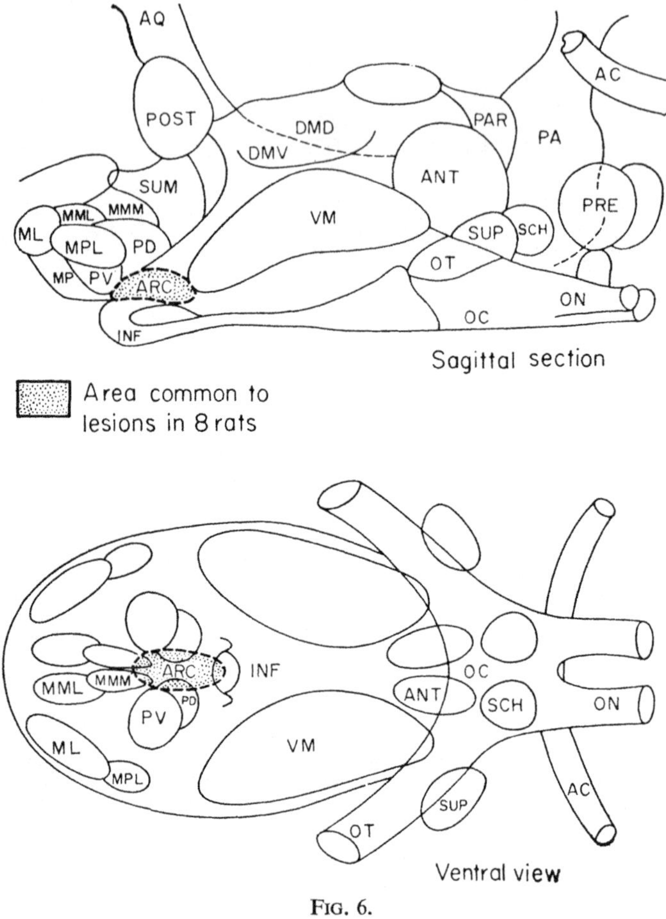

FIG. 6.

portion of the hypothalamus. In my laboratory, Mr. Gellert has been working on this problem for two years. Because true precocious puberty is properly defined as the early onset of otherwise normal sexual cycles, we have produced lesions in various parts of the brain in immature female rats, and then followed them and their controls until all were cycling. By serially sectioning the brains, we have located the lesion in each of the animals and then divided the animals into groups on the basis of common areas of destruction. In Fig. 5, the mean age for vaginal opening and onset of first estrus are shown for normal controls, animals with lesions in the anterior hypothalamus, animals with lesions elsewhere in the brain, and animals with a common area of destruction in the posterior tuberal region. There is no significant acceleration of puberty in any of the groups except the last, but there is a clear-cut and highly significant acceleration of puberty in the animals with posterior tuberal lesions.

Notice that there is a fair amount of variation in the time of onset of puberty in the rats with anterior hypothalamic lesions. A few individual animals in this group

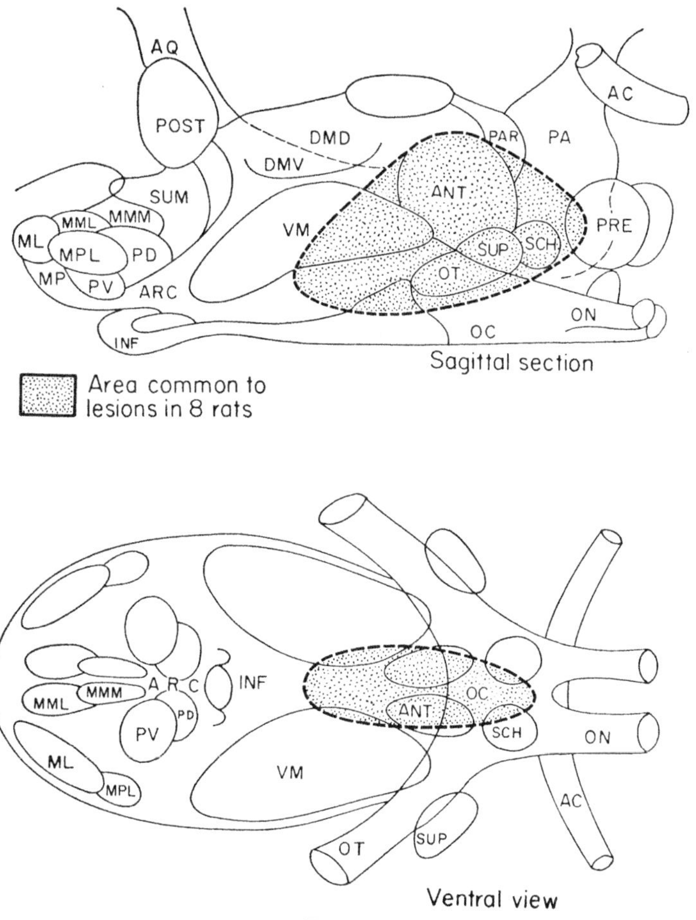

FIG. 7.

matured quite early. Accordingly, if we had analysed our data in the manner used by Harris and Critchlow, we might have called a few of these animals precocious; but the average for the group is not different from the controls.

The common area of destruction in the animals with posterior tuberal lesions is shown in Fig. 6. The inclusive area destroyed by lesions of the anterior hypothalamus is shown in Fig. 7. It seems quite clear that precocious puberty is a consistent finding when a small area in the arcuate nucleus, immediately above the infundibulum, is destroyed (Gellert and Ganong, *Acta Endocrinol.*, in press, 1960). In recent experiments we have also found precocious puberty after lesions of the amygdala, confirming Dr. Critchlow.

I must say that I am pleased that the site of effective lesions in our rats is in the same general area as the tumors associated with precocious puberty in humans. On the other hand, the findings raise important questions about the mechanism involved in the early onset of cycling in the experimental animals. Dr. Harris mentioned this morning, and I would like to emphasize it again, the possibility that the effects of these lesions are not due to interruption of some sort of inhibitory mechanism, but possibly the lesions are stimulatory in themselves. We know that the arcuate nucleus is involved in the regulation of gonadotropin secretion in the adult rat. Is it possible, therefore, that irritation around lesions destroying only part of this nucleus in immature animals stimulates the adjacent intact portions? Another unsettled question is why hypothalamic lesions are effective only in female animals. These are problems which can only be answered by future research.

M. C. Chang: I should like first to express my sincere thanks to our hosts for the invitation and to congratulate the previous speakers. Dr. Nalbandov presented beautiful photographs and interesting results on which I can only express my admiration. Then he concluded with the provocative idea that "ovulation is normally a process of physiological atresia which occurs as the result of absence of hormones rather than their presence and is thus comparable to menstruation" and that "LH (or another substance?) produces its effect on ovulation by initiating the process of atresia perhaps by initiating ischemia". It is very important for the progress of science to have theories to work on but I should like to pass a few comments for our discussion: (1) If ovulation occurs as a result of absence of hormones rather than their presence then hypophysectomy, the removal of FSH and LH should induce ovulation. But according to his results, a small amount of LH was still needed. (2) Using hypophysectomized animals to prove or to disprove a particular point is perfectly reasonable, but one must bear in mind that hypophysectomy may increase the threshold of one physiological process or decrease the threshold of another. How far the information obtained from hypophysectomized animals can be generalized to such an extent as a physiological process of ovulation in an intact animal is worthy of consideration. (3) Follicular atresia and menstruation, I think, are not comparable to ovulation because the former two processes are degenerative and regressive processes while the latter is an active and progressive physiological process. (4) Does ischemia play a part in ovulation? After reading Dr. Nalbandov's abstract, we ligated the left ovarian artery of two rabbits, then gave LH for the induction of ovulation. When examined subsequently the right ovaries were found to have ovulated normally while the left ovaries failed to ovulate. When we ligated the left ovarian artery about two hours before the expected time of ovulation the left ovaries again failed to ovulate. It seems that ovulation requires a normal supply of blood, and perhaps a larger than normal blood supply, at the time of ovulation and that severe ischemia would prevent ovulation rather than initiate ovulation.

Mr. Hammond gave us an excellent review on the artificial induction of ovulation in sheep and cattle. He mentioned the importance of nutrition in relation to the induction of ovulation. Here I should like to stress the influence not only of nutrition but also of environmental factors. Dr. Fernandez-Cano and I (*Amer. J. Physiol.* **196**, 653, 1959) have reported that in the rat following stress, such as brief changes of environmental temperature or reduced atmospheric pressure, there would occur inhibition of estrus and ovulation for a long time, about two to three estrous cycles. It seems to me that for the induction of ovulation by administration of hormones one should pay attention not only to ovulation but also to the proper estrous behavior, the transportation of sperm and eggs, the capacitation of sperm and the fertilization of eggs, and the proper implantation of eggs under the administration of hormones. If any one of these processes is upset by hormonal treatment the fertility of animals hardly can be improved.

Since this conference is mainly dealing with ovulation I should like to introduce here some results of my own. In 1944 Mr. Hammond, Jr. and I injected two groups of pregnant rabbits with 50 I.U. or 500 I.U. of HCG and we observed a large number of fresh corpora lutea in the ovaries (from 2 to 35). The majority of the animals ovulated a larger number of eggs than expected. In the accompanying table I present data collected more recently. It seems that ovulation can be easily induced in the pregnant rabbits and that about half of the pregnant animals superovulate; that is, ovulate a larger number of eggs than expected. The eggs are perfectly normal as shown by the presence of the first polar body and the second maturation spindle. They are physiologically normal because they can be fertilized either *in vitro* or after transfer to the fallopian tubes of mated rabbits. When a few pregnant rabbits were bred to males no ovulation occurred. Injection of gonadotropic hormone intraperitoneally into pregnant rats also induces ovulation, but only a small number of eggs were

TABLE 1. INDUCTION OF OVULATION IN THE PREGNANT RABBIT BY ADMINISTRATION OF SHEEP PITUITARY EXTRACT

	Total No. of animals	No. of animals failed to ovulate	Average No. of ovulation spots or eggs recovered
Estrous animals bred 2–3 times	51	4	9.3 (2–17)
Non-pregnant animals intravenous injection of 28–42 I.U. of pituitary extract	42	1	9.7 (1–15)
Pregnant animals (20–29 day) injection of 28–42 I.U. of pituitary extract	46	0	14.7 (4–31)

found from a few rats ovulated. You may recall that Burdick and Crump have reported that pregnant mice can be induced to ovulate by injection of chorionic gonadotropin (*Endocrinology* **48**, 273, 1951). I wonder whether the induction of superovulation in the pregnant rabbit could throw some light on the hormonal control of ovulation.

CHAIRMAN HISAW: Dr. Breneman, would you like to add something to the discussion?

DR. W. R. BRENEMAN: I have only one or two points to make relative to Dr. Nalbandov's paper. I like his ideas and in line with his conclusions and also at the suggestion of Dr. Fraps we have been attempting to inhibit one ovulation in hens by the administration of lithosperm. This material, an extract of the plant *Lithospermum ruderale*, will inhibit LH after mixture *in vitro* and will also inhibit the effect of LH on the testes of chicks *in vivo*.

Although Dr. Nalbandov did not point this out, most of you know that egg-laying in the hen usually occurs a little later on each succeeding day. It is possible to anticipate, therefore, the time of an ovulation and make lithosperm injections before ovulation occurs. When an injection is made approximately one hour before the anticipated ovulation, that ovulation is usually inhibited but succeeding ones occur normally. Originally we gave as much as 40 mg of lithosperm intraperitoneally but recently, with improved extracts, we find 1.0 mg is an ample amount to produce inhibition. That is, one ovulation is skipped.

Follicle growth continues when low dosages are given but is stopped with the high doses. Our current data indicate that it is possible to inhibit FSH *in vivo* with lithosperm but the dose required to inhibit FSH is many times that which is necessary to inhibit LH. It also requires much more lithosperm to inhibit FSH *in vitro* than it does LH.

DR. S. J. FOLLEY: I want to mention the case of the goat. Unlike what H. H. Cole showed many years ago for the ewe, in the female goat it is frequently possible, by a single injection of PMS, to induce not only ovulation but also estrus during the anestrous season. In such cases it is often possible to obtain a fertile mating. In some experiments we did ten years ago in our laboratory, we found that a single injection of 1200 I.U. PMS into anestrous goats was often followed by fertile mating. I think this occurred in about 22% of the females injected.

In other experiments on the quantitative effects of PMS on the ovaries of virgin goats, we found that small doses (about 400 I.U.) of PMS would cause ovulation without estrus, while it took between 1000 and 1200 I.U. to cause noticeable effects on follicular growth.

Thus the female goat seems to be somewhat different from her near relative, the ewe, in the following respect: there is, in many cases, no need to give two injections, spaced a cycle apart, in order to achieve out-of-season breeding.

DR. VILLEE: I should like to ask Dr. Nalbandov whether he believes the results he obtains are due to a direct action of the protein hormones on the hen's ovaries, or whether some steroid might intervene between the protein hormone and the tissue.

DR. NALBANDOV: May I start with Dr. Chang's comments. The references to the role of "atresia", "necrosis" and "ischemia" in the ovulatory process should be regarded as relative and not absolute terms. When I say that ischemia precedes the rupture of the follicle, I don't mean to imply complete cessation of blood flow but a reduction in the rate of flow and in the amount of blood. I agree that if one were to tie off the blood supply of an ovary or of an individual follicle these structures would invariably and inevitably disintegrate rapidly. This is not a physiological process and you cannot expect follicles or ovaries to continue normal function under these conditions. You next stated that if the proposed theory is correct, one should expect ovulation to occur in the hypophysectomized animal without exogenous hormone. According to the theory proposed ovulation does not follow a hormonal vacuum (as in hypophysectomy), but is caused by a relative reduction in the amounts of hormones made available to the follicle. This reduction in available hormone may be caused by a reduction in blood flow or, as Dr. Meyer suggests, may be due to the increase in the turgidity and fullness of the follicle which leads to a constriction of blood vessels and a reduction in the amount of blood flowing through. Referring to the slide shown by Dr. Meyer, I should like to suggest that his data support the contentions outlined by me, since the maximum ovulation rate occurs about 18 hr (and perhaps even later) after the injection of the ovulator, instead of occurring at the usually accepted time of about 10 hr after LH injection.

In reply to the last question I should like to confuse the issue by presenting a few preliminary observations on the role of progesterone in the ovulability of eggs. I remind you of the statement that in the normal laying hen it is never possible to induce the ovulation of obviously immature follicles with exogenous gonadotropins. However, tiny immature follicles can be induced to ovulate with relative frequency in intact hens if no treatment other than progesterone is given. Furthermore, hypophysectomized hens can be given a minimum dose of LH which is adequate to induce a single ovulation. If we now add progesterone to this minimum dose of LH, we can occasionally induce multiple ovulations. In this last experiment progesterone does not act on the missing pituitary gland, but it could act on the hypothalamus causing it to release ovulation-inducing substances which cooperate with exogenous LH to increase the frequency of follicles ruptured. It is, of course, also possible that in both experiments progesterone acts on the follicle directly and increases its sensitivity to LH. Which interpretation is the correct one, remains to be seen.

DR. ROBERT NOYES: I would like to raise a question concerning the mechanism of ovulation. Is it possible that LH acts by causing the dissolution of the granulosa? As you know one can grow granulosa cells of pre-ovulatory follicles in tissue culture but this becomes impossible after the granulosa cells have been exposed to LH.

DR. NALBANDOV: This observation seems to reduce the importance of the vascular system in ovulation and emphasizes the possible significanee of LH. It is obvious that a lot more work is needed before the process of ovulation is completely understood.

CHAIRMAN HISAW: The session is now open for general discussion of the papers of this morning.

However, if there is no objection I might start things rolling by mentioning one or two thoughts that have entered my mind. Several years ago Dr. A. Albert and I had an opportunity to make observations, of a rather general nature, on ovulation in the smooth dogfish (*Mustelus canis*). Ovulation occurs in the vicinity of Woods Hole, Massachusetts, during the last of June and the first of July. Approximately 6 to 12 mature follicles are situated far apart on a very large ovary and apparently one or two ova are ovulated at a time. The intervals between ovulations are probably quite long as each ovum must be provided with an elaborate membranous capsule. After ovulation has begun and one or more eggs have been released, hypophysectomy prevents further ovulation, which can be initiated by implanting pituitaries from other fish. I mention this with the thought that the smooth dogfish may be a suitable animal to use in the study of ovulation.

I also should like to mention some recent experiments by Mr. R. D. Lisk, a student in our laboratories, on effects of implanting fine needles containing estradiol-17β in different areas of the hypothalamus of sexually mature rats. The needles were fashioned from 27-gauge hypodermic needles. The estrogen was warmed to the point of melting and only the amount that could be drawn into the needle by capillary attraction was used. Under this condition the hormone available to the region in which the needle was implanted was the small amount that dissolved out from the tip end of the needle.

When such implants were made in the area of the arcuate nucleus estrous cycles ceased and after thirty days the uterus resembled that of a castrated animal. The ovaries contained no large follicles and the interstitial tissue was atrophic. Similar effects were produced in the male in which, after thirty days, the atrophy of testis, prostate and seminal vesicles approached that found about thirty days after hypophysectomy. It is of interest that such implants in other areas of the hypothalamus did not produce these effects in the male but in the female such implants in the mammillary bodies were about as effective as those in the arcuate nucleus.

DR. WILLIAM F. GANONG: These results are reminiscent of experiments reported by Flerkò and Szentagothai (*Acta Endocrinol.* **26**, 121, 1957) in which implants of ovarian tissue were made in the anterior hypothalamus in rats, and extreme atrophy of the uterus resulted. Control implants of other tissues were ineffective. These and other experiments suggest that estrogen feeds back to the anterior hypothalamus to inhibit FSH secretion. Maybe Dr. Harris would comment on his work on stilbestrol implantation in cats.

DR. GEOFFREY HARRIS: I believe the work you mention was that of Flerkò who transplanted minute fragments of ovarian tissue into the hypothalamus. If these transplants were placed near the paraventricular nuclei, atrophy of the uterus ensued. Similar transplants into the mammillary body or hypophysis, or liver grafts near the paraventricular nuclei, did not have this effect. From this and other experiments Flerkò concluded that the action of estrogens in inhibiting FSH secretion is on some nervous structure in the paraventricular region of the anterior hypothalamus.

The question of hypothalamic localization of endocrine functions can certainly be very difficult. Donovan and van der Werff ten Bosch, whose work was discussed this morning, were unable to localize their lesions to any precise hypothalamic structure. The effective lesions were, however, situated in the anterior hypothalamus. I think that the suggestion of Dr. Vaughan Critchlow, that these lesions may be interrupting some diffuse fibre system, such as the stria terminalis, may well be important in this respect. The problem of the site of lesion in the hypothalamus which results in precocious puberty was raised by Dr. Ganong this afternoon, while Dr. Sawyer this morning discussed the areas of the hypothalamus involved with patterns of sexual behavior.

In respect of estrous behavior in cats, Dr. R. P. Michael and myself found a few years ago (Harris, G. W. and R. P. Michael, *J. Physiol.* (*Lond.*) **142**, 26P (1958)) that implants of minute amounts of stilbestrol, fused onto the end of a needle which was inserted into the posterior hypothalamus, activated mating behavior in female cats. Similar implants in other parts of the brain did not produce this result. Since cats with mammillary body implants showed sustained mating behavior in the presence of persistently anestrous genital tracts, it was concluded that the hormone action was local and not general. Dr. Sawyer has, I know, found evidence that the region of the hypothalamus involved with sexual behavior in the cat lies more anteriorly. What the answer here is I don't know. The only thing that strikes me in this connection, and this I have discussed before with Dr. Sawyer, is that the production of a positive response by some experimental procedure involving the hypothalamus is probably more significant than the loss of a response. The hypothalamus is obviously concerned with many autonomic and endocrine functions. Therefore, the loss of a particular behavior pattern following a hypothalamic lesion might be brought about in many indirect ways, such as through failure in food intake, loss of control of body temperature or blood pressure, and so on. On the other hand the excitation of a behavioral pattern when it would not otherwise be present is probably much more specific.

DR. ERNEST KNOBIL: Mr. Hammond described a cystic ovary which, if ruptured mechanically, would undergo luteinization. Does this mean that there is normally a decompression of the follicle when luteinization occurs under hormonal influence?

MR. JOHN HAMMOND, JR.: The experiments were my father's, on the cow. After rupture of the cyst, you get another follicle to ovulate. You can induce this by injection of pregnancy urine; or, if you manually rupture the follicle, then you get luteinization of that same follicle. After luteinization, you can feel a great crack across the corpus, instead of an ovulation point. I have done this myself. I feel that you may stimulate a follicle to the point of being able to luteinize; but that luteinization may not follow unless the pressure inside the follicle is released.

I mentioned, I think, that when you express the corpus (following a PMS injection) you may get luteinization of ruptured follicles. I have in one or two cases bruised such a follicle and got a localized patch of luteal tissue in the wall of the follicle.

DR. ERNEST KNOBIL: I think most of us believe the hormone acts directly on the granulosa cells and transforms them into lutein cells.

DR. ROY O. GREEP: I should like to ask Dr. Harris to elaborate a little more on his concept of how the hypothalamic hypophyseal system works. He stated earlier that he makes an extract of the median eminence and does not include the hypothalamus on the basis that the active principle, whatever it might be, would thereby be diluted.

I should like to know how he visualizes the production of the active substance as a product of the nerve endings of fibres emanating from somewhere in the hypothalamus. I should like to know more about how this substance is produced in the median eminence, if indeed it is produced there. Or, does it migrate from somewhere in the hypothalamus? Surely, there must be some correction between the median eminence and the hypothalamus.

DR. GEOFFREY HARRIS: What I was trying to say this morning is this—the hypothesis is that nerve tract(s) pass through the hypothalamus and have their termination on the sinusoids of the primary plexus of the portal vessels in the median eminence. It is supposed that at this site some humoral substance is transferred from the nerve terminals into these vessels, and is then carried to the gland cells of the anterior pituitary where it exerts a regulating influence. Such a hormonal substance might well be present along the whole length of the nerve fibres, in the same way that acetylcholine is known to be present along the whole nerve fibre in the case of cholinergic neurons. It might then be argued that extracts of the hypothalamus would contain any active material involved with these nerve tracts but, on the other hand, such material would be expected to be greatly diluted by substances from nerve tissue adjacent to the tracts. In the case of the median eminence, however, we have here a minute piece of tissue in which the relative nerve tracts are focused. We might therefore expect to obtain more concentrated extracts, weight for weight of nerve tissue, from this area.

CHAIRMAN HISAW: Does that satisfy your curiosity?

DR. ROY O. GREEP: I should like to know whether he thinks the neural secretory material has anything to do with it, particularly that which has been identified in the supra-optico-hypophyseal tract.

DR. GEOFFREY HARRIS: I am a little bit doubtful about that for various reasons. One reason is that if the supraoptico-hypophyseal tract is stimulated electrically, ovulation does not necessarily occur. I am rather hesitant, therefore, about accepting this tract, or the innervation of the neurohypophysis, as being concerned in the neural mechanism underlying LH release in the rabbit. However, I think a polypeptide related to those known to be present in the neurohypophysis may well be concerned. If such a polypeptide is liberated at nerve terminals in the median eminence, the mechanism could I suppose be referred to as neurosecretory in type.

DR. ROY O. GREEP: I do not know of any other fibre tracts where there is thought to be movement of material. The idea of axial flow, of neurosecretory material in the tract, is now being questioned rather seriously.

There is another question I would like to ask Dr. Harris. Has he any evidence as to whether the active extract of the median eminence yields positive results by any of the classic tests for neurohypophyseal activity?

DR. GEOFFREY HARRIS: I think it is almost certain that such principles would be present in our extracts. The only thing I can say at the moment is that a rough calculation based on the amount of hormone known to be present in the posterior pituitary glands of rabbits and the proportion of the rabbit neurohypophysis formed by the median eminence, would indicate that only small amounts, of the order of 100 m U posterior pituitary hormone, would be present in the extract of one rabbit median eminence.

Referring to the idea of neurosecretion, the nerve fibres innervating the posterior pituitary would seem to be analogous to those presumed to exist on the present hypothesis. Posterior pituitary hormone does apparently exist, in one form or another, through the whole length of the neurons which innervate the posterior pituitary gland. Whether this material is in fact moving centrifugally along the nerve fibre is doubted by some workers, and it may be that what is liberated at the nerve terminal is actually formed at the terminal. I don't know what the answer is to this particular point, but it certainly seems as if the active material is present along the whole length of the fibre.

DR. WILLIAM F. GANONG: I should like to rise in defence of the median eminence. I admit that I have a vested interest. However, if we could switch for a moment to the regulation of ACTH secretion, the evidence here is that lesions in the mid-portion of the median eminence are the only ones which will block ACTH release. In stimulation experiments, ACTH secretion follows stimulation of the median eminence, the posterior tuberal region and the orbital surface of the frontal lobes. According to Mason (*Endocrinology* **63**, 403, 1958), stimulation behind the mammillary bodies, where the reticular fibres sweep into the hypothalamus, is also effective. Therefore, my concept is one of multiple inputs, coming down to a final, common pathway, the median eminence. I should like to ask Dr. Harris the same question he was asked by Dr. Folley this morning, but possibly with a slightly different emphasis. How do you feel about putting materials which are vasoactive directly into the pituitary? You recall this was a considerable problem some years ago, when people put materials directly on anterior pituitary transplants in the eye.

DR. GEOFFREY HARRIS: The only thing I can say about that is that we have infused other vasoactive materials into the pituitary without getting similar responses.

DR. GREGORY PINCUS: If there is a portal system present, can the blood flow back to the median eminence from the pituitary?

DR. GEOFFREY HARRIS: All the evidence indicates that blood flows only *from* the median eminence *to* the pituitary gland. This may be taken as established. There is no evidence that blood ever flows up the portal vessels to the median eminence.

DR. ROLAND K. MEYER: I shall describe data obtained in my laboratory by Mr. W. F. Strauss. The experiment was based on the publications of H. H. Cole (*Am. J. Physiol.* **119**, 704, 1937) who reported mating and fetal development prior to parturition in immature rats treated with pregnant mare serum gonadotropin (PMS). In our experiment female rats of the Holtzman strain were injected subcutaneously during the morning of the 30th day of life with one single dose of 0.4 Cartland–Nelson unit of Gonadogen (The Upjohn Company). Forty-eight hours later one or two females were placed with two adult males. Seventy-two hours after PMS injections, vaginal smears were taken; sperm or a vaginal plug was considered as evidence that mating had occurred.

He started with 144 female rats but many of these were used for other studies as the experiment progressed. On the basis of the data obtained from this group we predict that in a comparable group of 100 rats, 86 would mate, 81 would have an average

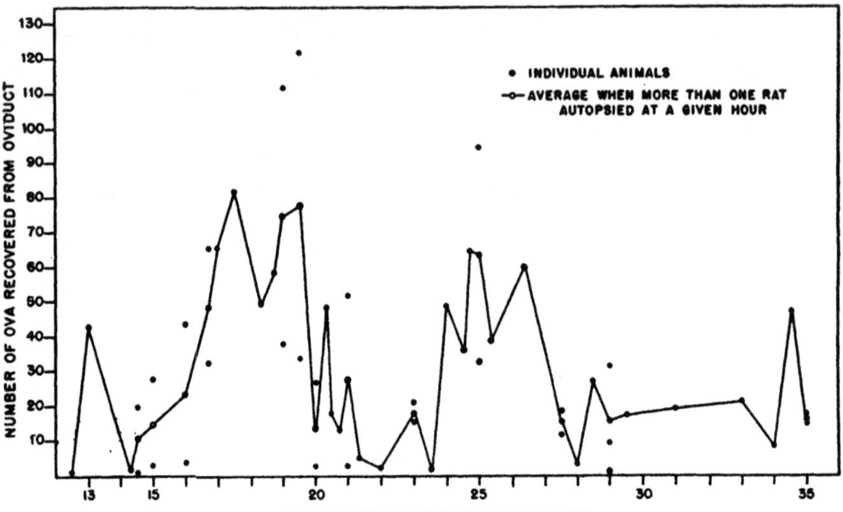

FIG. 1. Number of ova recovered from oviducts of immature hypophysectomized rats injected subcutaneously with a FSH preparation, and intravenously with a preparation containing both FSH and LH activity.

of 10 implantation sites on the 7th day after ovulation, and 75 would parturate an average of 8.5 young (average gestation 22.5 days). The young mothers would lactate and raise an average of 7.2 young to time of weaning.

Another group of immature females were treated with PMS as described for the first group, except that they were not allowed to mate. The time of the first and subsequent estrous periods was determined by use of vaginal smears. The first estrous smear after the one associated with vaginal opening occurred at an average of 40 days of life, compared with an average of 43 in untreated control rats. The succeeding cycles in the PMS-treated group were shorter and less variable than in the controls.

At this time I also would like to discuss a group of data from rats related to superovulation and tubal transport of ova. Although tubal transport is a topic outside the scope of this Conference, it can be an important factor in experiments concerned with the quantitative comparison of the effectiveness of ovulators. In these studies the usual procedure is to count the number of ova recovered from the tubes at a definite time after administration of the ovulator. The data which I will present are taken from the thesis of one of my students, Dr. Rae Whitney (Rae Whitney, Doctor of Philosophy Thesis, University of Wisconsin, 1944).

Sprague–Dawley rats were hypophysectomized when 29 or 30 days of age. They were injected subcutaneously with a FSH preparation made by trypsin digest method (W. H. McShan and R. K. Meyer, J.B.C. 132: 783, 1940). This preparation causes the development of follicles in the hypophysectomized rat, and when administered over a period of 10 days repairs ovarian interstitial cells and causes localized thecal luteinization and occasionally one to few corpora lutea. The FSH was injected once in the afternoon of the first day and twice daily for the next four days, a total of nine injections. At the time of the last injection, an intravenous injection was made of an unfractionated gonadotropic preparation, which was relatively rich in FSH and LH activity.

At varying times after the ovulator was injected, animals were killed and the ovarian bursa, oviducts, uterus and body cavity were flushed with saline. The number of ova in the washings was recorded.

The data are presented in terms of the number of ova recovered from the oviducts between 12 and 35 hr after the injection of the ovulator (Fig. 1). The maximum number of ova recovered was found between 16 and 20 hr. Between 20 and 24 hr the number of ova found in the oviduct was much smaller. It was during this time that one to five eggs were recovered from the body cavity of a few of the rats; ova were not recovered from the uterus before 48 hr after the ovulator was injected. We believe that when large numbers of ova are ovulated some of them accumulate in the bursa and are extruded through the bursal pore into the body cavity, thus accounting for the decrease found between 20 and 24 hr. A second peak in the number of ova was found between 23 and 26 hr. We do not have a satisfactory answer for this unexpected second peak. It has been suggested that ova found during this time are from a second group of follicles which were ovulated some hours after those which shed the eggs accumulating in the bursa and oviduct between 16 and 20 hr.

It is suggested that under the conditions of this experiment, and in similar experiments in which superovulation is experimentally induced in rats, the function of the oviduct is aberrant due to abnormal estrogen–progesterone levels. The practical implication of this concept is that in comparative studies of ovulators of different kinds the amount of gonadal hormones produced by different ovulators may vary, thus affecting the function of the oviduct, and the distribution of the ova in the different parts of the tract. It is also probable that when large numbers of ova are rapidly ovulated they accumulate in the bursa and many of them are forced through the bursal pore into the body cavity. This and/or the hormonally induced dysfunction of the oviduct are factors which should be considered in the development of methods which depend upon the recovery of ova for evaluating the effectiveness of ovulators.

THE INDUCTION OF OVULATION IN THE HUMAN BY HUMAN PITUITARY GONADOTROPIN

CARL A. GEMZELL

Department of Obstetrics and Gynecology, Karolinska Hospital and King Gustaf V's Research Institute, Sweden

THE clinical effects of gonadotropins, both pituitary gonadotropins and those obtained from extra-pituitary sources, such as pregnant mare serum or urine from pregnant, castrated or menopausal women, have been disappointing. In some cases, a polycystic enlargement of the ovaries has been reported but the finding is inconsistent. It is questionable whether the follicular growth induced results in maturation of an ovum to the graafian stage of development or whether an ovulation takes place when the luteinizing factor is added. The small number of pregnancies reported following such treatments indicates that an ovulation is brought about only occasionally or independently of the treatment.

The reason for the negative clinical results may be sought in the fact that gonadotropins obtained from other species have been used. Witschi (1) has shown that species specificity exists between gonadotropins of mammalian and amphibian origin and similar results in monkeys have been reported by Simpson and van Wagenen (2). An FSH preparation isolated from monkey pituitaries produced repeated ovulations in the monkey whereas FSH from sheep or pig pituitaries was less active. A similar specificity exists for other pituitary hormones such as growth hormone (GH). Li and Papkoff (3) have suggested that differences in biological activity result from differences in chemical structure. Human GH, for example, has a smaller molecular weight, an isoelectric point more on the acid side and different amino-acid end-groups than GH obtained from bovine pituitaries.

Antigonadotropic factors may also be the cause of the negative results. It has been noticed for a long time that the ovarian response to continued injections of gonadotropins gradually diminishes. Pregnant mare serum gonadotropins and those from sheep or pig pituitaries cause the appearance of antigonadotropic substances in blood as early as four weeks after the beginning of the treatment. Human chorionic gonadotropin or gonadotropin from the urine of castrated or menopausal women, however, does not give rise to antihormone formation, apparently because of its homologous origin.

These findings suggest that in order to obtain clinical effects with gonadotropin preparations from human pituitaries or urine should be used. Gonadotropins from the urine of castrated or menopausal women, which have mainly FSH activity, have been available for a long time, but the preparations are of low biological activity and their clinical effects are unsatisfactory. An FSH preparation obtained from human pituitaries was found to be quite active (4). When administered over long periods of time it did not evoke any formation of antigonadotropic factors.

A difficult problem in clinical practice is to prove if and when an ovulation takes place. Spontaneous ovulations do give rise to a number of signs that separately or together give rather good evidence—the rise in body temperature, the secretory reaction of the endometrium and the changes in vaginal smear and cervical secretion. These signs are all due to the release of free progesterone from a fresh corpus luteum.

In the case of ovulation induced by exogenous gonadotropins, however, these signs may not be valid. The normal physiological functions of the ovaries require certain ratios of FSH to LH and a slight change in these ratios may change the secretion of the ovaries. Administered in unphysiological doses, they may be effective in maturing the follicles without actually bringing about an ovulation. It is also possible that exogenous gonadotropins disturb the normal mechanism of ovulation in which a group of follicles are brought to a certain point of maturation and then undergo atresia while the favored one will continue to full development. Instead, the gonadotropins may bring several follicles to full maturation and thus bring hormone production to levels far above the normal.

The evidence for ovulation presented previously at this Conference is from carefully controlled animal experiments. Our results of gonadotropin studies in the human are somewhat less straightforward owing to the various conditions and the differences in the material. Clinical studies are often fraught with difficulties that are for the most part insurmountable. Every examination must be carried out in the interest of the patient and has to be justified from the point of diagnosis or treatment. Thus, in most cases, the proof of ovulation must rest on circumstantial rather than direct evidence.

The only absolute proofs of ovulation following the administration of gonadotropin are pregnancy or a fresh corpus luteum. To confirm a corpus luteum an abdominal exploration is usually necessary although sometimes culdoscopy may suffice.

We hesitate to employ surgical operations because the stimulated ovaries are very fragile and easily damaged. Furthermore, since surgical intervention is seldom justified, we have usually relied on circumstantial evidence such as an increase in pregnanediol excretion or secretory reaction of the endometrium.

SUBJECTS AND METHODS

Ovulation was induced in young women with primary or secondary amenorrhea with an FSH preparation obtained from human pituitaries and with a Swedish commercial preparation of human chorionic gonadotropins (Gonadex-Leo). All the patients were treated with human chorionic gonadotropin (HCG) several months before the administration of FSH in order to exclude the possibility that HCG alone could induce ovulation.

Preparation of human pituitary FSH. Human pituitaries obtained from autopsy cases were frozen and lyophilized. The dried glands were cut into small pieces and extracted in cold CaO-solution at pH 9.3 under continuous stirring. After centrifugation the clear supernatant was brought to 55% saturation by the addition of saturated ammonium sulfate. The precipitate was discarded and the clear supernatant was brought to 75% saturation by the addition of solid ammonium sulfate. The precipitate was collected by centrifugation, dissolved in water, dialyzed and lyophilized. This product was called human pituitary FSH and was used in the clinical trials.

Potency of human pituitary FSH. The human pituitary FSH was assayed against the provisional human menopausal gonadotropin (HMG-20A) standard preparation. On a weight basis the partially purified human pituitary FSH was thirty to fifty times as potent as the HMG-20A standard preparation when assayed by methods measuring total gonadotropin or FSH activities. In the ventral prostate test, which is considered to be specific for LH activity, the human pituitary FSH was only approximately 5 times as potent as HMG-20A.

Purification of human pituitary FSH. A further purification of the human pituitary FSH was carried out by Dr. P. Roos in Uppsala employing ion exchange chromatography and zone electrophoresis. A fraction was obtained which is more than 2000 times as active as HMG-20A.

Administration of human pituitary FSH. The human FSH preparation was administered in daily doses of 10 mg during a 10-day period. The 10 mg dose was chosen as it gave a significant increase in ovarian size and estrogen excretion in a hypopituitary dwarf. A dose of 1 mg per day had no effect and doses of 2 and 5 mg gave only a slight increase in proliferative endometrial activity. The 5 mg dose was tried in several cases without any effect. It may be suggested that a relatively large dose has to be administered in order to initiate the follicular growth; later a smaller dose may be enough. Thus, the effective daily dose of FSH corresponded to about 500 mg of the HMG-20A standard and the total dose during the 10-day period to about 5000 mg.

Repeated treatments with human pituitary FSH were performed in at least 10 women. All of these 10 women responded to the first treatment as well as to the subsequent ones. A young woman with primary amenorrhea was treated during a period of 2 years and received more than 1 gm of FSH.

Following each treatment a polycystic enlargement of the ovaries and an increase in the estrogen excretion were found. No untoward effects, such as fever or local reactions at the site of injections, were observed.

Criteria of ovulation. The following criteria of ovulation were employed: uterine biopsy, chemical determinations of estrone, estradiol-17β, estriol and pregnanediol.

TABLE 1. EVALUATION OF ENDOMETRIAL ACTIVITY

Atrophy	Proliferation			Secretion	
	Weak	Moderate	Intense	Early secretory phase (preparedness)	Full secretory phase
No glandular mitosis	>8*	<8–>2	<2	15–18 day of cycle†	19–28 day of cycle

* Number of glandular cross-sections studied, necessary to detect one mitosis (Tillinger and Westman, 1957).

† Basal vacuolization similar to the one found in normal cycles (Noyes *et al.*, 1950).

The endometrial activity was estimated according to Table 1.

The endometrium was *atrophic* (A) when no mitosis was found in sections of the glandular epithelium, *weakly proliferative* ($\bar{P}$) when more than 8 cross-sections were required to detect one mitosis, *moderately proliferative* (P) when less than 8 but more than 2 cross-sections were necessary and *intensely proliferative* ($\underline{P}$) when less than 2 were required to find one mitosis. Endometrial secretory activity was differentiated into *early secretion* (ES) with basal vacuolization, similar to that found in the 15th–18th day of the normal cycle and *full secretion* (S) representing the 19th–28th day of the cycle.

Urinary Steroid Assays. Estrogen assays were restricted to the estimation of the 3 "classic" estrogens—estrone, estradiol-17β and estriol. The method of Brown (5) was used, with a slight modification as described by Diczfalusy and Westman (6) and Brown *et al.* (7). The term "estrogen" will be used to denote estrone, estradiol-17β and estriol.

Pregnanediol was estimated according to the method of Klopper *et al.* (8), but the color correction equation of Allen (9) was used. The evidence in favor of this modification has been presented by Diczfalusy (10).

RESULTS

In evaluating the effect of human pituitary FSH it must be kept in mind that the preparation contains small amounts of LH and that the patients have their own pituitaries which may release FSH and/or LH. It would have been advantageous if hypophysectomized patients could be tested. We have only two who to a certain degree meet this requirement—a hypopituitary dwarf with advanced hypogonadism and a young woman who was recently operated upon due to a chromophobe adenoma. The other patients tested had a

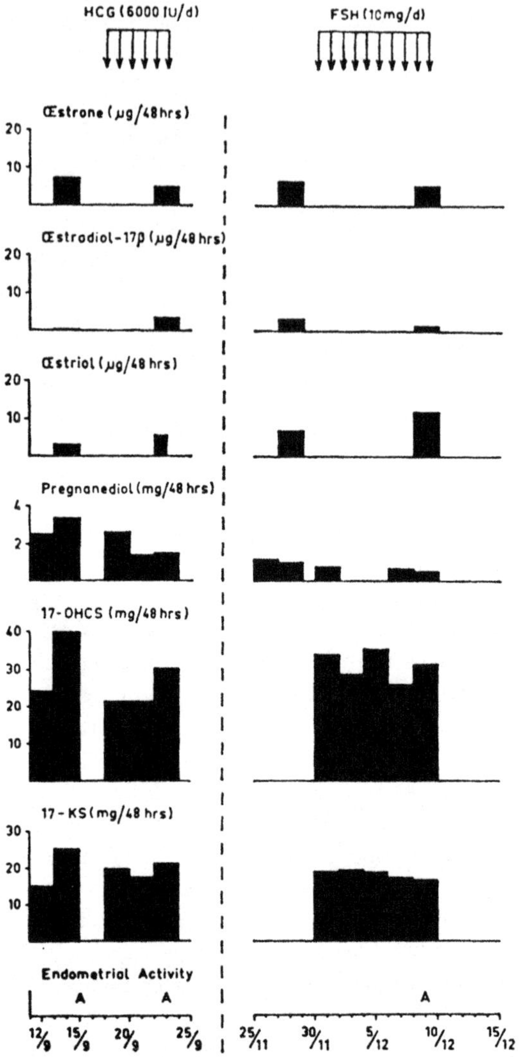

FIG. 1. Urinary excretion of estrone, estradiol-17β, estriol, pregnanediol, 17-hydroxy-corticosteroids and 17-ketosteroids before and following the administration of human chorionic gonadotropin (HCG) and—two and a half months later—of human pituitary follicle-stimulatin ghormone (FSH). Endometrial activity in biopsies: A = atrophic endometrium.

long-lasting amenorrhea with atrophic or weakly proliferative endometrial activity indicating little or no ovarian function.

Following the administration of 10 mg of human pituitary FSH over a 10-day period a polycystic enlargement of the ovaries was found in 27 out

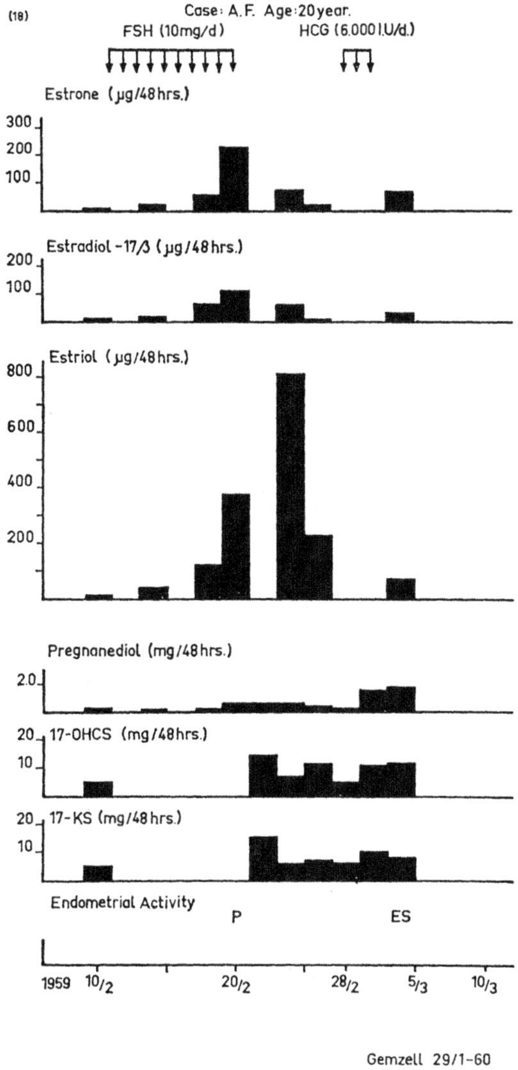

FIG. 2. Urinary excretion of estrogen, pregnanediol, 17-hydroxycorticosteroids and 17-ketosteroids before and following the administration of FSH and HCG. Endometrial activity: P = proliferative, ES = early secretory reaction.

of 40 women, an increase in estrogen excretion in 16 and an increase in pregnanediol excretion in 4 out of 30 women. Of 27 women with atrophic endometrium before the treatment 16 responded with proliferative activity, none with secretory reaction. Of 10 women with proliferative endometrial activity before the treatment 7 showed secretory reaction. However, 11 women out of 40 did not show any response to the administration of human pituitary FSH. Eight of these 11 women were operated upon and subsequent examination at operation revealed very hypoplastic ovaries entirely lacking germinative tissue. The 11 women who did not respond to human pituitary FSH had a pathologically elevated urinary excretion of gonadotropin while all the women who responded to human pituitary FSH had a low or normal gonadotropin excretion.

Figure 1 shows the effect of human pituitary FSH on the urinary excretion of estrogen and pregnanediol and on the endometrium of one of the 11 women in whom surgical exploration revealed ovaries without germinative tissue.

It follows from Fig. 1 that human pituitary FSH had no effect on the steroid excretion and the endometrium. Thus, it may be tentatively postulated that in order to obtain an effect with human pituitary FSH the ovaries must have germinative tissue (11).

Figure 2 shows the effect of human pituitary FSH and human chorionic gonadotropin (HCG) on a hypopituitary dwarf with primary amenorrhea and marked hypogonadism. Her endometrium was atrophic before the treatment.

FSH alone increased the urinary excretion of estrogen. The first increase was noticed in the urine on the 5th day of the treatment but already on the 2nd day the patient complained about tension in her breasts and an increase in vaginal discharge. After the last injection of FSH the urinary excretion of estrogen decreased. Pelvic examination revealed that the ovaries were enlarged, with diameters of about 6 cm. When HCG was administered 8 days after the last injection of FSH an ovulation took place probably within 24 hr as indicated by the rise in pregnanediol excretion and the secretory reaction of the endometrium.

Figure 3 shows the effect of FSH and HCG on a 24-year-old woman with secondary amenorrhea and atrophic endometrium.

HCG alone had no effect. After administration of FSH the urinary excretion of estrogen rose to very high levels, the size of the ovaries increased and the endometrium changed from atrophic to proliferative. When HCG was administered 24 hr after the last injection of FSH an ovulation occurred within 48 hr, as indicated by the rise in pregnanediol excretion, drop in urinary estrogen excretion and the secretory reaction of the endometrium. Figure 4 shows a similar effect in a 31-year-old woman with atrophic endometrium.

A very strong effect of human pituitary FSH was found in a 25-year-old woman with underdeveloped secondary sex characteristics, secondary amenorrhea and an atrophic endometrium (Fig. 5).

She was treated with HCG alone, with FSH followed by HCG and with FSH and HCG simultaneously. HCG alone had no effect. FSH caused a marked increase in the urinary excretion of estrogen, evident as early as after 5 days of treatment. The urinary excretion of estrogen reached a very

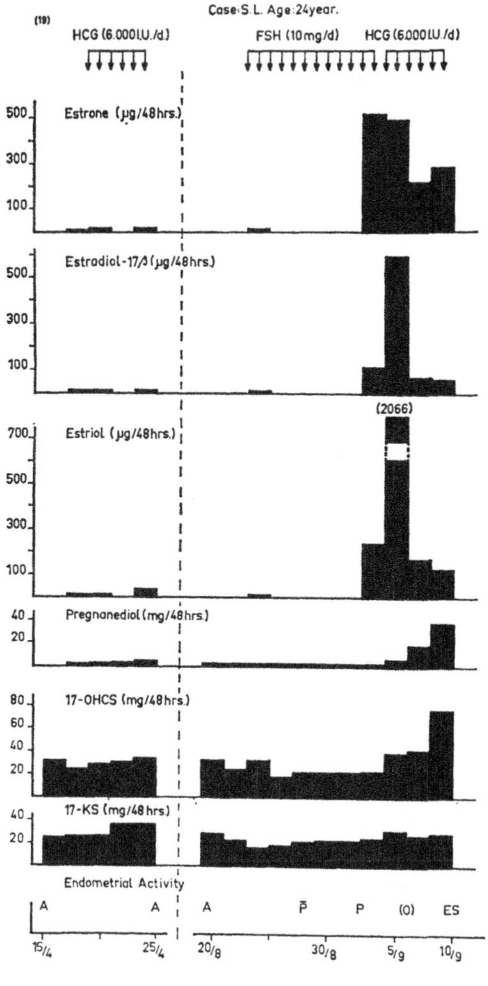

FIG. 3. Urinary excretion of estrogen, pregnanediol, 17-corticosteroids and 17-ketosteroids before and after the administration of HCG and FSH. (O) = day of ovulation.

high level, almost 5 mg per 48 hr. The ovaries increased in size during the same time, attaining a diameter of about 5 cm. When HCG was administered, 4 days after the last injection of FSH, an ovulation took place within 24 hr as indicated by the sharp rise in pregnanediol excretion and the secretory reaction of the endometrium. During the administration of HCG the ovaries increased further in size and reached the umbilicus. By a culdoscopy a large follicular cyst was evacuated and 750 ml of follicular fluid was collected and analyzed for estrogen. The fluid contained all three estrogens—estrone,

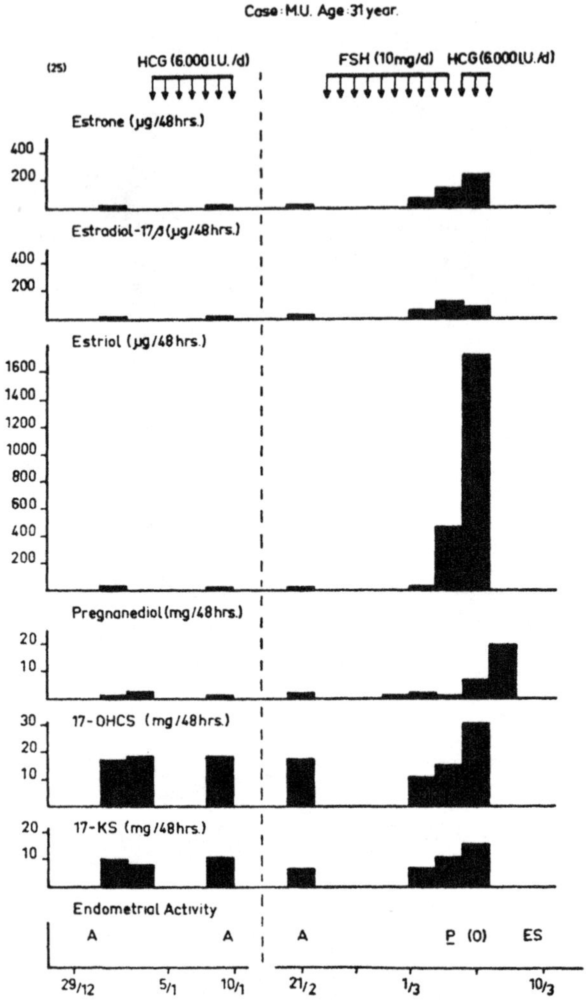

FIG. 4. Urinary excretion of estrogen, pregnanediol, 17-corticosteroids and 17-ketosteroids before and following the administration of HCG and FSH.

estradiol-17β and estriol. Following the withdrawal of the follicular fluid the urinary excretion of pregnanediol decreased from 140 mg to 60 mg per 48 hr. When FSH and HCG were administered together an ovulation occurred on the 6th day of treatment as indicated by the rise in pregnanediol

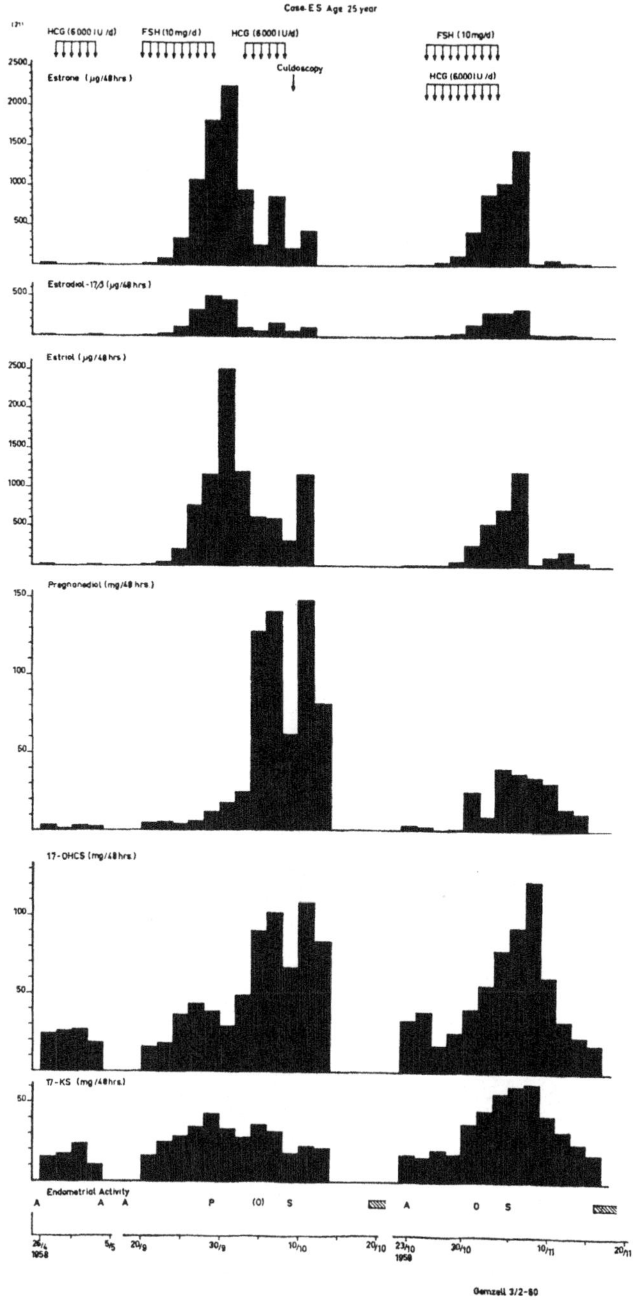

FIG. 5. Urinary excretion of estrogen, pregnanediol, 17-corticosteroids and 17-ketosteroids before and following the administration of HCG and FSH.

excretion and the secretory reaction of the endometrium. The elevated level of urinary pregnanediol lasted for about two weeks and a menstrual bleeding occurred when the excretion ceased.

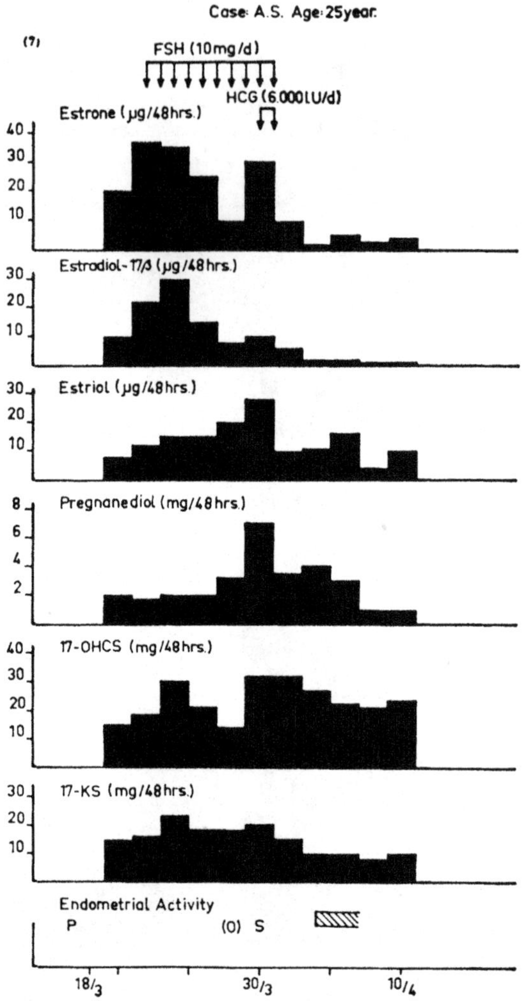

FIG. 6. Urinary excretion of estrogen, pregnanediol, 17-corticosteroids and 17-ketosteroids before and following the administration of FSH and HCG. The patient was operated upon April 1st.

The effect of FSH seemed to be a function of time. Following a 20-day treatment with human pituitary FSH in a 28-year-old woman with secondary amenorrhea, the ovaries reached a diameter of 12 to 15 cm and the urinary

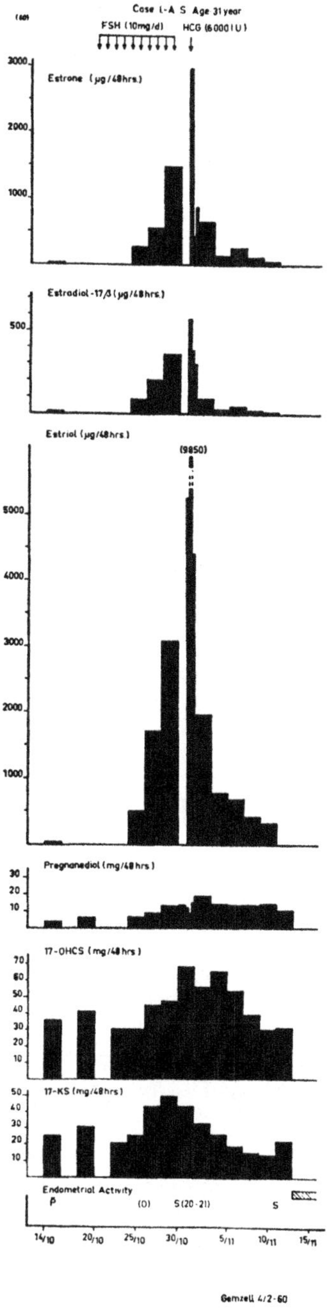

FIG. 8. Urinary excretion of estrogen, pregnanediol, 17-corticosteroids and 17-ketosteroids before and following the administration of FSH and HCG. Following the single intravenous injection of HCG the urine was collected in 3 8-hr samples.

excretion of estrogen an amount of 6.6 mg. A 10-day treatment in the same woman yielded ovaries with a diameter of approximately 5 cm and a urinary estrogen excretion of only 4.0 mg.

Figure 6 shows the effect of human pituitary FSH in an amenorrheic woman with proliferative endometrial activity indicating some ovarian function.

Following the administration of FSH a modest increase in ovarian size and estrogen excretion occurred. On the 6th day of treatment an ovulation took place, as indicated by the rise in pregnanediol excretion, the drop in estrogen excretion and the secretory reaction of the endometrium. The day after the last injection of FSH the patient underwent surgery and the ovaries were polycystic, enlarged and a single corpus luteum was found in one of them. An ovarian resection was performed and by histological examination the corpus luteum was found to be 4 days old (Fig. 7).

The low excretion of estrogen and pregnanediol found in this case was probably due to the fact that only one follicle matured and developed into a corpus luteum.

The effect of human pituitary FSH in an amenorrheic woman with secondary amenorrhea and proliferative endometrium is shown in Fig. 8.

As in the previous case, FSH alone caused an ovulation on the 6th day of treatment as indicated by the increased excretion of pregnanediol and the secretory reaction of the endometrium. Twenty-four hours after the last injection of FSH a single dose of HCG was administered intravenously. The urine was collected in 8-hr samples immediately following the injection. The HCG injection caused even during the first 8-hr period a very marked increase in the urinary excretion of estrogen; the excretion of pregnanediol, in marked contrast, was unaffected.

Of 50 amenorrheic women treated with HCG alone only 2 ovulated. The effect of HCG and FSH in one of these is shown in Fig. 9.

Following treatment with HCG an ovulation took place as indicated by the rise in pregnanediol excretion and a fresh corpus luteum observed by culdoscopy. When this patient, who had proliferative endometrium, was treated with FSH alone a polycystic enlargement of the ovaries and a marked increase in the urinary excretion of estrogen occurred, but there was no indication of ovulation.

The second amenorrheic woman, who ovulated following treatment with HCG, reacted in a similar way on the administration of FSH.

In five other amenorrheic women, repeated ovulations were induced at certain periods of time. Two became pregnant, each on the second attempt.

Figure 10 shows the successful result in a 29-year-old woman who had a secondary amenorrhea of about 7 years' duration and who had been married for 6 years.

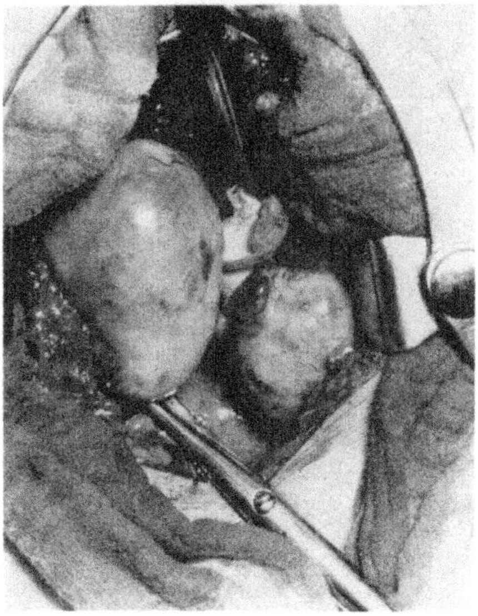

FIG. 7. Enlarged polycystic ovaries with a corpus luteum in the right one found at laparotomy.

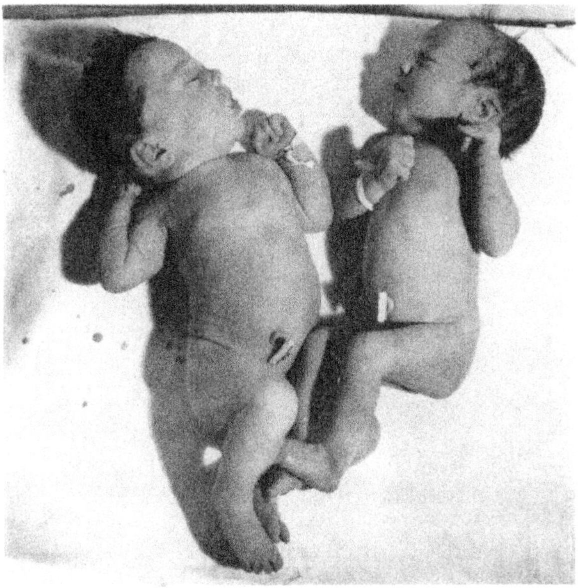

FIG. 11. The double ovum twins.

Human pituitary FSH was administered in order to prove that her ovaries responded. A schedule was prepared for induction of ovulation at certain points of time. The first attempt was a failure but the second one was successful. A rise in body temperature occurred at the time when ovulation was

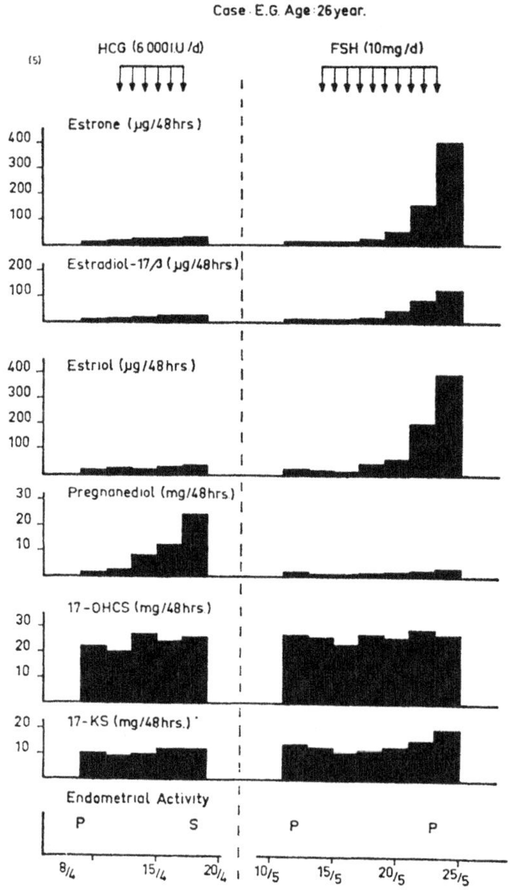

FIG. 9. Urinary excretion of estrogen, pregnanediol, 17-corticosteroids and 17-ketosteroids before and following the administration of HCG and FSH.

predicted to occur. When 2 weeks later no menstrual period appeared and the temperature was still elevated a pregnancy was suspected. Two weeks later positive pregnancy tests confirmed the diagnosis. The patient delivered double ovum twins 265 days later (Fig. 11).

Unfortunately, only in a few cases was it possible to examine the ovaries following treatment with human pituitary FSH and HCG. Following FSH alone the ovaries showed a great number of follicular cysts of various sizes.

The granulosa of these follicles was often damaged, probably due to rapid growth and the consequent change in intrafollicular pressure. Following FSH and HCG administration, polycystic, enlarged ovaries, either with a single

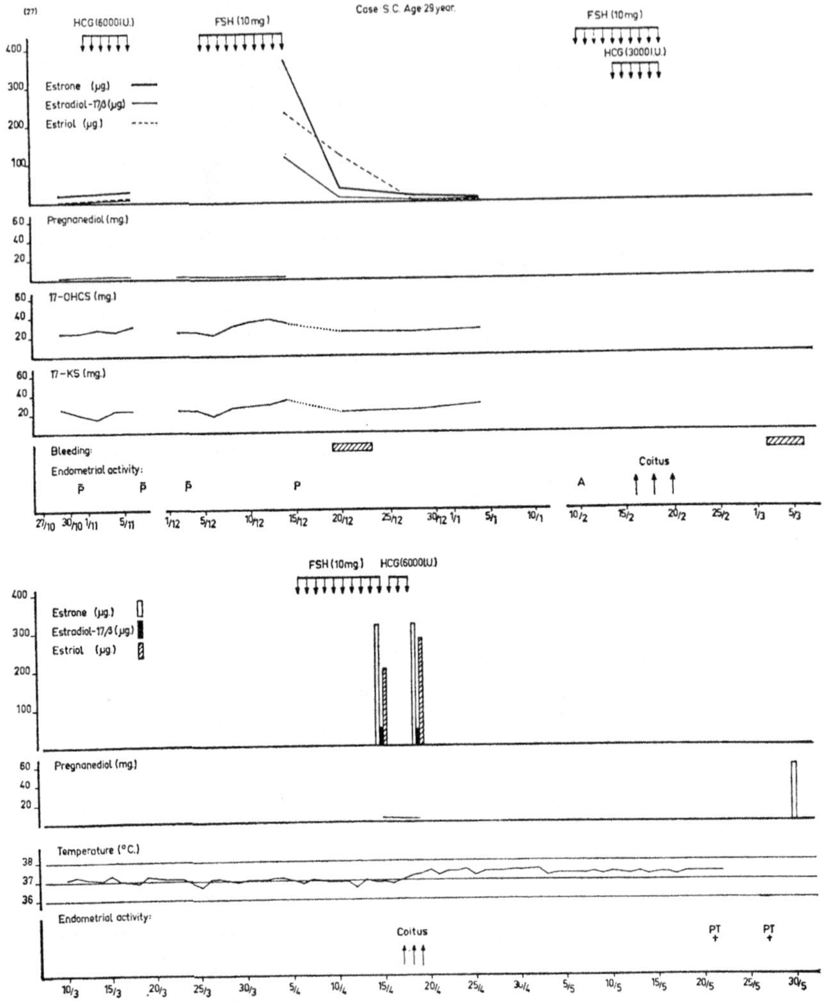

FIG. 10. Induction of ovulation and pregnancy in an amenorrheic woman. The second attempt was successful as is shown by the 2 positive pregnancy tests about 5 and 6 weeks after the time of ovulation.

corpus luteum or with a great number of corpora, were observed. In the latter cases the ovaries were hemorrhagic with follicles of various size filled with fresh coagulated blood. In the abdominal cavity hemorrhagic yellow fluid was often found, probably originating from the ruptured follicles. The stimulated ovaries were very fragile and ruptured easily upon handling. Two to three weeks later the enlarged ovaries were reduced in size and could not be felt by pelvic examination.

DISCUSSION

The enlargement of the ovaries and the high excretion of estrogen following the administration of FSH indicated that a large number of follicles were stimulated. During a normal menstrual cycle several follicles are brought to a certain point of maturation and then undergo atresia while a single one takes the lead to its full development. It was likely that the exogenous FSH disturbed this mechanism and brought all the stimulated follicles to full maturation. When these matured follicles were exposed to the luteinizing factor, luteinization occurred in all of them at the same time which resulted in several ovulations and corpora lutea formations. Whether these enlarged follicles were able to deliver normal ova was questionable. It might be suggested that the rapid growth and the changes in intrafollicular pressure distributed the normal development of the ova. However, at least in two cases the induced ova were fertilized and developed into normal fetuses.

The primordial follicles of the ovaries, as was shown in this study, have to be stimulated by the exogenous FSH for about 6 days before the luteinizing factor is effective. When the follicles reached this state of maturation luteinization took place very rapidly and a corpus luteum was formed within 24 hr. The luteinization of the ovaries was followed by a severe pain in the lower abdomen.

The strong effect of the exogenous FSH on the ovaries might indicate that the doses were too large or that the hormone was administered during too long a time. In several cases half the dose (5 mg) was administered without any effect. It was possible that the first doses of FSH have to be rather large in order to initiate follicular growth. After the follicles have been stimulated, smaller doses might be sufficient. Furthermore, the period of 10 days might also be too long, for the maturation necessary for the luteinization to occur was reached already within 6 days. After an ovulation has occurred the remaining follicles are still responsive to FSH stimulation and continue growing and produce large amounts of estrogen.

The tremendous rise in pregnanediol excretion seen in a couple of cases suggests that the amount of HCG administered might also be too large. In one case where a single corpus luteum was found, the pregnanediol excretion was 8 mg per 48 hr which was a quite normal level during the luteal phase. The high level of 100 to 140 mg per 48 hr found in one case might indicate that 10 to 15 corpora lutea had been formed. In a patient operated upon this suggestion was confirmed; the high excretion of 80 mg of pregnanediol was correlated with 5 corpora lutea. It seems also important that HCG was administered during a relatively short period of time, for HCG caused further enlargement of these ovaries which were stimulated by FSH.

TABLE 2. INDUCING OVULATION BY FSH (+LH) IN AMENORRHEIC WOMEN WITH VARIOUS ENDOMETRIAL ACTIVITY

Endometrial activity	No. of patients	Increase in ovarian size	Increase in estrogen excretion	Ovulation
Atrophic				
Without pituitary	2	2	2	0
With pituitary	16	16	16	0
Proliferative	10	10	10	7
Secretory	2	2	2	–

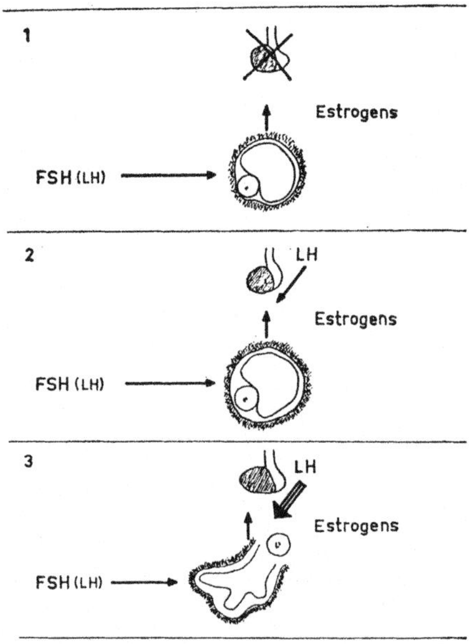

FIG. 12. The mechanism of ovulation in amenorrheic women with atrophic endometrium (1 and 2) and in those with proliferative endometrial activity (3).

The FSH preparation used in this study caused an increase in the production and release of estrogen even in a patient without a pituitary. A similar increase following the administration of a highly-purified preparation of FSH has not been observed in hypophysectomized animals. Only after small amounts of LH were added did the follicles produce and release estrogen. As the human pituitary FSH preparation contained small amounts of LH it was impossible to draw any conclusions on this subject. The problem will not be solved until a pure human pituitary FSH preparation is available and is injected into hypophysectomized individuals.

The response to human pituitary FSH was different in amenorrheic women with atrophic endometrium indicating no ovarian activity and in those who have proliferative endometrial activity indicating some ovarian function (Table 2). None of the women with atrophic endometrium ovulated following the administration of FSH alone while 7 out of 10 with proliferative activity ovulated.

It seems most likely to assume that the difference is at the pituitary level. The pituitaries of the first group of women lacked the capacity to release LH when stimulated by estrogen while the pituitaries of the second group released enough LH for an ovulation to take place (Fig. 12). It might also be suggested that the two amenorrheic women who ovulated on the administration of FSH had pituitaries which were insufficient in LH. One of them ovulated repeatedly during one year following the administration of HCG.

Acknowledgement.—This work has been done in collaboration with Dr. E. Diczfalusy and Dr. K.-G. Tillinger, Karolinska Hospital, Stockholm.

REFERENCES

1. Witschi, E. and C. Y. Chang, *Symposium on Comparative Endocrinology*, John Wiley, 1959.
2. van Wagenen, G. and M. E. Simpson, *Endocrinology* **61**, 316, 1957.
3. Li, C. H. and H. Papkoff, *Science* **124**, 1293, 1956.
4. Gemzell, C. A., E. Diczfalusy and K. G. Tillinger, *J. Clin. Endocrinol.* **18**, 1333, 1958.
5. Brown, J. B., *Biochem. J.* **60**, 185, 1955.
6. Diczfalusy, E. and A. Westman, *Acta endocrinol.* **21**, 321, 1956.
7. Brown, J. B., R. D. Bulbrook and F. C. Greenwood, *J. Endocrinol.* **16**, 49, 1957.
8. Klopper, A., E. A. Michie and J. B. Brown, *J. Endocrinol.* **12**, 209, 1955.
9. Allen, W. M., *J. Clin. Endocrinol.* **10**, 71, 1950.
10. Diczfalusy, E., *Acta endocrinol.* **20**, 216, 1955.
11. Gemzell, C. A., E. Diczfalusy and K. G. Tillinger, *Acta Obst. et Gyn. Scandinav.* **38**, 465, 1959.

DISCUSSIONS

Chairman: Astwood

Chairman Astwood: Thank you very much for that fine presentation, Dr. Gemzell. I think we might have a brief discussion, before going on to the next paper. Dr. Segal, do you have any remarks to make at this time?

Dr. Sheldon Segal: Dr. Gemzell's interesting studies and the results he has recorded speak for themselves so eloquently that there is very little left to question. I have but a few minor points of interest to raise. Until now, when pituitary gonadotropins have been extracted from animal glands, we have been shackled, to a certain extent, by the practical expediency of using whatever glands that could be obtained under slaughterhouse conditions. This has made it almost impossible to extract separately male and female pituitaries. Since the program of extracting human pituitaries for gonadotropins is still in its infancy, it might be possible to establish a collection procedure which would permit taking advantage of sex-specific characteristics. All would agree, on the basis of total gonadotropin assays, that quantitative differences exist and it is far from unreasonable to assume that qualitative differences might be uncovered which would play an important role in the biologic activity of human pituitary extracts. I would urge Dr. Gemzell to consider this possibility when making collections for future extractions.

The results indicate that there was a remarkable uniformity in the time required for ovulation after the supplementing dose of HCG was administered. In most instances it appeared to take approximately 10 hr. In a few cases, however, the evidence did seem to indicate a longer period of delay. This final maturation period of the follicle and enclosed ovum may be viewed as highly significant toward assuring the egg normalcy. The condition of the released egg is particularly important in these considerations since human gonadotropins will find widespread usage in cases of infertility in which induced ovulations will be given the greatest opportunity for subsequent fertilization and development. With this in mind, it would seem advisable to eliminate the use of HCG as the supplementary, ovulation-inducing substance and as soon as adequate supplies are available, establish the dosage levels required to complete with pituitary gonadotropins, the entire process of follicle stimulation, final maturation of the ovum and ovulation. The work reported by Dr. Simpson earlier in this Conference could be used to great advantage in determining the dosage ratios that would be required. In brief, I am contending that ovulation is a continuous process including the various steps mentioned above. The gametes released following the stimulation by human pituitary gonadotropin as an initial step followed by HCG stimulation to carry the process to completion may not have the same opportunity for normalcy as gametes that have developed completely under stimulation by pituitary gonadotropins.

My final comment is with respect to Dr. Gemzell's finding of multiple-follicle-stimulation following the administration of human pituitary FSH. It raises an interesting speculation on the possible phenotypic expression of a gene action known to exist in humans. Multiple or polyovular ovulations occur with familial and even racial distribution. For example, they occur less frequently among Japanese families than in Caucasians. To say that the phenomenon is controlled genetically, as all would agree, does not delve very deeply toward understanding the physiologic differences that exist at the level of the ovary. One could speculate in terms of gene penetrance, postulating that the greater the penetrance the greater restriction placed on the number of follicles stimulated at each cycle. The physiologic mechanism of the gene action is suggested by Dr. Gemzell's studies. He has overcome the genetic tendency for monofollicular development by increasing circulating levels and/or by altering ratios of pituitary gonadotropins to levels that are apparently out of the normally produced, genetically established range (I refer here to the frequent observation at laparotomy of multiple-follicle-stimulation and not to the single case of twinning, interesting though it may be). It would seem that the phenotypic expression of this character controlling multiplicity of ovulations may simply be in the normal gonadotropin levels for different races or families or, more likely, the sensitivity of the developing follicles to a given level of gonadotropins. The fact that no large differences in "normal" gonadotropin excretion levels have been found among various races may reflect the grossness of our present gonadotropin assays.

CHAIRMAN ASTWOOD: There are a couple of brief comments, I believe, that may be made at this time.

DR. DUNCAN E. REID: I would like to ask Dr. Gemzell whether he has attempted to prolong the normal menstrual cycle with human chorionic gonadotropin. Also, I should like to know if he has treated women, who might be classified as "chronic aborters", during the critical period of implantation and early placentation by administering human chorionic gonadotropin in the hope of prolonging the corpus luteum until such time as the syncytium began to produce sufficient amounts of sex steroids.

DR. CLAUDE A. VILLEE: May I ask a question? I would like to know whether Dr. Gemzell has used any of the LH, which is a by-product of his preparation of FSH, following the administration of FSH, instead of using the chorionic gonadotropin.

I noted in your preparation the LH does come out in a separate fraction.

The other question I have is this. Did this lady who produced the twins have any family history of twinning?

DR. JANET MCARTHUR: I was intrigued by the mention in Dr. Gemzell's abstract of an inhibitory action of progesterone given concomitantly with FSH. Would you be willing to discuss this a little further?

DR. CARL GEMZELL: In answer to Dr. Reid's question, we found that if FSH was administered after an ovulation was brought about, it was possible to prolong the cycle. As long as FSH was administered, there was an increase in follicular size and estrogen excretion and no bleeding occurred. When the administration of FSH ceased, a menstrual bleeding occurred, usually within one week.

We have speculated whether it is necessary to add something more for the corpus luteum to function and produce steroids. However, when we measured the urinary excretion of steroids there was always a large amount of progesterone produced. The corpora lutea produced in this way lasted about two weeks and when the pregnanediol excretion ceased, a bleeding occurred within one or two days.

It is difficult to state exactly when an ovulation takes place following the administration of FSH. In two cases we gave HCG intravenously 24 hr after the last injection of FSH and collected the urine in 3 8-hr samples. Unfortunately both of these women had already ovulated on the administration of FSH alone. We are planning similar experiments in order to find out just how long a time it will take to induce ovulation in ovaries which have been primed with FSH.

When HCG was administered to women who had been treated with FSH they consistently felt a severe pain in the abdomen about eight to ten hours later. It may be suggested that this pain indicates the luteinization of the ovaries.

We have not done any work on the purification of human pituitary LH but we are collecting the fractions which contain the LH activity.

The woman who delivered twins had had no previous record of twins in her family.

We have treated a number of amenorrheic women with progesterone and FSH in order to find out if the ovarian response was the same as following the administration of FSH alone. The first 5 women treated showed no ovarian response and we thought that it was possible to inhibit the effect of FSH on the ovaries by simultaneously administering progesterone (100 mg/day, intramuscularly). However, later experiments have shown that it is possible to obtain an increase in estrogen excretion with no change in ovarian size. The urinary excretion of estrogen following FSH plus progesterone is much lower than following the administration of FSH alone. These experiments are going on at the present time and I hope to be able to report on them at a later occasion.

FACTORS INFLUENCING OVULATION AND ATRESIA OF OVARIAN FOLLICLES

SOMERS H. STURGIS

THE human ovary at birth shows a cortex tightly packed with primordial follicles, and almost no interstitial tissue. We may estimate that there are upwards of five hundred thousand eggs in these newborn ovaries from somewhat meager evidence such as the finding of a Swedish investigator who counted four hundred and twenty thousand eggs in the ovaries of a 22-year-old normal girl who died suddenly (1). In the human as in other mammals, generally none are left after the age of sixty. If one ovulation were achieved with regularity every month of life from the age of twelve through fifty, then less than five hundred eggs in such a girl would ever achieve ovulation. By far the vast proportion, therefore, are lost in the process of atresia which begins at birth or before, and continues through to the menopause. The chance, then, that any given egg in the neonatal ovary will achieve ovulation is considerably less than one in a thousand. All the other eggs are wasted as their follicles degenerate, and eventually atrophy to an amorphous hyalinized scar. It is important to emphasize that atresia is the usual life story and course of the primate egg and follicle. It is only the unusual egg that matures in a ripening follicle and goes on to ovulate.

The study of ovulation control must embrace an understanding not only of the mechanisms behind the dramatic success of the unusual follicle that ovulates, but also of the background and physiologic causes for the much more common process of atresia. This process is going on constantly through the normal cycle in adult ovaries in follicles of various stages of development, but there are distinct waves of atresia related to certain times of the cycle. It is hard not to believe that there must be a functional element significantly added to the activity of the adult ovary by the dozens of follicles undergoing atresia at any given time. The reasons for this will be stated later. It is tempting to hope that the causes for atresia might be sufficiently understood so that one might also heighten or accelerate this phenomenon. If hormonal interactions are involved, these might offer a means for physiologic control of ovulation by some direct action on preovulatory follicles causing all to start dissolution before they reached full maturity.

The massive wastage of germ cells appears to be a rule of nature. Two results of this loss of follicles in the primate ovary are clearly recognized. In the first place, the interstitial tissue of the mature ovary is gradually built up by the theca of atretic follicles, and the fibrous organization of their remains. It seems likely that such an increase in bulk of interstitial tissue may be necessary before any one follicle in the ovary is enabled to achieve full maturation at or after puberty. The second, and perhaps much more significant aspect of the dissolution of eggs and follicles in mature life probably relates to the limitation of offspring to that which is typical for each species. At least in the monkey where the steps of atresia of the ovarian follicle have been studied in detail, it is apparent that this process wipes out all follicles of second rank in each cycle, the ones that ordinarily would be most likely next to mature and ovulate. Perhaps the most dramatic feature of nature's own control of ovulation in the monkey, and probably the human, is the induction of atresia in all but one of the ripening follicles each month.

Clearly this is not a local phenomenon such as one due to mounting intraovarian pressure associated with the rapid spurt of growth of the maturing follicle, because second rank follicles are wiped out equally just prior to ovulation in the contralateral ovary as well. Although atresia of lesser follicles continues unabated at all times of the cycle, yet this is a wave of dissolution that is significantly present during the ovulation phase.

It is important, then, to review the stages of atresia as seen in the monkey ovary in an attempt to fit these processes into what is known of gonadotropin stimulation and steroid response. The examples to be shown are from the beautiful collection of monkey ovaries in the Carnegie Institute of Embryology where a study was made through the courtesy of Dr. George W. Corner (2). Figure 1 shows the egg and surrounding cumulus on day 13 just before ovulation. The egg shows the first maturation spindle. The granulosa cells of the cumulus are beginning to separate with edema fluid. The theca interna layer is thin and delicate and hard to demonstrate. The diameter of this follicle was seven thousand microns. It was judged to be within 24 hr of ovulation. At the same time, in the same monkey, Fig. 2 indicates two follicles of second rank. These could be found by tracing down serial sections to measure in largest diameter nine hundred to twelve hundred micra. The striking features are first, the dissolution of the granulosa indicating the first sign of impending atresia, and second the dramatic thickening of the theca interna layer. To make the comparison of this theca hypertrophy with that of the maturing follicle more obvious, Fig. 3 shows the thin undeveloped theca layer of the maturing follicle and Fig. 4 shows in higher power the thick, juicy apparently secretory theca interna layer of the follicles going into atresia.

Within the next two or three days, these large follicles collapse rapidly and here in another specimen (Fig. 5) is seen, with Mallory's connective tissue stain, a follicle undergoing atresia with the egg already amorphous and degenerate. One can see the condensation of fibers between the cells of the theca interna forming the wavy line that will become the hyaloid membrane of later atretic follicles.

The same process probably occurs in human ovaries, although there is not yet available today sufficient material to follow the same stages as closely. The most striking feature of these observations for the present discussion is the hypertrophy of theca interna that appears coincident to the earliest sign of atresia in those follicles of second rank. This feature occurs coincidentally with the formation of the first polar body or second maturation spindle of the mature follicle about to ovulate. Incidentally, a careful study of rat ovaries under various stimuli fails to reveal any theca interna thickening coincidental to the cleavage of the ovum that typifies early atresia in this species. The absence of this theca interna thickening in an animal that can readily accommodate an average litter of nine in comparison with its presence as seen in the monkey in the eight to ten follicles wiped out each month, might lend suggestive support to the thesis that the factors causing this theca hypertrophy in the primate may be responsible in some way for the limitation of ovulation to a single follicle each month.

It is difficult to escape the probability that this clearly defined structure plays some endocrine role in the cycle. Other endocrine events of consequence are happening as well. The maturing follicle shows a tremendous spurt of growth from day 12 to day 14 of the cycle. This is simultaneous with the first high point in estrogen production during the menstrual cycle. In the last 24 hr before ovulation, there is also a sudden surge of production of the pituitary gonadotropin causing an LH effect. McArthur has documented such a peak in a normal cycle (3), and this has been confirmed by Taymor (4). There is considerable evidence to suggest that the surge in estrogen production by the spurting growth of the major follicle causes the release of this LH. It may not even be estrogens themselves, but breakdown products that have this result. Thus, if one castrates a rat and transplants one of the ovaries into the spleen, the steroids produced by the transplanted ovary will be brought in the portal circulation directly to the liver, and there become inactivated. The continuing atrophy of the uterus in such a preparation confirms that estrogens have not escaped into the general circulation from the liver. Yet, the transplanted ovary becomes converted into an almost solid luteal body. It seems probable in this case that the breakdown products of estrogen liberated from the liver are responsible for the LH and perhaps LTH coming from the pituitary that causes such luteinization of the transplanted gonad (5). Now, just as we have seen in the monkey that the period of theca hypertrophy in atretic follicles is short lived, about two to four days, so also have studies shown that the peak of LH is limited to the same time interval. It is unfortunate that we do not have any evidence of this LH peak yet available from the monkey nor do we have serial sections of sufficient human material to show that the theca proliferation in the human is similarly a transient phenomenon.

It seems probable, however, that the same time relationships apply both to monkey and human. As yet, we have no clear explanation for this wave of atresia, but before seeking to clarify this point it is worth noting some other aspects of atresia of the ovarian follicle.

As well as appearing as part of the normal life cycle of follicles in the ovary, there are other situations where abnormal atresia of ovarian follicles occurs. First, this has been noted to occur under instances of excessive and non-physiologic gonadotropin stimulation. Velardo (6) this month has reported follicle cysts, fragmented ova and degenerating follicles when large amounts of gonadotropins were given to hypophysectomized animals. Parkes has stated (7) that if one ovary is removed and a part of the other, then the remainder under the influence of the whole gonadotropic output responds with multiple cysts and follicular degeneration. Thus, follicles and eggs are rapidly "consumed". Two other situations in the human are also connected with the development of theca luteinization and cystic follicles. First, it is not uncommon in the newborn to see very marked theca luteinization in an immature cystic and degenerating follicle. A second abnormal situation is that seen in the polycystic ovary syndrome. It is to be noted that amenorrhea or anovulatory flows are characteristic of this clinical condition. The many small cystic follicles show characteristically the marked thickening of the theca interna. It is interesting that although spot checks of assays for LH in these so-called Stein–Leventhal cases have not always shown an elevation of LH, yet in McArthur's careful daily studies (3), a recurrent ebb and sway, up and down production with peaks every few days were documented throughout a month.

We have previously mentioned that the hypertrophied theca interna looks like endocrine tissue that is generally associated with steroid production. Ten years ago, we suggested (8) that this might be principally estrogens to support the level of these hormones in the circulation at the time of the cycle most important for many aspects of reproductive physiology. At the same time, there is considerable evidence that progesterone may be produced even before ovulation and the formation of the corpus luteum. In 1958 it was shown that human CG caused depletion of the ascorbic acid content of the rat ovary, and Parlow has demonstrated (9) the same effect from purified LH in the gonadotropin-primed, hypophysectomized rat. Using the histochemical staining techniques developed by Deane and others at Harvard, we have been interested to localize the concentrations of ascorbic acid in these ovaries. It is found that this substance is confined almost entirely to the corpora lutea where it is seen as a diffusely scattered fine, granular deposit. After a dose of LH to these animals, the ovary shows grossly a depletion of from 35 to 50%, and the ascorbic acid distribution changes to that of rather massive agglomerates of the granules. This effect is not well understood. Ascorbic acid is found also in interstitial cells of unprimed ovaries, but never

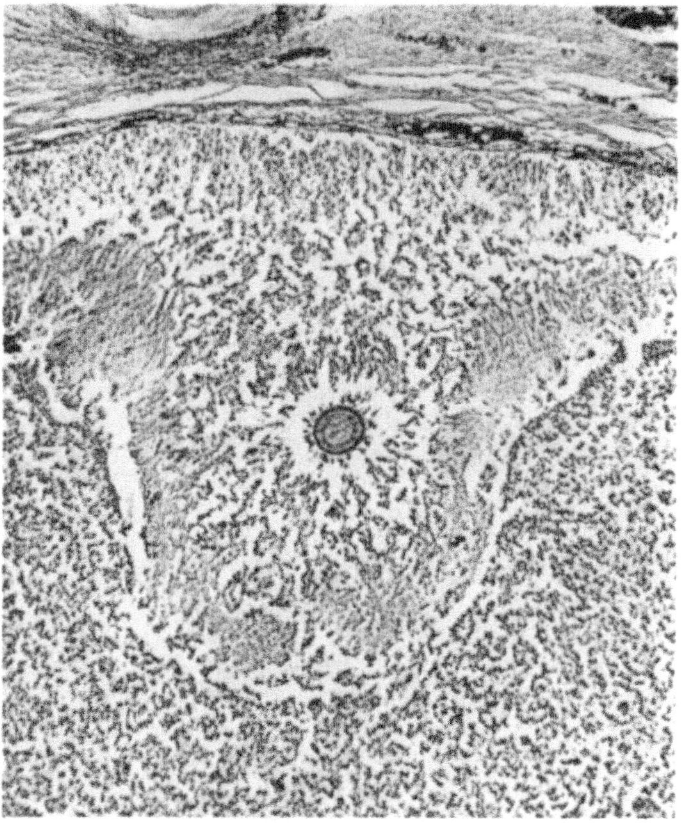

FIG. 1. Egg and cumulus of maturing follicle in the ovary of *Maccacus rhesus* on day 13. Under higher power the egg shows the first maturation spindle. The granulosa is beginning to show a loosening up due to the appearance of edema fluid. The theca interna is thin and delicate. The diameter of this normal follicle was seven thousand micra.

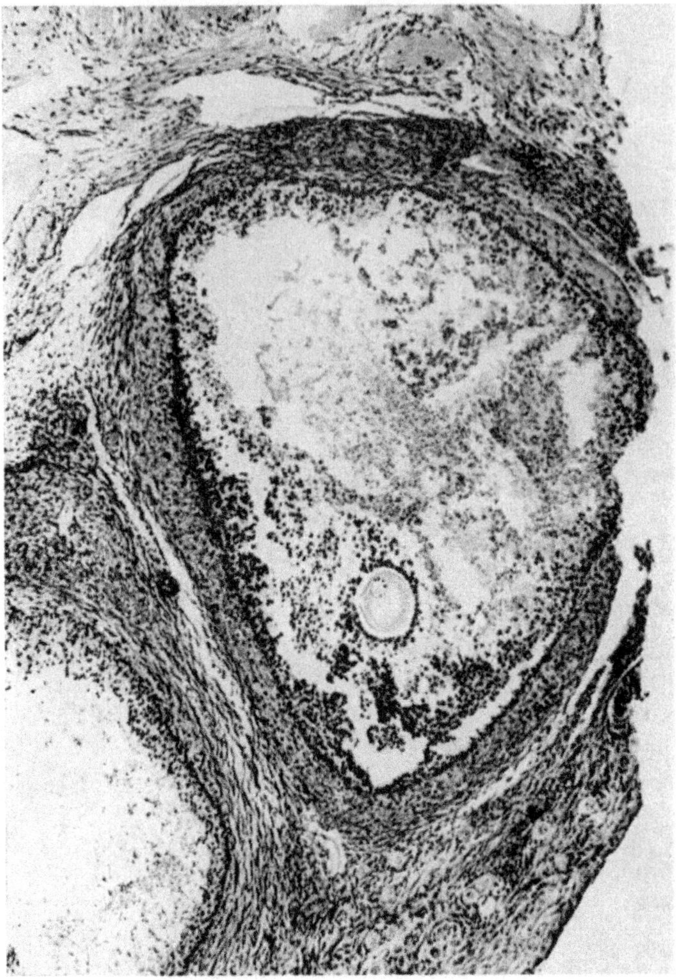

FIG. 2. Two more follicles in the ovary of the same monkey shown in FIG. 1. These measure approximately one thousand micra in diameter. Although the egg is relatively intact, the dissolution of the granulosa is apparent. The theca interna in both these second rank follicles is markedly thickened.

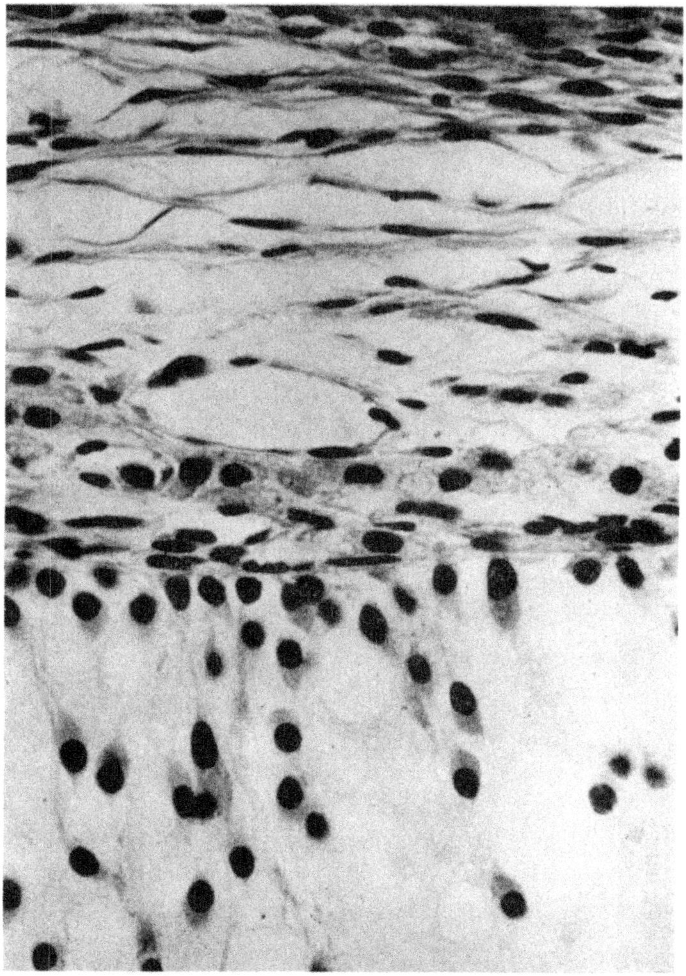

FIG. 3. High power of the thin and delicate theca interna layer of a mature follicle at ovulation time in *Maccacus rhesus*.

in healthy granulosa tissue. It is only seen in the granulosa of follicles that are starting to degenerate. It is tempting to believe that this substance might be mobilized as a precursor to progesterone production by thecaluteal or corporaluteal tissue. Let us now trace the sequence of events that appear to be validated by the evidence reviewed above. Throughout the first ten days or so of the proliferative phase of the menstrual cycle in the primate, many small follicles are developing and contributing in a minor degree to the slowly increasing level of circulating estrogen before they are lost in the process of atresia. By the eleventh or twelfth day of the cycle, perhaps a dozen or so follicles achieve a major degree of development, but only one of these generally proceeds with a tremendous spurt of growth towards maturation on day 14. A rapid increase in circulating level of estrogens is noted at this time, and coincident with this or shortly after it, there is found a first peak of gonadotropins producing LH effect. In this upsurge of follicular growth, only the major follicle survives and achieves maturation while all others of second rank are lost within twenty-four hours of ovulation by successive stages in the atretic process. One of the most striking features of this is the proliferation of theca interna which appears to coincide with the elevation in LH excretion and it subsides as this LH peak flattens out by forty-eight hours after ovulation presumably due to the inhibiting action of progesterone from the developing corpus luteum. The steps that lead the mature follicle to ovulate, a separation of cumulus and granulosa cells by intracellular edema, extrusion of the first polar body and development of the second maturation spindle, the migration of the follicle towards the cortex and actual extrusion of the egg through the stoma, all have been explained as functions of the peak of LH at mid-cycle. Possibly, these are steps that attend the fully developed follicle which may be relatively autonomous and independent of this gonadotropin by this time. Perhaps a more important effect of this peak of LH is that of instituting the process of atresia in the second rank follicles.

SUMMARY

The interplay between pituitary gonadotropins and the ovary of the primate at time of ovulation not only may insure that one follicle achieves maturation, but also may precipitate dissolution of the next largest follicles in both ovaries at that time. It is suggested that this is the mechanism through which ovulation is generally limited to one or two follicles each month. It has been emphasized that this atresia of contending follicles occurs prior to ovulation, and thus cannot be associated with the function of the post-ovulatory corpus luteum. The institution of atresia might well be due to the action of LH on these "second rank" follicles that are immature and unable to withstand such stimulation. It is at the time of the mid-cycle peak of LH effect that these show dissolution of granulosa and hypertrophy of theca interna. A striking example of this is sometimes seen in the neonatal ovary where theca luteinization of immature follicles occurs presumably in response to the LH effect of circulating maternal gonadotropins. Another example of theca proliferation of immature follicles associated with fluctuating LH peaks is also found in the polycystic ovary syndrome. The theca activity in these follicles that are destroyed lasts only a few days in the monkey, probably also in the human. It is highly probable as well that this tissue produces steroids during the transient phase of its existence. Since estrogens are of prime importance at this critical time in the cycle to stimulate optimal cervical secretions, tubal peristalsis and so on, it is a likely guess that this theca thickening helps maintain the level of circulating estrogens. The transient proliferation of theca in early atretic follicles may also be the source of progesterone production before ovulation occurs. Preliminary studies of concentrations of ascorbic acid, typically seen in fully formed corpora in rat and human, are noted in the rat in the theca and granulosa of unruptured follicles only when the latter show signs of early dissolution. It is possible that ascorbic acid appears as a precursor in progesterone production. The depletion of ascorbic acid caused by giving doses of LH in the presence of fully formed corpora is not clearly understood. However, this is a wholly unphysiologic experiment, since in the presence of functioning corpora lutea normally the pituitary does not excrete LH.

It may be theoretically possible to utilize the above reasoning to create a chronic state of anovulation such as exists in the Stein–Leventhal ovaries, by the correct timing and dosage of substances with LH effect. These would have to be given repeatedly to overstimulate each wave of developing follicles while they are still immature, before any one has reached that stage of maturity and developmental autonomy beyond which the further steps in maturation will inevitably lead to ovulation. Anovulatory cycles thus produced need not be considered necessarily damaging to the ovaries. The use of LH substances in this regard would only be an extension of a normal physiologic process causing the waste of one more follicle each month—a minor loss in relation to the tens of thousands degenerating through a lifetime. Whether or not if this scheme is successful it would eventually produce a persistent and relatively irreversible situation as is found in the polycystic ovary, is a matter of pure speculation.

REFERENCES

1. CORNER, G. W., *The Hormones in Human Reproduction*, Princeton University Press, 1946.
2. STURGIS, S. H., *Contributions to Embryology* **33**, 67, 1949.
3. MCARTHUR, J., F. INGERSOLL and J. WORCESTER, *J. Clin. Endocrinol.* **18**, 1202, 1958.
4. TAYMOR, M. L., *Fertil. & Steril.* **10**, 212, 1959.
5. STURGIS, S. H. and W. ACHILLES, *Endocrinology* **49**, 720, 1951.
6. VELARDO, J. T., *Science* **131**, 357, 1960.
7. PARKES, A. S., in Conference on *Mechanism of Ovulation* sponsored by the Planned Parenthood Federation of America, August 1959.
8. STURGIS, S. H., *J. Fertil. & Steril.* **1**, 40, 1950.
9. PARLOW, A., *Fed. Proc.* **7**, 402, 1958.

DISCUSSIONS

DR. McARTHUR: Dr. Sturgis has put histochemical techniques to good use in localizing the ascorbic acid present in the corpora lutea and interstitium of human ovaries, and has alluded to the fact that ascorbic acid may be implicated in steroid secretion. It is known that PMS, HCG and LH are all capable of effecting ovarian ascorbic acid depletion. However, it has proved difficult to establish a firm connection between this depletion and the secretion of any particular steroid or class of steroids.

Dr. Albert Parlow, who is working in our laboratory, has made an interesting new observation which appears to shed light upon this problem. Because of the similarity between the response of the rat ovary to LH and HCG, Dr. Parlow undertook to confirm and extend an important study by Dr. Greep. It will be recalled that in 1938 Greep (*Endocrinology* **23**, 154, 1938) found that adult female rats which were treated with pituitary extract and then hypophysectomized would respond to injections of chorionic gonadotropin by secreting estrogen, even after a post-hypophysectomy interval of as long as 15 days. The injection of LH, on the other hand, in the form available at that time, appeared to be without effect.

TABLE 1. THE INDUCTION OF ESTROGEN SECRETION BY MEANS OF HCG TREATMENT IN HYPOPHYSECTOMIZED PSEUDOPREGNANT RATS

Interval after hypophysectomy (months)	No. of rats	No. of rats showing vaginal cornification after HCG treatment	Length of period during which vaginal cornification could be maintained (days)
0.0	15	15	39
3.25	12	12	19
6.50	13	10	10
9.50	9	4	6

Dr. Parlow's first step was to treat rats with PMS and HCG in order to induce the formation of heavily luteinized ovaries and the state of pseudopregnancy. A single subcutaneous injection of PMS (50 I.U.) was given to 25–26-day-old female rats, and was followed, 56–65 hr later, with a single s.c. injection of HCG (25 I.U.). Five days after the HCG injection the animals were hypophysectomized and treated with 2.5 I.U. of HCG twice daily after the lapse of various time intervals, with results which are shown in Table 1. The secretion of estrogen was readily demonstrable by vaginal cornification. The appearance of such an ovary is shown in Fig. 1. It will be noted that there are no large antrum-containing follicles in the ovary, and that only primordial follicles, corpora lutea and interstitial tissue are identifiable. That the principal site of action of HCG is the corpus luteum is shown by the fact that 25–26-day-old rats which had not been pre-treated with PMS and HCG, and therefore possessed no luteal tissue, failed to respond to HCG 7 days after hypophysectomy.

Rats made pseudopregnant and subsequently hypophysectomized in the same manner secrete estrogen in response to stimulation with LH also. One week after hypophysectomy LH (NIH-LH-S1), 0.16 μg twice daily for 3 days, effected vaginal cornification 96 hr after the first injection; one month after hypophysectomy, LH 0.32 μg twice daily for 3 days was effective in 50% of the animals tested (Table 2). FSH, ACTH, GH and LTH were without effect.

Thus, from Dr. Astwood's experiments (*Endocrinology* **28**, 309, 1941) it would appear that the secretion of progesterone by the corpus luteum of the rat may be under the control of LTH, and from Dr. Parlow's study that the secretion of estrogen may be under the control of LH. This demonstration of a luteotropic action of LH in the rat tends to place the corpus luteum in physiologic alignment with the adrenal cortex and its response to ACTH.

TABLE 2. THE EFFECT OF LH AND FSH ADMINISTERED 80 DAYS AFTER HYPOPHYSECTOMY UPON THE SECRETION OF ESTROGEN BY CORPORA LUTEA PERSISTING IN THE OVARIES OF RATS WHICH HAD BEEN PRE-TREATED WITH PMS AND HCG.

Gonadotropin	Dose	No. of rats	No. of rats in which vaginal cornification was induced
NIH-LH-S1	3 μg	5	4
	2 μg	5	2
NIH-FSH-S1	400 μg	5	0

DR. ROY O. GREEP: I am very much interested in this observation. I well remember the experiments with HCG and the available luteinizing hormone in hypophysectomized adult female rats. I was greatly impressed with the fact that the LH then available would knock out the corpora lutea in 48–72 hr. Admittedly the LH was not pure and did produce some follicle stimulation. Later, at the Squibb laboratories we obtained a luteinizing preparation that was more highly purified. I tried the same experiment again and it did not work. I did not smear the animals and could very well have missed a response in terms of estrogen secretion as Dr. Parlow has now described.

Dr. Sturgis raised the point that it isn't the estrogens that cause the secretion of LH, but the metabolic product of estrogen. I would like to point out that under these circumstances described, you have essentially a "castrate" type of pituitary. It will contain a lot more luteinizing hormone, and there is evidence that it also secretes more. This would account for the spleen-implanted ovaries filled with corpora lutea. I don't think that one needs invoke metabolic products to account for ovaries of that appearance, under the circumstances.

CHAIRMAN ASTWOOD: We might limit our discussion, now, to five or ten minutes, and then go on with Dr. Rock's paper, and then take as much time as there is left for further discussion.

DR. CARL GEMZELL: Dr. Sturgis mentioned the polycystic ovary syndrome, and he also mentioned the excellent studies that Dr. McArthur has done with these patients.

We have treated a couple of cases with FSH, and in all these cases we obtained ovulation much earlier than the previous three or four days, which I think confirms the thought of Dr. McArthur that if there is too much delay it may induce FSH.

Regarding the question of progesterone production in these follicles that Dr. Sturgis brought up, we have no cases where the progesterone is produced in the follicles before ovulation or before the factor is added.

DR. ERNEST KNOBIL: I have a question to ask Dr. McArthur. What is the current status of the improved method, as far as assaying LH in biological fluids is concerned? Can this now be done successfully?

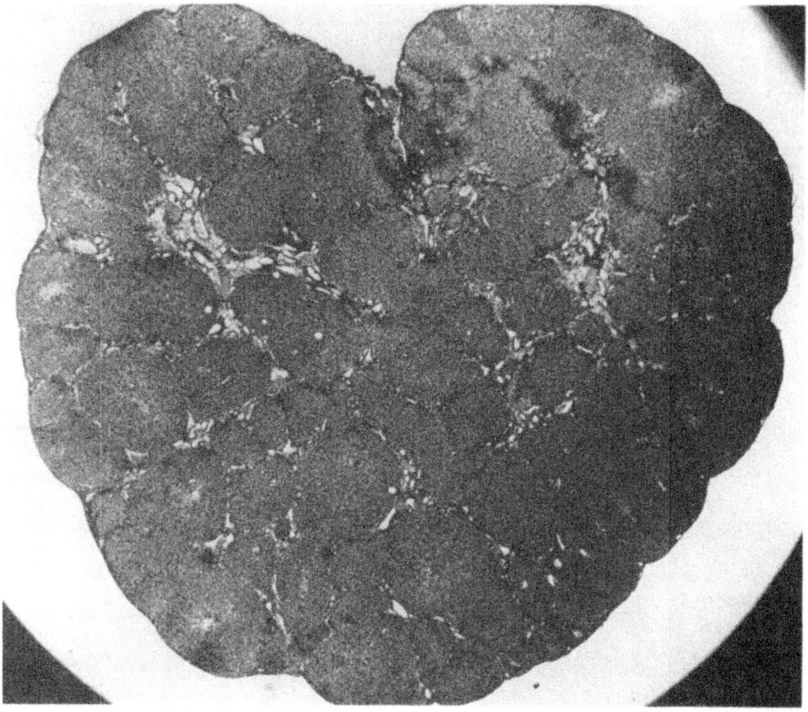

FIG. 1. Appearance of the ovary of an immature female rat which had been rested for 60 days after treatment with PMS and HCG and subsequent hypophysectomy, and which was actively secreting estrogen in response to HCG treatment.

DR. JANET MCARTHUR: Dr. Parlow discussed this recently at the N.I.H. Gonadotropin Workshop. He has found that the ascorbic acid depletion method is very satisfactory for the assay of pituitary LH. However, there appear to be interfering substances, both in plasma and urine, which prevent valid assays of the LH content of these fluids.

DR. ROY HERTZ: I want to thank Dr. Sturgis for his paper. There is, however, one phase of follicular development which I think is being largely overlooked.

You will recall that in that day-old ovary there was represented nothing but the primordial type of follicle, and we have very little knowledge actually of what transforms the primordial follicle into an antrum-containing follicle.

In the new-born rat, just as in the human ovary, the ovary at birth is made up entirely of such follicles in immediate juxtaposition to each other, with a very small, fine stroma between them, and there is no indication of any follicular organization in any part of the ovary at that time. It is not until about the eleventh day, post-natally, that one begins to see the beginning of granulosa cell development and an antrum formation. It is at that point that one gets the first responsiveness to gonadotropin. Up to eleven days, you can give massive doses of gonadotropin to the new-born rat, and get no response, until the follicle has become organized sufficiently to have an antrum of its own.

In the rabbit, this process takes ten weeks post-natally. So for ten weeks, during the post-natal period, we have this pre-pituitary process going on, with follicular differentiation, and the development of initial sensitivity to stimulation.

We became interested in what was involved in this process, and what role the pituitary may play in the process, and therefore grafted day-old ovaries under the kidney capsule of the mother of the young. She had just given birth to these babies. We then hypophysectomized the mother immediately. We found that this entire process of sensitization to gonadotropic hormone is independent of the pituitary. It goes along well, in a completely hypophysectomized female. It is not dependent upon any specific factor from the host; it seems to proceed quite independently of any known pituitary factors.

We do see that during this process there is a substantial mortality in the primordial ova. Their numbers progressively decline. There is something which they are contributing, or which their mortality is contributing, to the process.

This is an area which I feel, from a clinical standpoint, also, is being neglected. For instance, we now have four patients with ovarian hypoplasia, and biopsies of their ovaries show the identical histological picture that you have described for the ovary of the new-born.

It seems that in such individuals, this pre-pituitary process has gone up to the point of gonadotropin sensitization. These patients have ample gonadotropin in the urine, actually high levels, and yet the ovary has not gotten to the point of responsiveness.

DR. GREGORY PINCUS: We have also been conducting some studies with human pituitary FSH. The sample we used was prepared by Dr. Li and is very low in LH. With this we did not get an increase in estrogen production until HCG was also given. I would like to ask Dr. Gemzell whether he observed any estrogen production when he used his very highly purified FSH, which is probably more nearly free of LH.

DR. CARL GEMZELL: We have not done any experiments with the highly purified FSH as yet. The chemist who is woıking on it is more interested in finding out something about its physical–chemical properties; but I hope that when he is through we will be able to test it.

I don't know how much LH there is in Dr. Li's preparation of FSH. It is very likely that the contamination with LH is of great importance.

I haven't had any experience with the preparations of various activities, so I can't answer your question.

INHIBITION OF OVULATION IN THE HUMAN

JOHN ROCK

Free Hospital for Women, Massachusetts

I. AUTOGENOUS INHIBITION OF OVULATION

BEFORE discussing methods of suppressing ovulation in the human, it might be well to review briefly various aspects of autogenous failure of ovulation. We find this process inhibited not only in many different clinical conditions, but also in several physiological states (1, 2).

A. In Physiological States

There is physiological anovulation before puberty, as also after the climacterium. Moreover, oligo-ovulation is a comparatively frequent gynecological diagnosis among adults (1, 3). It denotes habitual failure of ovum release each year, for more than four weeks, or even for a few months, yet without discernible pathology. Of course in such cases we infer dysfunction of the "feed-back" or "push-pull" process, either as a weak "push" from gonadal hormones, or resistance to "push" in the hypothalamic-pituitary partnership. Furthermore, even in normally cyclic women, anovulatory cycles are occasionally interspersed among the usual ovulatory ones (1).

During the normal cycle, we have, of course, the postovulatory relative progestinism, the latter prevailing also in pregnancy with a hyperestrogeno-progestinism; and in lactation, we relate the usual anovulation to a similar prolactinism.

Anovulation may also occur as an accompaniment of a stress reaction disturbing hypothalamic function. The follicular inactivity of anorexia nervosa may be similarly indicted with probable assistance from dietary deficiency (4).

B. In Pathological Conditions

Leaving aside intrinsic ovarian insufficiency (hypoplasia ovarii) as an obvious cause of anovulation, other clinical conditions accompanied by failure of ovulation may be considered under two headings: those involving (1) extrapituitary pathology and (2) intrapituitary pathology.

1. *Extrapituitary pathology.* Extrapituitary pathology may cause sex hormone imbalance toward what one might rather vaguely term androgenicity —as with an arrhenoblastoma, or a hylar-cell tumor, or with hyperadrenalism —and thus hinder ovulation. In like manner, the ovulatory mechanism may

be deranged in what we could call conditions of relative estrogenicity, such as with cystic-stromal hyperplasia, as well as with granulosal cell tumor, or with dysthyroidism.

Yet another manifestation of extrapituitary pathology that inhibits ovulation is what clinicians might call progestinicity, such as is attributed to theca-lutein or corpus-lutein cysts, as if ever they do produce, for any length of time, a progestin—which I rather doubt. We also find anovulation with the chorionic gonadotropism incident to chorionepithelioma.

2. *Intrapituitary pathology.* Among diseases involving intrapituitary pathology, anovulation is associated with *Simmonds' disease* (hypophyseal cachexia), as well as with *Sheehan's disease* (postpartum pituitary necrosis), with *Cushing's disease* (basophilism), *Addison's disease* (hypobasophilism), and the *Chiari-Frommel syndrome* (pituitary adenomatosis), as also with inanition, doubtless made more harmful to the pituitary by coincident avitaminosis and contributory hypothalamic deprivation. (It is difficult to define the relative roles of nutritional deficiency and of stress reaction in the neurosis that manifests itself in *anorexia nervosa.*)

II. EXOGENOUS INHIBITION OF OVULATION

A. Reasons for Suppressing Ovulation

We might ask: "Why suppress ovulation?" It could be a simple exercise in biological research. We do not quite do that in humans, if we can help it. On the other hand, ovulation has been prevented therapeutically in order to relieve dysmenorrhea (5). Essential dysmenorrhea occurs only from what is improperly called a "secretory" and, more properly, a "progestational" endometrium. Furthermore, one might suppress ovulation to avoid Mittelschmerz, or even to prevent conception.

B. Means of Inhibiting Ovulation

With the latter aim in view, i.e. to control fertility, particularly in certain overpopulated areas, several methods of suppressing ovulation have been, and are still being, investigated (6–9). The requisites for ovulation have been reviewed by the previous speakers: the organs, the tissue systems, the hormones, and the various unctions. Thus one might find means of suppressing ovulation by disaffecting one or another of these numerous required cellular composites.

One can destroy the primordial follicles, as by radiation; or one can castrate. Specific thalamic function may be disturbed by scaring a woman "to death". Then she would not ovulate by virtue of stress reaction resulting in hormonal disturbance of thalamic neurones and their dependent pituitary cells. Normal cyclic function in these mid-brain nuclei may also be upset by direct medicinal modification of sex hormone concentrations. This will be discussed later.

Furthermore, in recent years there have been two lines of investigation with plant extracts, leading to reports of possible inactivation of gonadotropins by: (1) a postulated desensitization of the ovary to gonadotropins by lithospermum (9, 10); and (2) interaction of quinones from the Indian garden pea with gonadotropin so as to nullify the latter (9, 11).

III. INHIBITION OF OVULATION BY THE 19-NOR STEROIDS

Since none of the methods mentioned above seemed to offer a satisfactory solution to the problem of fertility control, and since, in harmony with the long-recognized ovulation-inhibiting action of progesterone recently reaffirmed (12–14)*, certain artificial progestins, the so-called 19-nor steroids, had also been found by Pincus and his associates (14, 17, 18) to inhibit ovulation in animals, Dr. García and I were fortunate to obtain these steroidal substances from Dr. Pincus. Oral administration in women on cycle-days 5 through 25 showed that these steroids had the same ovulation-suppressant effect as in laboratory animals (14, 19–23). Some of them, however, were more potent than others. One of them in particular, 17α-ethinyl-5(10)-estraeneolone, possessed such a high degree of ovulation-inhibitory, as well as other qualities, that it was chosen for use in large-scale field studies organized by Dr. Pincus, first in Puerto Rico and later in Haiti (8, 24–33).

It was unfortunate, perhaps, that we were supplied with the best preparations first. Our enthusiasm for some of the later, less effective ones was insufficient to encourage us to utilize our patients in the way animal experimenters so easily do their subjects. Possibly, therefore, some of the conclusions suggested by our negative results with the newer preparations derive only from a sample that is deficient in the number of cases as well as in variety of dosage. Presently, I shall discuss our experiences with several of these steroids of various degrees of efficacy.

First, I wish to state that Dr. Pincus provided not only the material and the motivation for these projects, but he also organized them. For the tables to be shown in connection with the field studies, Dr. Pincus compiled the data derived from the clinical observations which Dr. García and I, together with several physicians in the island areas, were able to supply.

A. Nature of the Ovulation-Inhibiting Steroidal Substances

Certain of these synthetic steroids, the so-called 19-nor steroids, are shown in Fig. 1 in relationship to the naturally occurring hormones, progesterone and testosterone.† The nortestosterones, norethindrone (*Norlutin*—Parke-Davis) and norethandrolone (*Nilevar*—Searle) were found to be very effective,

* The ovulation-inhibiting function of the corpus luteum had been recognized even long before the isolation of progesterone (6, 15, 16).

† Although ovulation is also inhibited by these naturally occurring hormones, as well as by estrogens in both natural and synthetic form, their use for this purpose is undesirable.

as was also norethynodrel, which by its molecular pattern is seen to be not a testosterone, but is more closely related to the classical estrogens. Details of the differences in molecular configuration among these three compounds, as well as the biological properties correlated with these differences, have been reviewed previously (34–36).

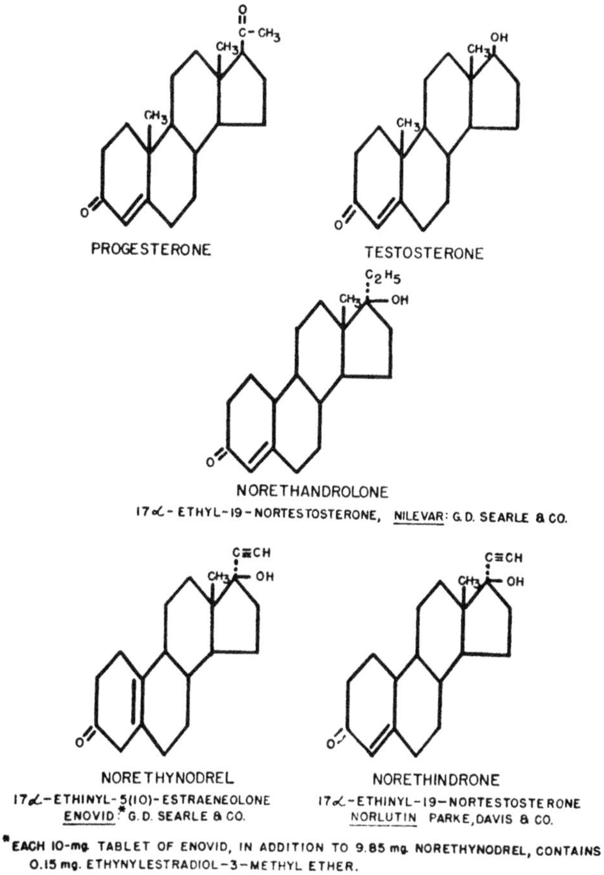

FIG. 1. Three commercially available synthetic 19-nor steroids are shown in relationship to the naturally occurring hormones, progesterone and testosterone. (After CROSSON, J. W., New Synthetic Steroid Progestins. *Fertil. & Steril.* **10**, 361–373, 1959.)

Norethynodrel (17α-ethinyl-5(10)-estraeneolone) is prepared and manufactured in combination with a small amount of 3-methyl-ether of ethynyl-estradiol. This estrogen component was found to be present in some of the original theoretically pure preparations of the 19-nor steroid. Since later products lacking the estrogen were not as effective, the 3-methyl-ether of ethynylestradiol is now purposely added to the norethynodrel. The 10-mg tablet marketed by G. D. Searle & Co., under the name of *Enovid*, contains 9.85 mg of norethynodrel and 0.15 mg of the 3-methyl-ether of ethynylestradiol.

Owing to its strong progestational effect, Enovid has proved of extreme value to the clinician in the treatment of certain gynecological disorders (35, 37). Furthermore, since Enovid is the 19-nor steroid most extensively utilized in the field studies relating to fertility control in Puerto Rico and Haiti (v.s.), most of my subsequent remarks will deal with this particular synthetic gestagen.

B. Nature of the Ovulation-Inhibiting Action of Enovid

It seemed of interest to determine which of the two components of Enovid, i.e. the norethynodrel or the 3-methyl-ether of ethynylestradiol, constitutes the active ovulation-depressing agent.

TABLE 1. EFFECTS OF THE 3-METHYL-ETHER OF ETHYNYLESTRADIOL ON NORMALLY CYCLIC WOMEN*

Patient	Dose (mg)	Rx cycle No.	Ovulation Index†		Pregnanediol (mg per day)	Cycle length (days)	Days of flow	Re-actions
			Body temperature	Endometrial biopsy				
F.M.	0.250	1	—	n.d.	0.1 = —	33	8	+
		2	—	n.d.	0.1 = —	35	7	+
		3	—	n.d.	0.2 = —	35	8	—
L.M.	0.125	1	—	—	0.4 = —	30	?	—
		2	10	12?	0.0 = —	23	8	—
		3	—	—	0.1 = —	26	8	—
R.P.	0.125	1	—	—	0.2 = —	36	5	—
		2	—	—	0.2 = —	37	6	—
		3	—	—	0.5 = ±	24	6	—
E.S.	0.125	1	—	—	0.2 = —	35	7	—
		2	8?	n.d.	0.6 = ±	23	6	+
		3	—	n.d.	0.1 = —	37	4	+
J.B.	0.050	2	17	—	0.1 = —	32	6	—
		3	39	—	0.1 = —	55	5	+

* Abbreviations: n.d. = not done; + = positive; — = negative.
† Figures = cycle-days when ovulation was indicated.

While some have attributed this role of Enovid to its estradiol component, we, on the other hand, are skeptical of this. For, as shown in Table 1, even though rather low pregnanediol values were found in patients with the use of the 3-methyl-ether of ethynylestradiol alone, it was not as regular and dependable in its ovulation-inhibiting action as is norethynodrel. Moreover, the clinical value of the 3-methyl-ether of ethynylestradiol was diminished, inasmuch as the flow following its withdrawal was uncertain both in time and in quality.

In an effort to discover the mechanism whereby Enovid exerts its ovulatory-inhibiting action, assays of urinary FSH were carried out on a few patients in Worcester under Dr. Pincus' (25) direction before, during, and after medication (Table 2).

TABLE 2. EFFECTS OF ENOVID ON URINARY FOLLICLE STIMULATING HORMONE

Subject	Age	Output (mouse units/24 hr)		
		Premedication	Medication	Postmedication
No. 1	56	144	60 [1]	
No. 2	54	24	7.2 [2] 0 [3]	79.2 [4]
No. 3	42 [5]	32	0	16 [6]
No. 4	60 [7]	39	69 [8]	48 [9]

(1) 20 mg/day for 4 days.
(2) 20 mg/day—collection on 6th day.
(3) 20 mg/day—collection on 10th day.
(4) Six weeks after medication.
(5) Premenopausal—collections at midcycle—received 20 mg/day.
(6) Next midcycle.
(7) 10 mg/day for 4 days.
(8) Collected on the 4th day of medication.
(9) Collected 10 days after last medication.

One patient, aged 56 (No. 1), who, before treatment, had excreted 144 mouse units of FSH per 24 hr, diminished her output to 60 mouse units following medication with 20 mg per day of Enovid for 4 days. In another woman, 54 years of age (No. 2), the FSH value decreased from 24 to 7.2 mouse units per 24 hr after she had taken 20 mg per day for 6 days; moreover, the urine collected on the 10th day of treatment showed no detectable FSH. Six weeks after cessation of medication, however, her FSH urinary content had risen to 79.2 mouse units per 24 hr. On the other hand, in a third menopausal patient, aged 60 (No. 4), treated with only 10 mg a day for 4 days, urinary assay of FSH on the 4th day of medication showed an elevation as compared to the pretreatment value. Moreover, in this case, the postmedication value, 10 days after cessation of therapy, was less than during treatment. The lower dose of Enovid administered to patient No. 4, or, possibly, a difference in threshold response, may account for the different result.

In a premenopausal woman, aged 42 (No. 3), who also received 20 mg per day of Enovid, collections were made at midcycle. Whereas the midcycle premedication value was 32 mouse units per 24 hr, and the postmedication sample, collected at midcycle 10 days after cessation of therapy, showed 48 mouse units per 24 hr, FSH was not detectable in the 24-hr urine specimen collected at the midpoint of the medicated cycle.

Because of the highly probable "feedback" of progesterone-suppression of LH, it seems very likely that the strongly progestational Enovid exerts the same influence. The gonadotropin-depressant action of norethynodrel, both in animals and in women, has been demonstrated by several other investigators (38, 39).

C. *Indices of Ovulation-Suppression with Enovid and Norlutin*

The effect of Enovid, as of Norlutin (norethindrone), on pregnanediol excretion is at least very suggestive of inhibition of ovulation. As shown in Table 3, the average premedication pregnanediol excretion in 40 ovulatory

TABLE 3. EFFECTS OF 17α-ETHINYL-19-NORTESTOSTERONE (I) AND 17α-ETHINYL-5(10)-ESTRAENEOLONE (II) UPON CYCLE LENGTHS, INDICES OF OVULATION, AND STEROID OUTPUT IN NORMALLY OVULATING WOMEN

Compound	No. of cycles	Mean cycle length (days)	Basal temperature (%−)	Endometrial biopsy (%−)	Vaginal smear (%−)	Pregnanediol (mg per day)	17-Ketosteroids (mg per day)
Control	40	27.2±0.51	6	0	0	3.4 ±0.27	5.2±0.47
I*	62	28.5±0.68	92	76	81	0.34±0.066	4.8±0.40
II**	34	26.7±0.48	82	93	72	0.30±0.074	4.5±0.47

* 10–40 mg/day. ** 10–20 mg/day.

cycles was 3.4 mg per day. With each of the two administered steroids, the average pregnanediol output was found to be only about 10% of this pretreatment value (20).

Absence of secreted progesterone is also reflected in the atypy of response in the other common indices of postovulatory corpus-luteum activity. Since in each of these tests the normal critical effect is due to progesterone, and the two artificial steroids are called "progestins" because of the fact that their action resembles that of progesterone, it is not surprising that inferences from temperature graphs, endometrial biopsies, and vaginal smears, although somewhat less exact, are similar to those from biochemical assay of an excreted product of progesterone itself (22).

In order to obtain more direct evidence of the effect of these steroids on ovulation, a careful study was made of the ovaries of women who had taken Norlutin (norethindrone) for one to 3 cycles before required laparotomy (20, 22). Whether operation took place late in the medicated cycle or early in the next untreated cycle, there was no evidence of corpus-luteum formation. More recently, these observations have been repeated with Enovid both by our own group (40) and by the Japanese investigator, Matsumoto (41). In neither of the two series was there any morphologic sign of recent ovulation.

D. Indices of Ovulation-Suppression with Other 19-Nor Steroids

Methylpregnone,* another 19-nor steroid more recently tested by us, did not give consistent results as far as ovulation was concerned (33). This is indicated in the normal pregnanediol excretion, as well as in the qualities of the endometrial specimens taken on or about cycle-day 21 (Table 4). The increase in basal body temperature might have been due to the thermogenic effect of the administered norsteroid.

TABLE 4. EFFECTS OF 17α-HYDROXY-6α-METHYLPROGESTERONE-17-ACETATE ALONE ON NORMALLY CYCLIC WOMEN†

Patient	Dose (mg per day)	Rx Cycle No.	Ovulation index‡		Pregnanediol (mg per day)	Cycle length (days)	Days of flow	Reactions
			Basal tempera-ture	Endo-metrial biopsy				
C. R.	1: days 5–21 2: days 22–25	1	25	—	0.3= −	39	7	Sp.
J. S.	1	1	19	10	2.6= +	29	6	—
		2	12	13	3.2= +	25	6	—
	4	3	15	15	1.5= +	27	6	—
E. D.	4: days 5–17	1	—	n.d.	n.d.	16	n.r.	B.T.
M. C.	6	1	—	9	1.2= +	22	4	B.T.
		2	—	8	0.8= +	21	4	B.T.
		3	—	14	1.2= +	26	5	—
G. S.	10	1	+	n.d.	0.2= −	27	n.r.	—
		2	+ ?	n.d.	2.4= +	28	3	—
		3	n.d.	n.d.	4.8= +	24	n.r.	—

† Abbreviations: n.d. = not done; Sp. = spotting during medication; B.T. = breakthrough bleeding; + = positive; — = negative; n.r. = no record.
‡ Figures = cycle-days when ovulation was indicated.

As shown in Table 5, still another 19-nor steroid, 17α-(1-methallyl)-19-nortestosterone, supplied to us by G. D. Searle & Co. as SC–8117, likewise was not too effective. It, also, was associated with an increase in basal body temperature. While this steroid does possess certain progestational qualities, it did not seem, in the dosage used, to suppress ovulation, except in rare instances.

IV. FERTILITY CONTROL WITH ENOVID

Table 6 shows the extent of the work organized by Dr. Pincus (30) up to November, 1958. The field work is at present supervised by Dr. Manuel Paniagua and Dr. Adaline Pendleton in Puerto Rico and by Drs. Rene Nicolas,

* 17α-hydroxy-6α-methylprogesterone-17-acetate (SC-9686—Searle and R-2076—Root Chemicals), the same as Provera (Upjohn).

TABLE 5. EFFECTS OF 17α-(1-METHALLYL)-19-NORTESTOSTERONE ALONE AND IN COMBINATION WITH ESTROGEN (ETHYNYLESTRADIOL-3-METHYL ETHER*) IN NORMALLY CYCLIC WOMEN†

Patient	Dose (mg)	Estrogen (mg)	Rx cycle No.	Ovulation index‡		Pregnanediol (mg per day)	Cycle length (days)	Days of flow	Reactions
				Body temperature	Endometrial biopsy				
T. H.	5	0	1	15	19	0.6 = ±	31	5	−
			2	17?	+	0.2 = −	32	5	−
			3	18?	+	0.7 = +	33	5	−
J. B.	5	0	1	12	n.d.	4.8 = +	24	5	+
			2	13?	17	1.8 = +	24	5	−
			3	—	15	3.1 = +	25	5	−
C. K.	5	0	1	13	12	1.2 = +	24	4	−
			2	14	13	0.3 = −	27	4	−
			3	7	13	1.6 = +	22	4	B.T.
A. K.	5	0	1	12	13	7.6 = +	25	6	+
			2	14	13	0.3 = −	27	7	−
			3	14	15	2.9 = +	26	6	−
A. N.	5	0	1	15	+	0.3 = −	29	3	−
			2	15	11	1.1 = +	27	4	−
			3	14	12	0.8 = +	27	4	−
M. J.	5	0	1	?	17	1.0 = +	27	6	−
			2	—	—	0.2 = −	29	4	−
			3	—	13	1.1 = +	27	4	−
S. Y.	10	0	1	13	n.d.	0.4 = −	28	7	−
			2	12	n.d.	3.3 = +	29	5	+
			3	11	n.d.	1.0 = +	25	7	+
A. P.	2	EE3ME 0.05	1	n.d.	+	0.4 = −	31	5	+
			2	—	—	0.6 = ±	18	—	B.T.
			3	—	—	0.2 = −	—	—	−
J. B.	5	EE3ME 0.05	1	21?	—	0.1 = −	35	5	−

* Designated in the table as EE3ME.
† Abbreviations: n.d. = not done; + = positive; − = negative; B.T. = breakthrough bleeding.
‡ Figures = cycle-days when ovulation was indicated.

TABLE 6. FERTILITY CONTROL WITH ENOVID: DESCRIPTION OF PROJECTS

Project	Date begun	Total No. of subjects to November 1958	No. of active cases	Total No. of cycles of experience	No. of woman-years
San Jaun	April 1956	438	211	4988	382
Humacao-R	April 1957	117	105	1410	115
Humacao-P	June 1957	126	95	658	51
Haiti	Dec. 1957	149	108	1077	87
		830	519	8133	635

Raymond Borno, and Vergniaud Pean in Haiti. Dr. Celso-Ramón García, who largely planned the clinical aspects of these projects, makes periodic visits to Puerto Rico and Haiti for consultation, collection of biopsy material, and examination of patients.

The regimen adopted in the island projects entails cyclic medication with 10 mg per day of Enovid from cycle-days 5 through 24, inclusive, i.e. a total of 20 pills a cycle, or one less pill than in the schedule first followed in the local cases (v.s.).

As of November, 1958, 830 subjects had participated in the experiment (Table 6). Of this number, there were 519 who were still using the medication. In all, there were 8133 cycles of experience, the sum total of which added up

TABLE 7. FERTILITY CONTROL WITH ENOVID: MEAN AGE OF SUBJECTS AND PREGNANCY RATES BEFORE AND DURING MEDICATION IN THE FOUR PROJECTS

Project	Mean age (years)	Pregnancy rate per 100 woman-years			Per cent reduction	
		Before medication		On medication		
		Marriage years	Exposure years		In pregnancies	In fertility
San Juan	27.2	60.9	244	3.2	95	98.7
Humacao-R	26.9	68.0	272	0.9?	99	99.7
Humacao-P	28.4	55.8	222	2.0	96	99.1
Haiti	30.7	60.2	241	3.4	95	98.6
All	28.0	61.2	246	2.7	96	98.9

to 635 woman-years. In Table 7 are seen the pregnancy rates before and during medication in the four projects. Whereas the mean pregnancy rate before treatment had been 61.2 per 100 woman-years, it decreased during medication to 2.7, representing "a 96 per cent reduction in the pre-medication rate, and in terms of years of exposure to the chances of conception (i.e., eliminating pregnancy times in pre-medication years) a 98.9 per cent reduction in fertility" (30). It should be noted that the frequency of coitus remained essentially the same during medication as it had been prior to treatment (Table 8).

With the most recent survey, as of November, 1959, the number of cycles had increased to more than 12,000; and the total number of women treated to about 1200. We think we have a fairly dependable picture of what this material will do. The pregnancy rates, as of November, 1959, are shown in Table 9.

Here we see more than 10,000 cycles during which no tablets were missed. Within this group, there is one questionable case of a pregnancy in a social worker who at first said that she took all the tablets but later, when the figures were brought to her attention, admitted that she may have forgotten some.

When patients missed tablets, follicles were sometimes ready to rupture, and not much of a release was required to enable some of them to do so.

TABLE 8. FERTILITY CONTROL WITH ENOVID: MEAN FREQUENCY OF COITUS REPORTED PER MONTH IN PREMEDICATION AND MEDICATION CYCLES

Cycle No.	Humacao-R	Humacao-P	Haiti
Premed.	6.2	8.7	8.6
1–2	6.5	9.0	8.1
3–4	6.5	9.4	9.5
5–8	6.7	9.9	10.1
9–12	6.5	8.9	10.7
13–16	6.4	—	—
17–20	6.2	—	—
% increasing	50	50	52
% decreasing	42	34	41
% no change	8	16	6

TABLE 9. FERTILITY CONTROL WITH ENOVID: PREGNANCY RATES ACCORDING TO NUMBER OF PILLS MISSED VS. POSTMEDICATION PREGNANCY RATE
(All Projects Combined: Data Tabulated as of November, 1959)

Pills missed	No. of cycles	Pregnancies	
		Number	Rate*
0	10,705	1 ?	0.12
1–5	1,116	4	4.6
6–19	422	14	42.9
	12,243	19	2.8
Postmedication rate*		186	

* Pregnancy rate per 100 woman-years.

There were some 1500 cycles in which medication was intermittent. In the group in which tablets were omitted on not more than 5 days, 4 pregnancies occurred. There were 14 pregnancies when medication was missed on more than 5 days.

V. OTHER EFFECTS OF ENOVID

A. Effects on the Menstrual Cycle

1. *Cycle length.* One almost indispensable clinical quality in an ovulation-suppressant is its capability to be used effectively without disrupting the

pattern of normal cyclic menstruation. Women throughout the world seem to value what they otherwise call "the curse". In Table 10 are shown the mean lengths of cycles recorded in the different areas of the field study where the most numerous observations were made (30).

TABLE 10. FERTILITY CONTROL WITH ENOVID: MEAN MENSTRUAL CYCLE LENGTHS (DAYS) IN RELATION TO THE NUMBER OF TABLETS MISSED

Project	Mean cycle length (days) according to number of tablets missed		
	0	1–5	6–19
San Juan	28.0±0.05	26.3±0.27	30.2±0.53
Humacao-R	29.7±0.10	30.7±0.84	33.6±1.56
Humacao-P	28.6±0.14	28.1±0.97	20.5±1.52
Haiti	29.3±0.	30.1±0.43	29.0±1.75

We find that the ordinary interval of about 28 days is generally maintained if the patient takes the tablet, as directed, from day 5 through day 24. Those who occasionally omit the tablets, or take them a little longer than prescribed, will menstruate earlier or later, according to the modification of the prescribed regimen. This will change the mean cycle lengths. The more the regimen is modified, the greater will be the variation in the mean cycle lengths.

2. "*Breakthrough bleeding*." Suppression of ovulation by use of the "pill" under consideration is not completely without minor disturbances. There is occasionally slight to moderate pink or red discharge from the endometrium during medication: a little of what we term "breakthrough bleeding" (Table 11).

TABLE 11. FERTILITY CONTROL WITH ENOVID: INCIDENCE OF BREAKTHROUGH BLEEDING AS % OF TOTAL CYCLES ACCORDING TO CYCLE OF MEDICATION

Cycle No.	San Juan	Humacao-R	Humacao-P	Haiti
1	4.8	6.0	11.9	6.7
2	3.8	0.9	4.9	0.0
3	2.0	2.0	2.5	1.6
4	1.5	1.0	1.5	2.5
5–9	2.3	0.6	0.0	2.2
10–14	1.9	0.9	3.3	4.2
15–19	0.9	0.0	0.0	
20–24	1.1	0.0		
25–29	2.9			
30–37	1.0			
Mean (all cycles)	2.0	1.2	3.8	2.7

This is rather easily controlled by increasing the dosage. If the daily dose is 10 mg, a per diem increase of 5 mg usually stops the bleeding. We have seen that such staining occurs more often in the early than in the later cycles of treatment. This is clearly shown in Table 11. A contributory factor in this connection may be the patient's tendency in earlier cycles to fail to adhere to the regimen as prescribed. However, it must be remembered, in considering these tabulated figures, that some of the women who have this early bleeding drop out of the treated group; this naturally leaves a lower average number of affected patients in the later cycles.

TABLE 12. FERTILITY CONTROL WITH ENOVID: INCIDENCE OF AMENORRHEA IN VARIOUS CYCLES OF MEDICATION

Cycle No.	San Juan	Humacao-R	Humacao-P	Haiti
1	0.2	0.9	0.8	2.0
2	1.0	0.9	1.0	5.1
3	0.0	1.0	2.5	4.8
4	0.6	0.0	0.0	1.7
5–9	1.2	0.4	1.9	2.8
10–14	0.5	0.6	0.0	0.5
15–19	0.5	0.5	0.0	
20–24	0.5	0.0		
25–29	0.0			
30–37	0.0			
Mean (all cycles)	0.7	0.6	1.2	3.2

3. *Amenorrhea: "Occult regression of the endometrium."* One interesting observation, so-called "occult regression of the endometrium", sometimes incorrectly termed "silent menstruation", shows that menstruation is not in essence a breakdown, but only a regression of the endometrium. This may be complete, yet without bleeding. The sudden occurrence of amenorrhea after perhaps a number of regular cycles during treatment usually disturbs the patient. When menstruation fails to appear after she stops the medication as prescribed, she believes she must be pregnant, but she is not. The temperature graph descends to the premedication level. Then, after about 10 to 20 days, without intervening catamenia, ovulation will again take place.

Hence patients who are using these steroids for contraceptive purposes must fix the regimen entirely on the occurrence of menstruation. If this does not follow within 6 days after the end of one cycle of medication, pill-taking must be resumed by the 10th day at the latest, or ovulation is very likely soon to occur. The incidence of this interesting and physiologically instructive phenomenon is suggested in Table 12. It happens, in fact, on the average in less than 2% of all cycles (30).

B. Effects on the Endometrium

The effect of Enovid on the endometrium shows other very interesting and striking aspects. After only 3 or 4 days of medication, we observe the glandular changes which are found 3 or 4 days after ovulation in a normal, untreated cycle.

Typical are mobilization of the nuclei toward the luminal border of the cells and beginning edema of the stroma. If the medication, started on cycle-day 5, is continued for 8 days, we get a postovulatory 8-day tissue, with

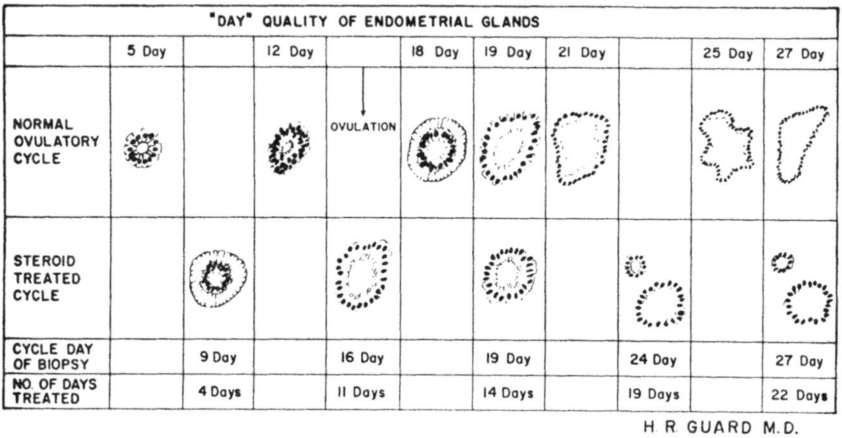

FIG. 2. Time differential in development of endometrial glandular epithelium in steroid-treated vs. untreated women. (Reproduced by permission from PINCUS, G., J. ROCK, C.-R. GARCÍA, E. RICE-WRAY, M. PANIAGUA and I. RODRIGUEZ, Fertility Control with Oral Medication. *Am. J. Obst. & Gynec.* **75**, 1333–1346, 1958.)

decrease of secretion by the cells. We used to think that the presence of secreted material in the dilated glands, characteristic of this phase, indicated continued secretory activity. We are now taught by Bartelmez (42) that this material is not being actively secreted but is merely the accumulation in the glands of previously secreted material unable to pass out because progesterone has inactivated the formerly contractile myometrium. This phase, then, as pointed out by Bartelmez, is properly designated "progestational", not "secretory".

Dr. H. R. Guard of Bombay, who was working here as a Research Fellow with us, as well as with Dr. Pincus, made a schematic drawing (Fig. 2) from some of our slides to illustrate the characteristic sequence of changes in the glands during the normal ovulatory cycle. These changes, worked out by a number of investigators, including our own group (43–45), are compared in the schema with changes during medication with Enovid. This comparison has been published previously (26, 27).

1. *The normal, untreated cycle.* In the classical 28-day cycle, the pseudocuboidal lining of the early proliferative gland (cf. Fig. 2, *day* 5) gradually changes to pseudostratification as ovulation approaches (Fig. 2, *day* 12). Next is depicted the 4-day postovulatory gland with mobilization of the nuclei toward the lumen. Then the nuclei promptly recede toward the bases of the cells at about 5 days after ovulation (Fig. 2, *day* 19). In the 21-day gland, i.e. at about 7 days after ovulation, the secreted material begins to accumulate so that the glands dilate and subsequently become "saw-toothed" on day 25 of the normal cycle. The succeeding premenstrual secretory exhaustion, characteristic of day 27, is also depicted.

2. *The treated cycle.* Now let us consider what occurs during a treated cycle. When medication is started on day 5, the entire process is accelerated. Already on the 9th cycle-day, pills having been taken for 4 days, we find the same sort of active gland that, in the normal, untreated cycle, is observed not until 4 days after ovulation, i.e. on about day 18.

At this stage in the medicated cycle, the speed of epithelial change decreases. On cycle-day 16, the 11th day of treatment, we get a gland which resembles that typical of only the 5th day after ovulation (day 19). Even so, its secretory progress is more advanced than would be the case with a 2-day-old corpus luteum (day 16 of the normal, untreated cycle).

From then on, the glands regress faster and also further than they do in the ordinary progestational phase of the normal cycle. Many of them become very small, like the postmenstrual glands. We find numerous simple, hypotrophic glands in the thinned-out endometrium, accompanied by some glands that are characteristic of secretory exhaustion. The reticular stroma of the proliferative and early postovulatory phases also more rapidly and completely progresses toward a predecidua.

At about the 21st day of the cycle, when the patient has had 16 days of treatment, the pathologist who does not know this consisted of norethynodrel may render a diagnosis: "consistent with beginning pregnancy". This is excusable, for, commonly, the tissue closely resembles that in which progestational stromal mutation has been prolonged; and easily unnoticed is the fact that some of the glands fail to show the regression which is so characteristic of pregnancy decidua.

It is noteworthy that this progestin may extend its influence in 15 days to the stroma of the lower uterine area and even into the upper cervix where, in the normal, untreated cycle, we ordinarily do not find the characteristic signs of autogenous progesterone even just before menstruation (Fig. 3).

VI. EFFECTS OF LONG-TERM USE OF ENOVID

A. *Effect on Ovulation in Postmedication Cycles*

Since Enovid evokes endometrial changes reminiscent of pregnancy, it seemed as though it might be of value in endometriosis for, during pregnancy,

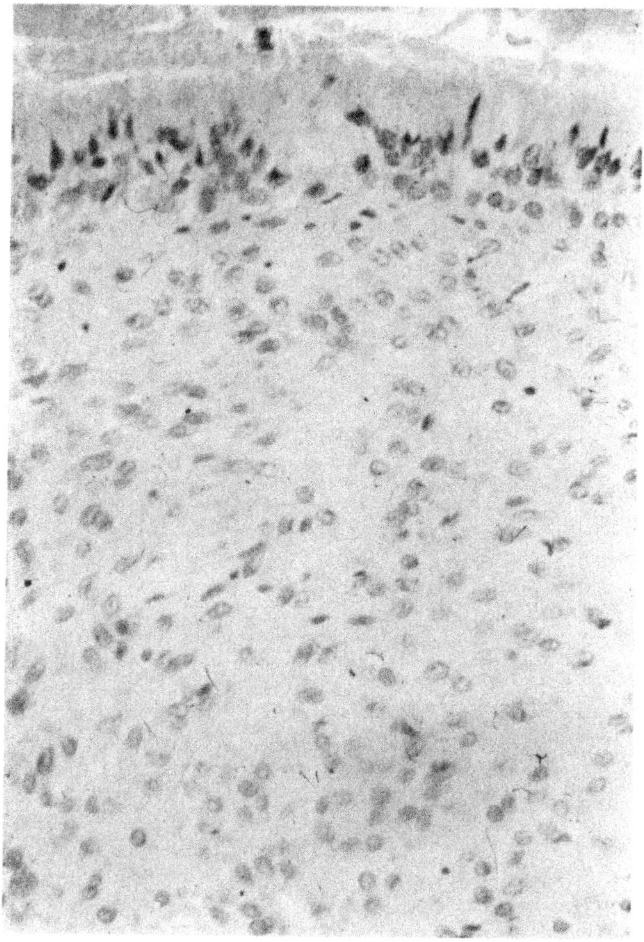

FIG. 3. Effect of Enovid on endometrial histology. Biopsy on 15th day of treatment. Decidua-like stroma of cervix, probably at internal os. (Magnif. ×400.) Reproduced by permission of ROCK, J., C.-R. GARCÍA and G. PINCUS, Synthetic Progestins in the Normal Human Menstrual Cycle. *Recent Progress in Hormone Research*, Volume XIII (Edited by G. Pincus), pp. 323–346, Academic Press, New York, 1957.

ectopic endometrium not uncommonly regresses. Dr. Robert W. Kistner (37) has already published extensively on his successful use of Enovid in endometriosis. At the Reproductive Study Center, Dr. García gave continuous Enovid medication to patients in their twenties and thirties for time intervals ranging from 2 to 9 months. This continuous administration afforded an opportunity to evaluate the effects on ovulation after discontinuance of such long-term therapy.

TABLE 13. EFFECT ON RECURRENCE OF OVULATION FOLLOWING CESSATION OF LONG-TERM ENOVID* THERAPY FOR ENDOMETRIOSIS

No. of patients followed up	Postmedication cycle (No.)	Mean cycle length (days)	% Ovulating
13	First	36	70
7	Second	27	100

* The regimen was as follows: 10 mg/day for 2 weeks; 20 mg/day for the 3rd and 4th weeks; then 30 mg/day for 2 to 3 months.

As seen in Table 13, even after treatment with 10–20 mg per day for one month and then 30 mg a day for 2–3 months, no permanent damage was done to ovulation potential. In the first postmedication cycle, ovulation occurred in 70% of 13 patients; and in the second postmedication cycle, all of 7 patients tested were found to have ovulated. Fairly prompt recurrence of ovulation is a constant finding after intermittent consumption of this material, as has been pointed out previously (22).

B. Effect of Enovid or Norlutin on the Ovaries

The question arose: How about the effect of long-term use of these substances on primordial follicles? Do these steroids, norethynodrel and 3-methyl-ether of ethynylestradiol (Enovid) or norethindrone (Norlutin), cause atresia, not only of the ripe follicles or the second-grade ones, but do they also cause destruction of the reserve ova?

This was difficult to determine. Dr. Richard R. Thornton, then a medical student, was kindly permitted to search through the pathological material at the Massachusetts General Hospital and to collect all the normal ovaries he could. These contributed largely to the untreated control material. For comparison, some ovaries were obtained from our own patients treated with Enovid before required oophorectomy. They were supplemented by ovarian biopsies from the Puerto Rican study, most of which were supplied by Dr. Pendleton.

As shown in Fig. 4, the treated and the control cases were divided into age groups: 18–21; 22–25; 26–29 years of age, etc. Serial sections were made at 10 μ in thickness and every twentieth section was mounted and stained for study. Most of the specimens supplied from 10 to 25 such selected sections. More were available in the control group than could be obtained from biopsy material.

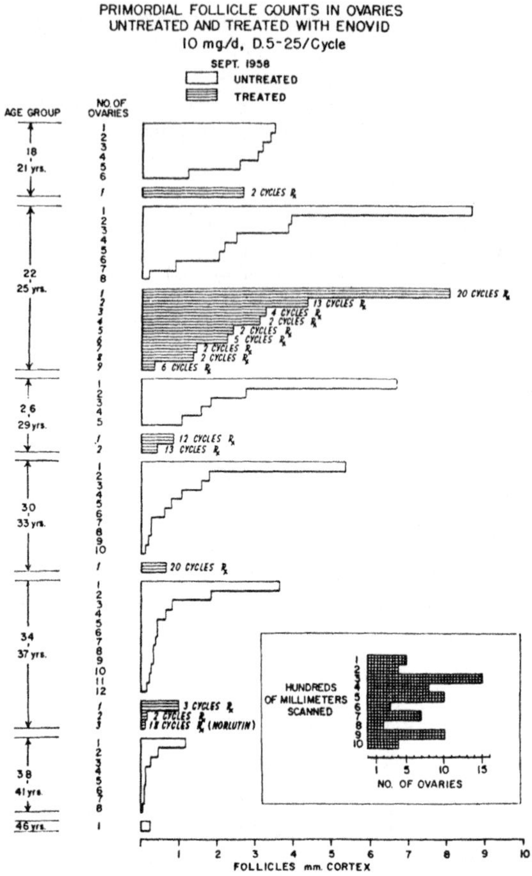

FIG. 4. Effect of Enovid (and Norlutin) on the number of primordial ovarian follicles in women of different age groups.

The stained slides were then projected on a screen for accurate measurement of curvilinear distances along the ovarian cortex, and the number of primordial follicles per millimeter of cortex was computed. The values for the untreated and the treated specimens were then compared. Statistically, there was no significant difference between untreated and treated ovaries in the number of primordial follicles present. Even in one woman who had received medication for 20 cycles, the number of normal primordial follicles was not less than the control value.

Although not as many treated ovaries as we could wish have been studied so far, the indication is that undeveloped ova are not damaged by Enovid.

C. *Effect of Enovid on Future Reproductive Potential*

The innocuousness of Enovid to the ovaries is also evidenced by the fertility of patients following cessation of medication. That Enovid does no harm to the reproductive potential is shown by a follow-up study of women in San Juan who, after treatment for even as long as 34 cycles, manifested, after cessation of therapy, a fertility rate that differed only slightly from their premedication performance (Table 14). Moreover, even among those using contraceptives of some other sort after discontinuance of Enovid, we find that many pregnancies occurred.

TABLE 14. FERTILITY CONTROL WITH ENOVID: PREGNANCY RATES OF 84 WOMEN USING NO CONTRACEPTIVES FOLLOWING WITHDRAWAL FROM SAN JUAN PROJECT (Medication for 1–34 Cycles)

No. of patients followed up	No. of medication cycles	Pregnancy rates per 100 woman-years
36	1–5	181
16	6–10	159
11	11–15	258
13	16–25	200
8	26–34	189
84	—	Mean: 186

Hence we believe that ovulation potential is not diminished by long use of these steroids that prevent its expression.

D. *Other Effects of Enovid*

Appropriate studies revealed no evidence of liver damage in patients participating in the field projects who had used the material cyclically without interruption for as long as $2\frac{1}{2}$ years (30–32). In our own local cases, 10 individuals, who had been on Enovid therapy for more than a year, also failed to show any sign of liver dysfunction. Furthermore, no deleterious effects on the blood (26) or on general health and well-being (31, 32) could be detected.

COMMENT

I have reported that 10 mg a day was selected as the standard dosage of Enovid. The material is expensive; the present retail price in this country is about 55 cents per 10-mg tablet; and so we have tried 5 mg and even as little as 2.5 mg per day. While, with lower dosage, there is a slightly higher incidence of breakthrough bleeding, the % of untoward reactions, such as transient nausea, which at 10 mg per day is experienced by about 10% of patients, is definitely decreased. Moreover, ovulation is equally well inhibited at lower dosages.

In conclusion, it may be stated that in norethynodrel we have a substance that suppresses ovulation and seems to be quite harmless. I believe that, with availability of material and with the proper motivation, large numbers of fairly illiterate people can be encouraged to use it. There is good reason to conclude that Enovid will do no damage either to the woman herself or to her future reproductive potential.

REFERENCES

1. García, C.-R. and J. Rock, Ovulation. Chapter II in *Essentials of Human Reproduction. Clinical Aspects, Normal and Abnormal* (Edited by J. T. Velardo), pp. 22–54, Oxford University Press, New York, 1958.
2. Sommers, S. C., The Pituitary and Hypothalamus. Chapter V in *The Endocrinology of Reproduction* (Edited by J. T. Velardo), pp. 59–97, Oxford University Press, New York, 1958.
3. Rock, J., M. K. Bartlett and D. D. Matson, *Am. J. Obst. & Gynec.* **37**, 3–12, 1939.
4. Sturgis, S. H., III. Functional Disorders. 1. Amenorrhea: Classification and Treatment. In *Progress in Gynecology*, Volume II (Edited by J. V. Meigs and S. H. Sturgis), pp. 163–175, Grune & Stratton, New York, 1950.
5. Sturgis, S. H. and F. Albright, *Endocrinology* **26**, 68–72, 1940.
6. Henshaw, P. S., *Science* **117**, 572–582, 1953.
7. Gordon, J. E., J. B. Wyon and T. H. Ingalls, *Am. J. Med. Sci.* **227**, 326–357, 1954.
8. Hoagland, H., Population Problems and the Control of Fertility. *Daedalus* (*Journal of the American Academy of Arts and Sciences*), pp. 425–443, Summer, 1959. (Issued as Vol. **88**, No. 3, of the *Proceedings of the American Academy of Arts and Sciences.*)
9. Jackson, H., *Pharmac. Revs.* **11**, 135–172, 1959.
10. Noble, R. L., Chapter VI. Plenary Session: Oral Methods of Fertility Control. Antigonadotrophins in Plants. *Report of the Proceedings of the Sixth International Conference on Planned Parenthood*, 14–21 February, 1959, pp. 243–250, New Delhi, India. The International Planned Parenthood Federation, London, 1959.
11. Sanyal, S. N., Chapter VI. Plenary Session: Oral Methods of Fertility Control. Oral Contraceptive for Use by Both Males and Females. *Report of the Proceedings of the Sixth International Conference on Planned Parenthood*, 14–21 February, 1959, pp. 254–257, New Delhi, India. The International Planned Parenthood Federation, London, 1959.
12. Pincus, G. and M. C. Chang, *Acta Physiol. Latinoamericana* **3**, 177–183, 1953.
13. Slechta, R. F., M. C. Chang and G. Pincus, *Fertil. & Steril.* **5**, 282–293, 1954.
14. Pincus, G., *Acta Endocrinol.* **23** (Supplement XXVIII), 18–36, 1956.
15. Beard, J., *The Span of Gestation and the Cause of Birth*, Jena, 1897. (Cited by Asdell, S. A., *Physiol. Revs.* **8**, 313–345, 1928. Citation is on page 325.)
16. Macht, D. I., *Surg., Gynec. & Obst.* **66**, 732–747, 1938.
17. Pincus, G., M. C. Chang, E. S. E. Hafez, M. X. Zarrow and A. Merrill, *Science* **124**, 890–891, 1956.
18. Pincus, G., M. C. Chang, M. X. Zarrow, E. S. E. Hafez and A. Merrill, *Endocrinology* **59**, 695–707, 1956.
19. Rock, J., G. Pincus and C.-R. García, *Science* **124**, 891–893, 1956.
20. Rock, J., C.-R. García and G. Pincus, Synthetic Progestins in the Normal Human Menstrual Cycle. *Recent Progress in Hormone Research*, Volume XIII (Edited by G. Pincus), pp. 323–346, Academic Press, New York, 1957.

21. ROCK, J. and C.-R. GARCÍA, Observed Effects of 19-Nor Steroids on Ovulation and Menstruation. *Proceedings of a Symposium on 19-Nor Progestational Steroids*, pp. 14–25, Searle Research Laboratories, Chicago, 1957.
22. GARCÍA, C.-R., G. PINCUS and J. ROCK, *Am. J. Obst. & Gynec.* **75**, 82–97, 1958.
23. ROCK, J., C.-R. GARCÍA and G. PINCUS, Chapter VI. Plenary Session: Oral Methods of Fertility Control. Clinical Studies with Potential Oral Contraceptives. *Report of the Proceedings of the Sixth International Conference on Planned Parenthood*, 14–21 February, 1959, pp. 212–214, New Delhi, India. The International Planned Parenthood Federation, London, 1959.
24. RICE-WRAY, E., Field Study with Enovid as a Contraceptive Agent. *Proceedings of a Symposium on 19-Nor Progestational Steroids*, pp. 78–85, Searle Research Laboratories, Chicago, 1957.
25. PINCUS, G., Long Term Administration of Enovid to Human Subjects. *Proceedings of a Symposium on 19-Nor Progestational Steroids*, pp. 105–118, Searle Research Laboratories, Chicago, 1957.
26. PINCUS, G., J. ROCK, C.-R. GARCIA, E. RICE-WRAY, M. PANIAGUA and I. RODRIGUEZ, *Am. J. Obst. & Gynec.* **75**, 1333–1346, 1958.
27. PINCUS, G., J. ROCK and C.-R. GARCIA, Effects of Certain 19-Nor Steroids Upon Reproductive Processes. *New Steroid Compounds with Progestational Activity. Ann. N.Y. Acad. Sci.* **71**, Art. 5, 677–690, 1958.
28. PINCUS, G., *Postgrad. Med.* **24**, 654–660, 1958.
29. PINCUS, G., *Studies on Fertility* **10**, 3–26, 1959.
30. PINCUS, G., J. ROCK and C.-R. GARCÍA, Chapter VI. Plenary Session: Oral Methods of Fertility Control. Field Trials with Norethynodrel as an Oral Contraceptive. *Report of the Proceedings of the Sixth International Conference on Planned Parenthood*, 14–21 February, 1959, pp. 216–230, New Delhi, India. The International Planned Parenthood Federation, London, 1959.
31. PINCUS, G., C.-R. GARCÍA, J. ROCK, M. PANIAGUA, A. PENDLETON, F. LARAQUE, R. NICOLAS, R. BORNO and V. PEAN, *Science* **130**, 81–83, 1959.
32. PINCUS, G., J. ROCK, M. C. CHANG and C.-R. GARCÍA, *Fed. Proc.* **18**, 1051–1055, 1959.
33. PINCUS, G., Progestational Agents and the Control of Fertility. *Vitamins and Hormones*, Volume XVII, pp. 307–324. Academic Press, New York and London, 1959.
34. CROSSON, J. W., *Fertil. & Steril.* **10**, 361–373, 1959.
35. ROCK, J., C.-R. GARCÍA and G. PINCUS, *Am. J. Obst. & Gynec.* **79**, 758–767, 1960.
36. DRILL, V. A., *Fed. Proc.* **18**, 1040–1048, 1959.
37. KISTNER, R. W., *Clin. Obst. & Gynec.* **2**, 877–889, 1959.
38. SAUNDERS, F. J. and V. A. DRILL, Part I. Biological Activity in Animals. Some Biological Activities of 17-Ethynyl and 17-Alkyl Derivatives of 17-Hydroxyestrenones. *New Steroid Compounds with Progestational Activity. Ann. N.Y. Acad. Sci.* **71**, Art. 5, 516–531, 1958.
39. EPSTEIN, J. A., H. S. KUPPERMAN and A. CUTLER, Part III. Biological Activity in Man. Comparative Pharmacological and Clinical Activity of 19-Nortestosterone and 17-Hydroxyprogesterone Derivatives in Man. *New Steroid Compounds with Progestational Activity. Ann. N.Y. Acad. Sci.* **71**, Art. 5, 560–571, 1958.
40. GARCÍA, C.-R. and J. ROCK, Unpublished data.
41. MATSUMOTO, S., Cited by PINCUS (33).
42. BARTELMEZ, G. W., *Am. J. Obst. & Gynec.* **74**, 931–955, 1957.
43. ROCK, J. and M. K. BARTLETT, *J. Am. Med. Assoc.* **108**, 2022–2028, 1937.
44. ROCK, J., *Am. J. Surg.* **48** (New Series), 228–237, 1940.
45. NOYES, R. W., A. T. HERTIG and J. ROCK, *Fertil. & Steril.* **1**, 3–25, 1950.

DISCUSSIONS

DR. FREDERICK HISAW: I notice that we have only a few minutes before closing time so I shall be as brief as possible.

First, I should like to call Dr. Sturgis' attention to two papers, if he is not already acquainted with them. One is by Dr. I. G. SCHMIDT (*Am. J. Anat.* **71**, 245, 1942), who made a thorough study of follicular development during the estrous cycle of the guinea pig, and the other is a similar study of the rat by Dr. CHARLES E. LANE and F. R. DAVIS (*Anat. Rec.* **73**, 429, 1939).

In connection with Dr. Rock's discussion I should like to mention some unpublished observations by F. L. Hisaw, Jr. on the effects of progesterone on the menstrual cycle and ovulations in monkeys. We have several adult monkeys (*Macaca mulatta*) whose menstrual cycles have been carefully recorded for several years, and these were used in the experiments. The object was to find the minimal subcutaneous dose of progesterone which, when given daily, would not disturb the length of a normal cycle, and to determine the effect of such treatment on ovulaton. Briefly, it was found that 0.25 or 0.5 mg progesterone daily, starting soon after conclusion of a menstrual period, did not influence the time of appearance of the next expected menses, nor was there an effect on subsequent normal cycles. However, 0.75 mg daily seemed to produce an increase in length of the cycle. Laparotomies performed at a time corresponding to the middle of the luteal phase of a normal cycle showed that one animal out of six given 0.25 mg progesterone ovulated, and ovulation did not occur in eight animals given 0.5 mg. This seems to suggest that it might be possible to give progestational compounds to women in amounts sufficient to inhibit ovulation and not modify the length of the normal menstrual cycle.

Dr. Rock and Dr. Pincus have mentioned that in their experiments better results were obtained when estrogen was given concurrently with their progestational compounds. By this they mean, as I understand, that breakthrough bleeding during a treatment is less likely to occur under these conditions. This probably is due to two different effects, depending of course on dosage. It is well known that small doses of estrogen greatly facilitate the action of progesterone on the endometrium, and also these two hormones, when given concurrently, more effectively inhibit secretion of pituitary gonadotropins than either alone. Castrated monkeys on 10 μg of estradiol daily rarely show breakthrough bleeding even though the treatment is continued for a period of months, and the daily dose of progesterone is approximately 1.5 to 2.0 mg. Such treatments do not prevent the appearance of "castration cells" in the pituitary, and gonadotropin content is correspondingly high. However, at the conclusion of such treatments, if both hormones are given at the same dosage for an additional twenty days, the gonad-stimulating capacity of the pituitary is almost depleted. (SALHANICK, H. A., F. L. HISAW and M. X. ZARROW, *J. Clin. Endocrinol. & Metab.* **12**, 310–320, 1952.)

DR. WARREN O. NELSON: In these closing minutes I should like to devote discussion primarily to Dr. Rock's presentation. There are, however, two other points that I should like to make in connection with the earlier papers.

During this meeting, we have considered occasionally, but only occasionally, the important question of the relationship between the gonadotropic hormones and estrogen production. This point arose this morning in connection with Dr. Gemzell's presentation and it was evident, I believe, that the question as to whether FSH or LH or a combination of the two is involved in the secretion of estrogen by the ovary remains unresolved.

I think this relationship is much clearer in the case of the testes, where there seems to be little doubt that LH is the factor important in the production of the steroid hormones. There should no longer be serious doubt that steroid hormone production in the testes occurs in the Leydig cells. These are influenced by LH (or ICSH) and by the same token, then, LH would be expected to be the factor that stimulates the production of estrogen, and also of androgen in the ovary as well as the testis. Since recent evidence indicates the source of estrogen production probably occurs by way of an androgenic precursor, it follows that LH is the probable factor of importance.

I believe all of us should have liked to have heard more from Dr. Gemzell about the direct effect of steroids on ovarian function. The evidence that he did present suggests that there may be a direct inhibitory effect of progesterone on ovarian response to FSH, but perhaps it might also be interpreted on the basis of progesterone inhibition of endogenous gonadotropin. It must be remembered that the subjects had pituitaries and that their pituitaries contributed to the total response or lack of response.

Finally I should like to comment on some of the interesting compounds discussed by Drs. Rock and Pincus. We have had reason to be concerned with them because of our interest in procedures that interfere with fertility, and in one way or another we have examined all of these compounds.

A consideration that has commanded our interest has been their gonadotropin inhibiting properties. Our evaluation of this activity has involved a procedure that we believe gives a fairly good idea about the relative inhibition of FSH and LH. We have used the 30-day-old male rat, treated 30 days. The 30-day-old male rat is immediately pre-pubertal and during the next 30 days would normally become an adult male. However, by suitable treatment with an effective inhibiting compound, he can be kept in the immature state, so far as reproduction is concerned, for 30 days or as long as might be desired.

As I have said, we can obtain a good index of the relative suppression of the two gonadotropins. The weight of the testes provides excellent evidence of the effect, or lack of effect, of FSH. The accessory organs, such as the prostate, seminal vesicles, and epididymis, reflect the presence or absence of adequate amounts of LH.

In general, we have found that effective gonadotropin inhibiting compounds require about twice the dose for FSH inhibition that they do for LH suppression. This has been a consistent finding.

The one point that I should like, finally, to make with regard to the gonadotropin inhibiting effects of these compounds is that the important point in the inhibition of ovulation may not be so much a matter of relatively complete inhibition of total gonadotropin production as it is the relative inhibition of FSH or LH. Since LH appears to be inhibited more readily by the steroids in question, it would seem likely that ovulation might be interfered with by reduction in LH without detectable reduction in total gonadotropins.

This consideration recalls the studies that Dr. Rock and Dr. Pincus made with progesterone in the inhibition of ovulation. In the women so treated, about 80% of the cycles were believed to be anovulatory. Where highly effective gonadotropin inhibitors, such as Enovid and Norlutin, are concerned, gonadotropin inhibition may be so complete that the question of relative inhibition is of little importance. In the case of progesterone inhibition, I daresay that total inhibition was not obtained and that the question of relative inhibition assumes importance. In all likelihood the partial reduction of LH secretion was sufficient to prevent ovulation in some cases.

CHAIRMAN ASTWOOD: Our time schedule has now run out, and I am afraid I shall have to turn the meeting back to Dr. Villee, who wants to make a few remarks. Before so doing, I want to voice the opinion of those present that Dr. Villee has done a marvellous job in arranging the Conference, and we are all sufficiently grateful to him to acclaim this event. (Applause.)

DR. CLAUDE VILLEE: Thank you very much, Dr. Astwood, for your very kind remarks.

I want to express on your behalf our deep appreciation to the Association for the Aid of Crippled Children and to Mrs. William FitzGerald, who is here, for making this Conference possible. Many of you have told me how much this Conference has meant to you, and I hope that Mrs. FitzGerald will take back to her Board the consensus of opinion that it was a most worthwhile way to spend a pleasant week-end.

SUBJECT INDEX

Adenohypophysis, 59, 68, 98
— activation of, 115, 116
— activity of, 57, 67
— avian, 143
— control of, 66
— functions of, 101, 113
— infusions, 67
— stimulation of, 82, 109
Adrenergic agents, effects of, 67, 146
Adrenolytic blocking agent SKF-501, effect of, 146
Adrenocorticotropin (ACTH) (*see also* Hormones)
— effects of (in animals), 8, 20, 52, 84, 182, 220
— secretion of, 67, 113, 189
Adynamia, 84
Amygdaloid complex (*see also* Glands)
— lesions, effect of, 60, 61, 76, 77, 82, 115, 183
— pathways, 81
— role of, 75, 78, 115
— stimulation of, 82, 101
Androgenicity in women, 222
Androgens, effect of, 113, 115–117, 120, 121, 243
— potency of, 39
— secretion of, in hens, 147
Antifertility agents, effect, in rabbits, 94, 95
— — in women, 229–234, 239
Atropine, effect of, in hens, 146
— — in rabbits, 124
— — in rats, 102, 104, 107–111
— — in ruminants, 99

Barbiturates, effect of, 113, 145, 146

Chlorpromazine, effect of, 50
Cholinergic blocking agents, effect of, in hens, 146
Chorionic gonadotropin (HCG) [*see also* Hormones, Gonadotropins *and* Pregnant Mare Serum (PMS)]
— effect of, in monkeys, 1, 19, 20, 22, 52
— — in rabbits, 84, 92
— — in rats, 16–20, 25–29, 185, 216, 219
— — in women, 192, 194, 197–208, 210, 211
Conception, rate of, in ruminants, 172, 173, 174
Corpus luteum (*see also* Ovaries, Ovulation)
— ascorbic acid content of, 216–219, 221
— cysts, 99, 223
— formation of, in rabbits, 29, 170
— — in rats, 3–5, 26, 46, 47, 76, 113, 116, 218
— — in ruminants, 98, 99, 177
— — in women, 193, 216–218
— function of, 217
— maturity of, in rats, 5
— occurrence of, in rats, 76, 77
— regression of, in ruminants, 164, 165, 177
— removal of, in ruminants, 169, 170, 173
— resorption of, in rats, 47
Corticoids (*see also* Steroids)
— effect of, 120
Cortisone (*see also* Steroids)
— effect of, 25, 50

Delalutin (*see* Progesterone derivatives)
Diencephalon, centre, 178
— lesions, effect of, 151, 178
Dysthyroidism, effect of, in women, 223

EEG patterns and characteristics, in rabbits, 82–86, 88, 91, 93–95, 98
— reactions in rabbits, 85–93, 95, 98, 100
Endometrium, activity of, in ruminants, 99
— — in women, 195, 197, 208, 209
— atrophy of, 196–198, 209
— development of, 235
— extracts, effect of, in ruminants, 99
— reactions of, 202, 204
Enovid (*see also* Norethynodrel), as fertility control agent, 229–234, 239
— effect of, on "break-through" bleeding, 233, 234
— — on control of amenorrhea, 234
— — on endometrium, 235
— — on future reproductive potential, 239
— — on liver disfunction and blood, 239

Enovid, effect of, on ovaries, 237, 238
— — as ovulation inhibitor, in rabbits, 93
— — — in women, 50, 226, 227, 240, 243
— — ovulation suppressant, in women, 228
— — in post-medication cycles, 236, 237
— — on preganediol excretion, 228
— preparation of, 226
Estradiol, assay, 195
— effect of, in monkeys, 242
— — in rabbits, 90
— — in rats, 187
— occurrence, 53
Estriol, assay, 195
Estrogens, assay, clinical, 195
— effect of, in monkeys, 216, 218
— — as ovulation inhibitor, in hens, 132, 154, 159
— — — in rabbits, 37, 81, 82, 89–95
— — in rats, 46, 48, 50, 110, 120
— — in ruminants, 118, 163, 164, 166, 169, 173, 174, 179
— — *in vitro*, 51
— — in women, 216, 218, 242, 243
— excretion, in women, 195–205, 207, 211, 212
— implants, 51
— in invertebrates, 49
— levels, 154, 155, 158, 190
— production of, 48, 51, 207, 208, 215, 242
— release of, in women, 208, 209, 215, 219, 242
— secretion of, in animals (misc.), 56, 79, 119, 178
— — in hens, 147, 158, 159
— — in monkeys, 52
— — in rats, 52, 113, 219
— stimulation, in hens, 154
Estrogenicity, in women, 223
Estrone, assay of, 195
Excitation hormone (progestagen?) (*see also* Hormones)
— concentration of, in hens, 153, 154
— effect of, in hens, 155
— occurrence of, in hens, 156

Fetus, development of, in rats, 190
— — in women, 207
Follicles, activation of, 70
— aggregates of, in hens, 159
— atresia, 24, 29, 30, 184, 186
— — in hens, 125, 126, 128–130, 132, 142, 147, 160, 214, 217, 218
Follicles, atresia, in monkeys, 214, 215, 217
— — in rats, 50, 215
— — in women, 193, 207, 213, 215, 216, 237
— atrophy of, 65, 213
— cell wall of, 35, 48, 51, 124, 129, 132
— cysts, 167, 216
— degeneration of, in rats, 26, 27, 33
— development of, general, 1, 52–54, 56, 59, 61, 221, 242
— — in hens, 123, 128, 130, 133, 134, 153, 158, 185
— — in rats, 2, 3, 6, 8, 9, 13–15, 17–19, 20, 24–27, 30–35, 49–50, 113, 242
— — in ruminants, 98, 164, 169, 170, 173, 186
— — in women, 192, 207, 217
— enlargement of, 26, 33, 56, 207
— ischemia of, 129, 132, 184, 186
— maturation of, general, 27, 35, 134, 170, 210, 214, 215, 217
— — in hens, 133, 134, 137–143, 151, 153, 156, 160, 161
— — in rats, 26, 27, 30, 33
— — in women, 204, 207, 213
— meiosis of, 24, 26, 30
— overgrowth, in hens, 147
— resorption of, in hens, 156
— release of, in hens, 153
— rupture of, 56, 63, 122–124, 186
— — in hens, 124, 130, 141, 146, 147, 156
— — in rabbits, 53, 70
— — in women, 207
— sensitizing substances, 123
Follicle stimulating hormone (FSH) (*see also* Hormones)
— assay, 6, 139, 227
— effect of, in animals (misc.), 123
— — in hens, 127–130, 132, 138, 143, 153, 154, 158, 185
— — in monkeys, 1, 19, 20, 22, 23, 52, 192
— — in rabbits, 84
— — in rats, 2, 4, 5, 7–12, 14–20, 49, 54, 190, 220
— — in ruminants, 163, 165, 168, 169, 171, 173, 180
— — in women, 193–195, 197–208, 210–212, 220, 242
— estrogen excretion effect, 36
— inhibition of effect, 184, 185, 187, 243
— occurrence of, 35, 53
— potency of, 6–9, 19, 20, 193, 194
— preparation of, 6, 7, 138, 194

Follicle stimulating hormone (FSH), purification of, 6, 7, 20, 194
— secretion in animals, misc., 59, 61, 63, 65, 66
— — in hens, 156, 177

Gestagen, effect of, in hens, 156
Gestation in rats, 190
— in women, 192, 205, 206
Glands (*see also* Amygdaloid complex, Gonads, Optic glands, Pituitary)
— activity of, 57, 59
— endocrine, maturing of, 56
Gonadotropins [*see also* Hormones, Chorionic gonadotropin (HCG), Pregnant Mare Serum (PMS)]
— assay, 19, 120, 121, 181, 210, 211
— effect of, in animals, misc., 79, 124, 216
— — in hens, 124, 128, 130, 139, 140, 144, 154, 155, 158
— — in monkeys, 2, 52
— — in rabbits, 70, 91, 95, 185, 221
— — in rats, 2, 14, 19, 24–28, 33, 50, 57, 58, 111, 221
— — in ruminants, 98, 163, 165, 168, 169, 179
— — in women, 192, 193, 211, 216, 224
— excretion, in women, 198, 211
— inactivation of, 224
— levels, 27, 33, 211
— occurrence of, 56, 57, 180
— production of, 2, 3
— release blocking, in ruminants, 167
— release of, 79
— secretion of, in hens, 143, 144, 151, 152, 153, 156–158, 160
— — in rabbits, 84, 95, 98, 99
— — in rats, 57, 58, 61, 63, 75, 78, 113, 115, 116, 119–121, 184
— — in ruminants, 118, 173, 178
— — suppression of, 157
— specificity, 192
— stimulation, in monkeys, 182, 214
— — in women, 216
Gonads (*see also* Glands)
— activity of, 57, 58
— atrophy of, 62
— effect of environment on, 59
— — light, in birds, 144
— enlargement of, 58
— function, 133, 144
— stimulation of, 59
Growth hormone (*see* Somatotropin, Hormones)

Hamartomata, effect of, 58
Heats, in rabbits, 87, 89, 90
— in ruminants, 165–171, 174, 177
Hormones [*see also* Adrenocorticotropin (ACTH), Chorionic Gonadotropin (HCG), Excitation Hormone (Progestagen), Follicle Stimulating Hormone (FSH), Growth Hormone (Somatotropin), Human Menopausal Hormone (HMG), Interstitial Cell Hormone (ICSH), Luteotropin (LH), Melanophore Stimulating Hormone (MSH), Neurohypophysis Hormone, Ovulation Inducing Hormone (OIH), Oxytocin, Posterior Lobe Hormone, Pregnant Mare Serum (PMS), Sex Hormone]
— balance, in hens, 158
— disturbance, 223
— effect of, 123, 184, 188
— — in hens, 132, 152
— — in monkeys, 22
— — on ovulation, 79
— — on rats, 3, 4
— endogenous, elimination of, 3, 95
— — production of, in ruminants, 163
— exogenous, effect of, 95, 125, 128
— as fertility control agents, in ruminants, 163
— interaction with other hormones, 52
Human menopausal hormone (HMG) (*see also* Hormones)
— effect of, in women, 194
Human pregnancy urine (PU), effect of, in ruminants, 163, 165, 168–170, 188
— — in women, 192
17-Hydroxycorticoids (*see also* Steroids)
— excretion of, in women, 196, 197, 199, 200–203, 205
— levels of, in ruminants, 179
Hypophysectomy, effect of, in hens, 125, 126, 129, 130, 144, 149, 186
— — in rats, 3, 110, 184, 219
Hypophysis, activation of, 84, 91
— blocking action, 110
— effect of lesions, in hens, 151
— portal veins of, 66, 101
— role of, 79
— transplants, 79
Hypoplasia in women, 222
Hypothalamus, activation of, 67, 113, 115, 151
— assay of, 69
— centres of, 94, 95, 146, 179
— effect of lesions, in animals (misc.), 61–63, 181, 187, 188
— — in hens, 146–149, 177
— — in rats, 57, 58, 75, 76, 117, 182–184
— — in ruminants, 174, 178–180

Hypothalamus, effect of lesions, on FSH secretion, 62
— — implants, 187
— extracts, effect of, 68, 69, 100
— function of, 56, 65–67, 82, 98, 109, 222
— preoptic region, activity of, 149
— — effect on ovulation stimulation, 59, 64, 101, 102, 104–106, 108, 109, 111, 115
— — lesions, effect of, in hens, 147–149, 151
— sex centres, 101, 118
— stimulation of, 64, 81, 98, 101, 103, 104, 113, 115, 117
— supra-optic region, avian, 151, 152, 189
— — function of, in hens, 152

Insemination, artificial, effect of (ruminants), 165, 167, 168, 171, 184
Interstitial cell, ascorbic acid content, 216
— atrophy of, 187
— evolution of, 187
— repair of (rats), 3, 4, 6, 8, 9, 190
— stimulation of, 13, 36
Interstitial cell hormone (ICSH) (*see also* Hormones, Gonadotropins)
— assay and purification of, 8, 9
— effect of, in frogs, 123
— — in rats, 2, 3, 5–8, 12, 14–20, 49
— occurrence, 181, 243
— secretion of, in rats, 113

Ketosteroids (*see also* Steroids)
— excretion of (animals), 118
— — (women), 196, 197, 199–203, 205

Lithosperm, effect of, in hens, 185
— — in women, 224
Luteotropin (LH) (*see also* Hormones, Prolactin)
— activity levels, in hens, 141, 154, 160
— — in monkeys, 215
— — in ruminants, 180
— assay of, 156, 216, 221
— content in pituitary, in rats, 120, 121
— effect of, in hens, 122, 123–130, 132, 138, 139, 147, 154, 157, 185, 186
— — in monkeys, 49, 52, 53
— — in rabbits, 84
— — in rats, 56, 177, 190, 216, 218–221, 243
— — in ruminants, 163, 168, 173, 174, 179
— — in women, 193, 194, 209, 211, 228, 242, 243
— excretion of, in women, 217
— mechanism, in the rat, 111, 157
— preparation of, 138
Luteotropin (LH), secretion of, in hens, 124, 125, 132, 138, 145–147, 156, 157, 160
— — in rabbits, 64–67, 69, 122
— — in rats, 71, 113, 122
— — in ruminants, 98, 99, 174

Median eminence (*see also* Tuber cinereum)
— avian, 143, 144, 147, 149
— lesions, effect of, 61
— stimulation of, 65, 101, 104, 110, 111, 113, 115
— structure of, 66–69, 189
— tissue extracts, 67–72, 119
Melanophore stimulating hormone (MSH) (*see also* Hormones)
— effect of, 52
Myometrium, development of, 132

Neurohypophysectomy, effect of, in hens, 144
Neurohypophysis, avian, 143, 152
— innervation of, 189
— structure of, 68, 189
Neurohypophysis hormone (*see also* Hormones)
— effect of, in ruminants, 98
Nilevar (*see* Nortestosterones)
Norethindrone (Norlutin), effect of, as ovulation inhibitors, in rabbits, 93–95
— — — in rats, 46, 48
— — — in women, 224, 237, 238, 243
— — ovulation suppressant, in women, 228
— preparation of, 225
Norethynodrel (*see also* Enovid), effect of, as ovulation inhibitor, in rabbits, 93
— — — in rats, 46–48
— — — in women, 225, 227, 228, 237
— — ovulation suppressant, 240
Norgestagens, effect of, 93–95
Norlutin (*see* Norethindrone)
Norsteroids (*see also* Steroids)
— derivatives: 17α-(1-methallyl)-19-nortestosterone (SC 8117), 229, 230
— — methylpregnone, 229
— effect of, as ovulation inhibitors, in women, 44, 48, 224
— properties of, 225
Nortestosterones (incl. Nilevar)
— derivatives, 41, 44
— — as ovulation inhibitors, in rabbits, 41, 44, 93
— — — in women, 224

Optic gland (*see also* Glands)
— enlargement of, 59
— lesions, effect of, 57
Ovaries, activation of, 104, 130
— atresia, in monkeys, 214
— atrophy of, 56, 61, 65, 81, 125, 178
— avian, 124
— — development of, 133
— development of, 57, 58
— enlargement of, in animals, 58, 188
— — polycystic, in women, 188, 192, 195, 197, 198, 200, 204, 206, 208, 216, 218
— function of, 134, 193
— hypoplastic, in women, 198
— implants in, in rats, 50
— insufficiency (hypoplasia), 222
— ovum content in, 213
— regression of, 151, 170
— removal of, in ruminants, 171
— rupture points, 71
— stimulation of, 207
— superovulation, in rats, 30, 192
— transplants, 24–28, 30, 33, 56, 79
— — regression of, 26
— — relation to iris and cornea, 26
— — vascularization of, 25, 26, 33, 56, 66
— — viability of, 26
Oviducts, regression of, in hens, 151
Ovulation, general: blocking agents, 84, 98–100, 102, 104, 107–111, 113, 124, 130
— cycle, diestrous, 102, 104–106, 109–111, 115, 116
— — effect of environment, 59–61, 98, 109
— — effect of operations, 60, 61
— — cycle, effect of pharmaceutical compounds, 87, 115, 116, 119
— — induction of, 118
— — proestrous, 102–107, 111, 115, 116
— effects of hormones on, 79
— — pre-optic region, 101, 109
— induction of, 81
— non-spontaneous, 63
— reflex, 79
— spontaneous, 25, 63
Ovulation in hens: accelerators, 124
— blocking agents, 146
— cycle, 134, 137–139, 152, 154
— — induction of, 177
— — mechanism, 156
— — threshold response, 153, 154
— frequency, 134, 135, 137–139, 153
— induction of, 128–133, 139, 140, 143, 145, 148, 149, 151, 157
Ovulation in hens: inhibition, 145, 146, 185
— inhibitors, 142, 159
— interruption of, 147, 148, 151, 158
— lag, 134–139, 152–155, 158–160
— lapse, 141–143, 145, 147, 152–154, 157, 159
— — effect of barbiturates, 146
— — effect of photoperiod, 144, 145, 154, 155, 157, 158, 160, 161
— mechanism, 122, 124, 128, 129, 132, 134
— multiple, 130, 186
— premature, 141, 145, 146
— resumption of, 143, 144, 151
— sequence, 134–143, 153, 154, 157–159
— stimulation, 140, 152, 159
— super-, 130
— suppression of, 147, 148
Ovulation in monkeys: control, 242
— mechanism, 213, 217
Ovulation in rabbits: control, 37, 48
— induction of, 81, 82 101
— "reflex", 101
— spontaneous, 70, 71, 90
— super-, 185
Ovulation in rats: control of, 37, 113, 115, 117
— inhibitors, 113
— mechanism, 215
— spontaneous, 71, 101, 104, 105, 113, 121
— super-, 2, 5, 25, 190
Ovulation in ruminants: "asynchronous", 160
— blocking agents, 167
— cycle, control of, 163
— — effect of lesions, 177
— — effect of photoperiod, 164
— — effect of transplants, 119
— — follicular phase, 164
— — induction of, 166
— — length, 164, 168, 171–174
— — luteal phase, 164, 167, 168, 175
— interference, 166
— mid-cycle, 168, 169
— multiple, 99, 164–166, 168, 169, 171, 172, 173, 175
— rate of, 166, 167, 169–171, 173–175
— "shock", 168, 169
— "synchronous", 165
Ovulation in women: anovulation, 218, 222, 223
— control of, 214

Ovulation in women: criteria, 195
— cycle, factors, 213
— — length of, 228
— — luteal phase, 207
— — prolongation of, 211
— failure, 222
— indices, 228
— induction of, 192–194, 198, 204–206, 210
— inhibition of, 222, 223, 225, 243
— mechanism, 193, 208, 222
— mid-cycle, 217
— multiple, 211
— oligo-ovulation, 222
Ovulation inducing hormone (OIH) (*see also* Hormones)
— effect of, in animals, misc., 19, 32, 62, 122
— — in hens, 144, 154, 155, 159, 161
— — in rats, 19, 105, 107, 109, 220
— occurrence of, 19
— release of, in hens, 138–147, 149–155, 157–159, 161
— — effect of light on, in rats and rabbits, 146
— — — pharmacological agents on, in hens, 146
— — — in rats and rabbits, 145
— — interruption, in hens, 151
— release, in rabbits, 84
— release-mechanism, in hens, 153, 154, 157, 158, 161
— — -stimulus, in hens, 152, 159
— — -suppression, in hens, 147, 158
— secretion of, in rabbits, 79, 80
Ovum, atresia, 25
— degeneration, 25, 26, 170, 214
— fertility of, of rats, 31, 33
— fertilization of, in rats, 25, 31, 54
— — in ruminants, 165, 167, 169, 171, 172
— — in women, 207
— implants, in ruminants, 164, 168
— maturation of, 24–26, 30, 33, 35, 50, 54
— — in women, 192, 213
— meiosis, 26, 30, 33, 36, 54
— recovery of, 31, 168, 171, 191
— release of, in animals, misc., 50, 56, 123
— — in hens, 125, 129, 132
— — in rats, 2, 4, 9–11, 15, 19, 105
— — in ruminants, 168, 169
— survival of, 31, 171
— transplants, 31–33
— transport of, in rats, 190
— — in ruminants, 168, 170, 172
Oxytocin (*see also* Hormones)
— effect of, 67, 98, 99, 118, 119, 124
— secretion of, 118

Pituitary (*see also* Glands)
— activation of, general, 63
— — in hens, 146, 147, 154
— — in rabbits, 82, 87, 89, 95, 98
— activity of, 66, 68, 98, 143, 149, 209
— development of, 57
— — effect of, in hens, 142, 143
— extracts, infusions, effect of, 68, 69, 71, 119, 210, 219
— function of, 66, 67, 143, 144, 152
— general systemic circulation, 65
— hypophyseal portal circulation, 65
— implants, 187
— nerve-supply of, 65
— removal of, 147, 149
— secretion, effect in ruminants, 166, 179
— — effect of, 56, 58
— stalk, hypophyseal portal vessels, 59, 61, 63, 66, 67–69, 79, 179
— — stimulation of, 65
— — transplantation, effect of, 65, 119, 123
Pituitary hormones (*see also* Hormones)
— effect of, in monkeys, 2, 19, 49, 51, 52
— — in rabbits, 80, 84, 95, 189
— — in rats, 2, 13, 14, 49, 51
— — in ruminants, 168, 173
— release, 67, 80, 82, 95, 98, 100, 122, 123, 167, 209
Polydypsia, in hens, 151
Posterior lobe hormone (*see also* Hormones)
— effect of, 19
Pregnanediol, assay, clinical, 195
— excretion of, 196, 198–205, 207, 211, 228, 229
— levels, 202
Pregnant Mare Serum (PMS) (*see also* Hormones, Gonadotropins)
— effect of, in hens, 128, 158
— — in rabbits, 84
— — in rats, 25, 27–29, 33, 52, 190
— — in ruminants, 163, 165, 166–174, 185, 186
— — in women, 192, 219
Pregnenolone, effect of, 50
Progestagen, effect of, in hens, 155
— occurrence of, in hens, 156
Progesterone (*see also* Steroids)
— assay, 53, 155, 156

Progesterone, derivatives of:
17α-hydroxyprogesterone (Delalutin), 41, 45, 93
17-acetoxyprogesterone and derivatives, 41, 42, 45
— effects of, general, 53, 79, 217, 243
— — in frogs, 51, 123
— — in hens, 94, 126, 132, 140, 142, 143–149, 151, 155, 156, 186
— — in invertebrates, 49
— — in mice, 50
— — in monkeys, 52, 242
— — in rabbits, 87–90, 93, 109
— — in rats, 102, 104, 109, 110, 115–117, 120, 220
— — in ruminants, 100, 118, 166, 169, 172, 173, 174, 179
— — in women, 39, 41–46, 51, 224, 228, 243
— levels, in rats, 190
— precursors, 217, 218
— secretion of, 79
Progestinicity, 223
"Progestins", effect of, 228
Prolactin (LTH) (Lactogenic hormone) [*see* also Hormones, Luteotropin (LH)]
— activity levels, 215
— effect of, in frogs, 156
— — in hens, 123
— — in rabbits, 84
— — in rats, 5, 8, 20, 91, 119, 220
— function of, 118, 119
— secretion of, 118, 119
Protein hormones (*see also* Hormones)
— effect of, in hens, 186
Pubertas praecox, in humans, 182–184, 187
Puberty, onset of, in animals, 56–59, 62, 76
— — in humans, 58
Pyometra, in ruminants, 168

Reproductive patterns, in ruminants, 163
Reserpine, effect of, 50, 99, 119

Sex hormones (*see also* Hormones)
— concentration of, 223
Sex hormones, imbalance, 222
— secretion of, 57
Somatotropin (Growth Hormone (GH)) (*see also* Hormones)
— effect of, in animals, 22, 23, 84, 192, 220
— properties of, 192
Sperms, transportation of, 184
Steroids, as ovulation inhibitor, 37, 45–47, 49, 50, 53, 80, 228, 234, 243
— — stimulants, 48–50
— effect of, in hens, 146
— — in rats, 120
— — in ruminants, 173
— excretion of, in women, 211
— production, *in vivo*, 215, 218
— secretion of, 79, 219, 228
— urinary assay, clinical, 195
Stilbestrol, effect of, 50, 51, 109, 187
Stimulation, electrical, 79, 99, 101, 189
— — in rabbits, 64, 66, 67, 80, 81, 85–87, 89, 91
— — in rats, 100, 103–106, 110, 111, 113, 115, 117, 120
— — parameters, 105–108, 111, 113
— sensory, 63
Stimulation–lesion experiments, 80

Testicles, atrophy of, in animals, 152, 180, 187
Testosterone, effect of, in rabbits, 90, 91, 95
— — in rats, 62, 113
— — in ruminants, 166, 167
— — in women, 224
Thalamus, effect of lesions in, 58, 60, 61, 76, 77, 151
— function, disturbance of, in women, 223
Thyrotropin (TSH) (*see also* Hormones)
— effect of, 8, 20, 84, 182
— secretion of, 67, 69
Tuber cinereum (*see also* Median Eminence)
— effect of lesions, 58
— stimulation of, 64

Uterus, atrophy of, in rats, 187, 215

Vasopressin, effect of, 84
— infusions, effect of, 119

Printed in Dunstable, United Kingdom

88528529R00167